Cancer: A Healing Crisis

DEDICATION

To the memory of my dear friend, Michael Lombardi;
and — with deep affection — to his beloved wife, Iris.

Cancer
A Healing Crisis

The Whole-Body Approach
to Cancer Therapy

Jack Tropp

CANCER RESOURCE CENTER

JACK TROPP
Co-Director

G.R.D. CLINIC
5880 San Vicente Blvd. #103
Los Angeles, CA   90019   (213) 933-8457

FIRST EDITION

© 1980 by Jack Tropp

Library of Congress Catalog Card Number: 80-65682

ISBN 0-682-49583-2

Printed in the United States of America

Contents

PART 1: THE WHOLE BODY

PART 2: DR. MAX GERSON

Preface

In the crucible of suffering emerges revelation and truth. For six heartrending months, from January to June 1973, I saw my beloved wife, Dyna Min Hong Tropp, waste away in quiet desperation as she suffered the mounting pain of spreading ovarian carcinoma. When, in January, the surgeon emerged from the operating room and coolly pronounced that she had but a few months to live, I felt like I, myself, had just died.

With a hopeless prognosis facing me, I panicked and started running, searching for panaceas—a quest utterly doomed to failure from the start. We were set helplessly adrift by a sea of literature—books and articles by writers of the so-called alternative press, most of them terrifyingly fragmented, often tenuous, and just as often confusing. Flying on wings of fear, we were tossed about in the whirlpools and eddies of one country and clinic after another—hoping against hope. On June 29, 1973, the day of Dyna's death, I was still hoping and still not believing we had reached the end.

If courage and love could have been equated with survival, then Dyna would have lived a thousand years. In a land of strangers, this unassuming Oriental soul remained undaunted. Never did a murmur of recrimination or regret pass her lips. The only words I ever heard (whispered weakly in my ear one afternoon as I leaned over her hospital bed) were, "Our bad luck!" She was willing to go with me to the ends of the earth—and did—but to no avail. She passed away bravely, with her heart full of faith and full of love—the physical pain less grievous than her tender concern for me.

Her spirit has provided the impelling force that kept me persevering during five demanding years of commitment to writing *Cancer: A Healing Crisis*. If I had had access then to the information contained in this book, it would have made our decisions more viable and the path clearer; it would have helped our peace of mind, too, no matter what the end result might have been. I will go further: I am convinced that Dyna's life would have been considerably extended, with even the possibility of remission and recovery if the information that lies between the covers of this book had been available to me then. At the very least, it would have given a brave, dear woman a fighting chance.

I hope, dear reader and friend, that you will be helped by what I have written in *Cancer: A Healing Crisis*.

God Bless,
JACK TROPP

Acknowledgment

Mr. Raphael J. Cheatham originally proposed this book project to the author and then made office space and facilities available for this purpose. It was a privilege to have been his friend and to have had the benefit of his great personal warmth and encouragement through sometimes very difficult days—until his death on July 14, 1977. I cannot overestimate Mr. Cheatham's contribution to this book. Certainly, it could not have been written without his invaluable support. The many discussions that we had; his close-in moral support and assistance; his vast storehouse of personal knowledge, friends, and connections; his priceless library—all were generously made available. I hope that his contribution to the American Natural Hygiene movement will bear good fruit.

The author owes a debt of gratitude to others who helped him along the way. I ask forgiveness in advance for errors of omission, which, assuredly, will be many, and start now with dear, supportive old friends: Mary and Murray Sprung; Charles and Kanchan, warm humans; Hugh McCormick, always being; Elaine Miller, warmthful; Dr. Jeffrey L. Fine, sparking and sparkling; Ruth and Eugene Kennedy, quietly real; Helen Knigge and Jessie Alm, helping in the wings; Janet Legunn, with the light of her friendship.

Charlotte Gerson Straus proved an exceptional friend and counselor over the years, cheerfully providing needful facts—especially valuable biographical notes about her father, Dr. Max Gerson, that enriched the content of his life and works. I owe a heartfelt debt of gratitude to both Dr. Rita Leroi and Dr. Josef Issels. Dr. Leroi was, throughout, a rock of inspiration and helped me through many trials with her sage, practical advice and perceptive encouragement. Dr. Issels, too, contributed generously in many ways, often beyond just the book's necessities. Dr. Bernard Jensen and Dr. Liechti-von Brasch were quietly helpful and encouraging.

My exploited daughters, Dale, Roberta, and Marcia, were compelled to listen to my bucolic rhetoric about Dr. Max Gerson as much as twenty years ago; but they stoically continued to encourage my efforts to bring his story into print.

Sister Maureen Hunt of the Franciscan Center in Tampa was a

shining light, always selflessly available. My dear friend, Father John Keane, provided a special quality of spiritual support and friendship that meant a lot to me and carried me over many hurdles.

A few abiding friends also proved helpful in practical ways: Murray Schwarzman, Otto E. Roethenmund, Jacob Shapiro, Irwin Beutel, and Yukie and John Dillenburger.

There were literally scores of doctors, clinics, and governmental agencies that responded generously to my requests for information; their offices harbored scores of sympathetic and helpful, but unsung and anonymous, librarians and secretaries. To all of these I am indebted and owe a note of thanks.

I received exceptional assistance from my publisher, Mr. Ed Uhlan, whose humanity, empathy, and courage in undertaking a controversial work was inspiring, especially in the occasional "hard-times" days. I am grateful, also, to the editor, RoseEllen Sanfilippo, who skillfully guided the book through the gauntlet of the production process.

The writings of Paramahansa Yogananda continually sustained me, as did the personal example, life, and works of Father Matteo Ricci. Over the years, Dr. Hiroshi Motoyama of Japan played an important role in hardening my resolution to venture the book and to continue it through to completion.

I thank them all for being my friends. I hope, trust, and believe that this book will be well received and, thus, in a small way, constitute some reward for their confidence and faith in me.

Introduction: The Wounded Physician

On September 21, 1951, on the Tegernsee, at Rottach-Egern, in the quiet fastnesses of the Bavarian Alps, occurred an event of momentous proportions, one that may very well shake the foundations of modern medicine.

In front of a tiny hospital staff, newly recruited, an ambulance rolled up ominously in the late afternoon, to disgorge its lone occupant.

This was at the newly christened Ringberg-Klinik, patched together only one week earlier from the remnants of a rundown hotel. The ambulance had brought the clinic its first patient.

The white-clad figure of a physician looked on anxiously as the patient was wheeled in. A flash of concern crossed his dark eyes, but quiet resolve lay in the set of his shoulders.

The still form on the stretcher struck the assembled group like a clap of thunder in a cloudless sky. Their faces blanched at the sight of the wasted body so obviously near death.

White-faced with shock at the patient's condition, the clinic's nurse went up to the doctor and said, "I cannot touch her. This is a death house." He quietly replied, "I know how you feel, but our job is to help people."

The ambulance men carried in a body ravaged by cancer in its last stages: bald, from repeated courses of radiotherapy; blind, deaf, and dumb as the direct result of a massive, rapidly growing, and inoperable brain tumor; totally paralyzed in both legs and right arm; bladder and rectum no longer functioning. The dying patient lay in the pitiable posture of a spastic.

Lydia Bacher was that dying patient. She had been previously declared by her doctor as no longer "responsive to further radiation therapy." Her consultant physician, Professor Adolf Reimer, confirmed that no further treatment would help. Pain-killing drugs were recommended, to be administered at home. On September 3, 1951, Mrs. Bacher had been discharged from the hospital by her doctor—to die at home.

It was in this condition that Mrs. Bacher arrived at Ringberg-Klinik on September 21. Treatment began at once.

On October 1, she was able to urinate.

On October 10, her overall feeling of well-being was better.

On October 20, her speech had returned. She could now also read the headlines of newspapers; her hearing was improved: she could hear noises at a distance of three feet, and distinguish words at closer range.

On November 30, the spastic nature of her movement had decreased; the entire arm could move by itself now; incontinence was lessened; and she had control over her bowel movements.

By December 12 there had been a general improvement in her entire condition.

On December 15 she walked for the first time since her admission into the hospital three months earlier.

On January 20, 1952, she had a relapse; she could not walk, and was very depressed. But the immunotherapy and the entire regimen were continued.

On February 13 she had overcome the crisis; there were daily signs of lasting improvement.

On March 1, she walked and spoke very clearly; she read well; hearing was good. All limbs were normal.

On March 17, Mrs. Lydia Bacher was discharged from the Ringberg-Klinik.

When she presented herself for examination to the doctors who had originally treated her, they could not believe their eyes. It *had* to be an apparition! They were stunned. Their minds could not—would not—grasp the fact that she had survived. The trauma of such an experience threatened their very sanity.

It was—they unanimously declared—a "spontaneous" remission!

The conditioning structured by their education and training in orthodox medical practice could not survive a rational search for causes. They could not tolerate even the *idea* of an investigation into the kind of therapy that had been used to bring Lydia Bacher back from the grave.

But the earth *had moved*—and the smoke today is only just beginning to clear, with the advent of doctors who are today practicing "metabolic therapy" or "biological medicine," which incorporates an increasing number of the components of *Ganzheitstherapie,* or the "whole-body treatment," which Lydia Bacher had received.

Josef Issels, an *"Auslander"* to the villagers of Rottach-Egern, was the country doctor who snatched Lydia Bacher from the jaws of death. When he accepted Lydia Bacher as his patient that fateful day, he was the living embodiment of "the wounded physician" so poignantly described in Carl G. Jung's moving passage: "As a doctor, I constantly have to ask myself what kind of message the patient is bringing me. What does he mean to me? If he means nothing, I have no point of attack. When the doctor wears his personality like a coat of armor, he has no effect. The doctor is effective only when he himself is affected. Only the wounded physician heals."

German medical orthodoxy of that time, operating by the doctrine of *"Stahl und Strahl"*—steel and radiation—had suffered a mortal wound in the corridors of history. Past was indeed prologue, and this pronouncement by the doctors, unconscious of its portent, was—in fact—the foreboding Mayday message of orthodox medicine as we know it. Echoing loud and clear in the crisp Alpine air, it was a broadcast programmed to carry its message of ultimate requiem to the doorstep of posterity, where we now stand.

This "happening" in the Bavarian Alps presaged a period of glacial flow in medical annals that has precipitated cold shakes and shivers in all sectors of the Establishment. Ganzheitstherapie is moving implacably on a collision course toward the Chinese Wall of insulation that surrounds the medical community. When it reaches ground zero, it may very well resolve the issue of what happens when an irresistible force meets an immovable body.

Dr. Josef Issels was not a clown or juggler in a medical circus doing a precarious balancing act with patients' lives; not a charlatan in Indian headdress dispensing snake oil from the back of a prairie wagon. His proven record of success with terminal cancer patients stands unparalleled in the history of medicine, he having seen and personally treated more patients in the last stages of the disease than any other clinician in medical history. Working with the patient's natural defense system—and less with drugs, surgery, and irradiation—he achieved partial remissions, control, and cure rates straining the credulity of the most notable cancerologists of our time. This record will probably stand as long as medical orthodoxy maintains its death grip on the old order.

In one study of survival where whole body treatment was applied to 252 patients who had undergone conventional surgery and irradiation, 16.6 percent were alive and fully fit for work 5 years after treatment, and, of these 42, 39 were alive and well and showed no signs of cancer 10 years after that, making in all a total survival time of 15 years.

In another impressive study of 370 patients in all types and stages of cancer, an unbelievable 87 percent were alive and well after a period of 5 years, with no relapses or detectable metastases. (World statistics show a relapse rate of 50 percent.) The follow-up methods employing Ganzheitstherapie reduced the dangers of reactivation of the malignancy to 13 percent, an unheard-of achievement, and a record not likely to be challenged in the immediate future.

Dr. John Anderson, M.D., Professor of Physical Medicine, Kings College Hospital, London, a cancer specialist with a brilliant academic background—also consultant to the World Health Organization—speaks

from personally having visited with Dr. Issels, in February 1969, and
from having examined his patients and inspected his medical records:

> I accept his findings of a long remission rate of nearly 17 percent
> in terminal cases. I am of the considered opinion that this is a new
> approach to cancer treatment and appears to be a considerable im-
> provement on what is usually offered. My overall opinion is that the
> Issels approach to the treatment of cancer is a unique and pioneering
> solution to a very difficult problem. He is undoubtedly producing
> clinical remissions in patients who have been regarded as hopeless.
>
> Dr. Issels is an able physician, a shrewd and penetrating clinician,
> whose principles and practice of medicine I admire. He is a shrewd
> observer of clinical conditions and has probably had more clinical
> experience with his six thousand patients at medically treating cancer
> than anyone else.
>
> There can be no doubt that he is genuine in what he does and
> the results he gets. . . . My overall impression is that the clinic is
> well ordered and fulfills the best tradition of medicine.

Dr. Robert J. C. Harris, Head of the Department of Environmental
Carcinogenesis at the Imperial Cancer Research Field, London, England—
hardly an Issels fan—preferred (as did other stalwarts of the Establishment) to close his eyes to Issels's accomplishments. In one unguarded
interview, he quite naively gave the devil his due: "Why Issels's patients
don't die is beyond me. His definition of terminal patients is accurate;
the figures he gets are remarkable by any standards."

Then, Dr. Harris made a revealing statement: "But you must remember
that millions of pounds are spent on cancer research every year, and
you can't expect anybody in the field to seriously believe that somewhere
in Bavaria there is a man who's got hold of something which has escaped
the rest of us."

Why Issels's patients didn't die had already been answered by
Ganzheitstherapie, and by his unsurpassed record of success in the treatment of terminal cancer patients, but he was deliberately boycotted by
and isolated from the medical community. It was heartbreaking to
exemplify the highest precepts of his profession, performing the role of
the Good Samaritan to the hilt, yet to an empty theater. Medical orthodoxy
stayed away in droves. But there were a few who paid him homage, and
this, somehow, made up for the dark days.

In December 1956, Dr. Josef Issels was invited to Rome by Pope
Pius XII for a private audience. On December 14, 1956, Pope Pius and
Dr. Issels held a long and memorable meeting. Pope Pius had long been
deeply interested in cancer research. Impressed with Issels's work, he
questioned him closely on every aspect of his treatment, especially his
ideas bearing on the religious and ethical considerations involved in the
management of the so-called "incurables." Issels was illuminated by this

meeting because he found here a strong community of interest and thinking on the philosophical and religious levels. He was deeply pleased when he realized that he was already practicing, in his therapy, the moral and humane precepts, with marked benefits to the patients and their families. He found himself, happily, in an area of complete agreement with the Pope, who had himself suggested to an international medical conference the desirability of eliminating the words "incurable" and "inoperable" from the traditional thinking of orthodox medicine. The audience ended on a high inspirational note, when Issels received the holy blessings of Pope Pius XII, and encouragement to continue his good work.

This meeting reinforced Issels's conviction that there was a higher power guiding him. It strengthened his dedication and resolve to continue on course. His spiritual insights were also shared to a very large extent by another great medical doctor in the field of cancer, Dr. Denis Burkitt, who said, "I am a religious man, and I am not at all surprised to learn that Dr. Issels believes at times that he, too, can be guided by God when it comes to making what conventional cancer researchers would dismiss as no more than an intuitive guess at how to handle a patient."

Dr. Josef Issels, the Dean of Ganzheitstherapie, epitomized—to our minds—the genius who captured the essence of a rich medical inheritance, and organized the diverse elements into a viable system—a true healing science—while at the same time, with wise discrimination, incorporating within it the invaluable contributions of our modern medical technology. Issels was the standard-bearer, the Prometheus who carried the flame from his venerable ancestors of truth in medicine, to illuminate the modern medical environment. On that memorable day, September 21, 1951, when Lydia Bacher was wheeled into his pitifully small hospital, he raised his beacon on a lonely Bavarian mountaintop, broadcasting a message of hope.

PATHFINDERS

From a broad array of notables working with biological methods (sometimes referred to as "alternative therapies"), we have chosen in this work to examine comprehensively the clinical modalities of just three "wounded physicians" who worked with, primarily, terminal cancer patients, and who exemplify, to the highest degree, the revolutionary content and practice of holistic medicine.

Josef Issels is, of course, the first one, and we shall speak of his methods and medicaments more exactly in a moment. The other two are Dr. Max Gerson and Dr. Rita Leroi of the Lukas-Klinik. Their work will be discussed in detail later in this book.

It may be appropriate at this point to mention briefly that, although there will appear certain differences in some methods and agents used (as will be brought out in the course of our discussion), there is present a solid commonality characterized by their basic precepts. For all of them, holism, or totality, underlies the clinical management process, and their common fount has its wellsprings in viewing cancer as a systemic disease rather than as a localized phenomenon. Their communion with integral medicine lies further in the fact that Issels, Gerson, and Leroi all demonstrated an enlightened understanding of humanics, and so brought into play potent psychological and spiritual influences in the physician-patient relationship. All of these preponderant elements that constitute successful clinical management are detailed in later chapters, so that the reader, especially the involved professional, can take note of the impelling common denominators that form the dynamics of the true art of healing.

Before detailing Dr. Issels's regime, let us pause a moment to note that, apart from its emphasis upon the emotional and psychological factors, he gives somewhat greater emphasis than either Dr. Leroi or Dr. Gerson to medical therapeutics, especially in the life-and-death crises attending typically hopeless cancer patients received at the Ringberg-Klinik. Most of his therapeutics, however, lie closer to the outer fringes of orthodox medicine—if not actually beyond these parameters. Issels does not passionately embrace orthodox methodology as a matter of routine, but neither does he deplore it. Highly individualistic immunotherapeutic measures characterize his main thrust, but, as he himself indicates, he uses "surgery where possible, chemotherapy where indicated (although very sparingly, and then only for a short period), and radiotherapy where necessary." It is immunotherapy, however, that remains the spine of his treatment, to which all of the other components are subordinated.

As for Dr. Rita Leroi of the Lukas-Klinik she—to the greatest extent—utilized predominantly natural approaches, and mild homeopathic remedies, relying more emphatically than the others upon a strong nutritional program—all contained within a reinforcing spiritual framework.

Dr. Max Gerson employed an almost total dietary regime. Basing his work upon vast clinical experience, Gerson was supersensitive to the emergent needs of his desperately ill patients—most in the last stages of cancer. In the early period of treatment, he would include some relatively mild medical agents and specified extracts and solutions—having a closer identity with food supplementation and detoxifying activity—than with drugs in the precise sense. But even these gentle medicaments were used only to surmount the crisis stages and were later discarded altogether in favor of a total nutritional regime when the patient was out of the woods, so to speak.

These devoted healers are not alone; there are others, most without honor in their own country, who can surely be cited as wounded physicians, eligible perhaps for some medical equivalent of the Purple Heart. Out of the many deserving of recognition, we have chosen a few to be described in these pages, hoping that all worthy exponents of signs and wonders in the healing arts will by their very works be known—and so identified, also, as worthy of appreciation and regard.

Ganzheitstherapie, the mysterious catalyst—in one guise or another—is at work. A new breed of doctor is looming on today's scene. These stalwarts uniformly display an exceptional though unenviable talent for being carted off to jail via the dubious courtesy of their local medical chapters. Their crime? Administering "metabolic therapy," the current parlance in America for whole body treatment of their patients.

}❧ ❧{

This book is intended as a chronicle of medicine in our times, distinguished by its accent on cancer therapies that appear to be of urgent consequence to those who are themselves afflicted, or who are concerned for family or friends near and dear to them. Because health and disease—like life and death—form a continuum, the problem of prevention and treatment presents itself simultaneously. The point at which the precancerous or cancerous state may intersect the line of good health, remains one of the most challenging problems of our times, although, as will be seen, optimism is warranted, because this, too, has its very positive solutions via a number of tests and diagnostic procedures that are available, although not all are generally known or practiced.

In learning about whole-body treatment, therefore, a clear insight into prevention emerges. The reader is here supplied with the components of Ganzheitstherapie and practice. Using these directional signs, caution signals, and topographic configurations as a road map, he is free to plot his own course as inclination and conviction dictate.

We fervently hope and believe, too, that members of the medical fraternity will also find some kernels of wisdom tucked away in these pages that may provide food for thought.

Our own satisfaction lies in opening a door that for diverse reasons has been kept partially or completely closed, and in knowing that we have tried—and, we hope, succeeded—in lighting a candle.

There is a new fury in the sounds of healing blowing in today's wind. It is this message and inspiration that we wish to bring you in this portrait of the "Wounded Physician"—he who symbolizes Faith, Hope, and Love —but the greatest of these is Love.

Part 1
The Whole Body

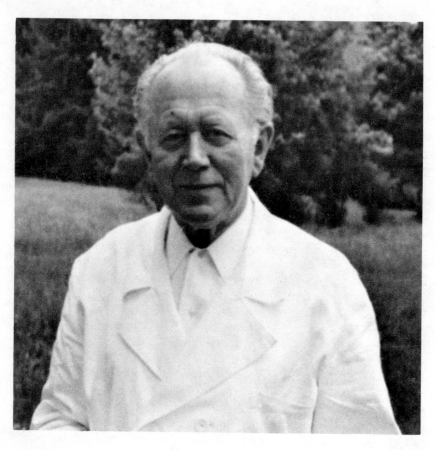

DR. JOSEF ISSELS

1

Dr. Josef Issels and Ganzheitstherapie

At first glance, the constituent agents and methods of Issels's "whole body approach"—Ganzheitstherapie—will appear a complex and highly diversified medical-type regime. The differentiating features (i.e., from traditional modes) are the introduction of the alternative variants—which Issels lumps into the general category of "immunotherapy" and which, for the most part, must be classified as "unorthodox." It is these that play the major role in his double-edged therapeutic program—directed against the tumor milieu itself, and concurrently designed to rehabilitate the body's defense mechanisms. Dr. Issels gravitated on an oblique path toward the treatment of cancer. He received his first training as a surgeon and then decided on general practice so that he could get at the roots of illness. He became heavily involved in the pathology of chronic diseases because these cases represented the heaviest part of his patient load. Sometimes he observed illnesses that would develop over generations and noted occasional correlations with hereditary factors, i.e., the grandfather had gastritis, his son an ulcer, and then the grandson, cancer of the stomach—his point of least resistance. Dr. Issels's finely honed scientific mind, fertilized by this rich experience, eventually led him to the formulation in 1953 of his combination therapy—his whole-body treatment of cancer. The aim of Dr. Josef Issels's basic therapy was to eliminate all causal factors such as dental and tonsilar foci, and fields of neural disturbance; abnormal intestinal flora, faulty diet, exogenous chemical and physical factors, and psychic stress; also, treatment of secondary damage and tumor milieu to restore normal functions of organs and organ systems. This is achieved by general measures, and by what he calls "substitution therapy"—and rehabilitation of the body's immunological defenses. (See Figure 1.)

His is a complex and diversified approach, and is so closely tailored to the individual requirements of the patient that it would need most careful instruction for any physician to become adept, particularly one without Dr. Issels's exceptionally broad background in clinical practice, especially cancer treatment. Nevertheless, in time, inherent modes of

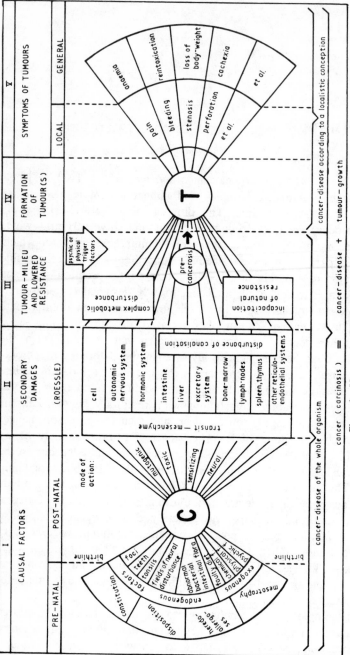

Figure 1. Hypothesis of Pathogenesis of Cancer[6]

Pre- and post-natal endogenous and exogenous causal factors (I), by mutation, toxicity or neural effects, via the "transit mesenchyme", produce secondary damage (II), in cells in control mechanisms (nervous and hormonal systems), in the detoxifying, excretory and defence systems.

Affects on excretory canalization lead to complex metabolic disturbances which lower natural resistance and produce an imbalanced condition gradually developing into a "tumour milieu" (III).

From such primary, pre-cancerous condition (III), a secondary, pre-cancerous condition may develop at a place of least resistance, and when defence potency is lowered further an oncogenous condition may result in a malignant growth developing at the site of least resistance.

"Localistic conception" with respect to malignant disease means the tumour and its local and general symptoms, the tumour being regarded as the *cause* of the disease. "Holistic conception" means latent oncogenic disease. Complete malignant disease, therefore, includes latent malignancy of the whole organism (I, II and III) and the cancerous growth (IV) with its symptoms (V). This conception regards the tumour as the *symptom* of the disease.

practice and therapeutic constituents could be codified, and standards established for a practical medical regime that could be followed by the average oncologist, and the interested physician. Issels himself clearly recognizes the problems present and has more than once expressed an impassioned desire to enter lecture and instruction work, where he could teach his methods to medical students and doctors at the universities, clinics, and hospitals.

In the following, we will include the most important agents and treatment methods that can be said to dominate Josef Issels's clinical management program of the cancer patient—apart from orthodox methods of treatment—which are not excluded, but which do not control the healing modality. As we will observe, the so-called alternative agents and methods dominate his program of clinical management.

Issels's preference was to avoid conventional approaches whenever possible, using them only circumspectly. His Ganzheitstherapie was anchored more in therapeutic agents and modalities that dealt very gently with the body—allying themselves with the flow of the body's natural healing powers, and avoiding the harsh abuses intrinsic to orthodox procedures. And Issels always used, as a firm adjunct, supportive nutritional therapy, which complemented his "whole body" program of treatment.

Following are the primary therapeutic agents and modes that he employed:

1. *Pyretotherapy or Hyperthermy*—the induction of high fever under clinical conditions, which alerts the defense mechanism of the body. Issels induced two kinds of fever: one, which he called "active," by the injection of bacterial substance to which the body would react; and the other a "passive" fever, that is, a febrile reaction provoked artificially, usually from outside the body. "Active fever," Issels said, "may be induced by injection of the drug Vaccincurin, or Pyrifer, an ethical preparation. Made from coli bacteria specially treated, it irritates the fever control mechanism in the midbrain, and in about four hours, the body temperature is raised.

"I generally induce passive fever by placing the patient inside a custom-built cylinder containing electrodes which emit ultra-short waves. Completely enclosed, the body is bombarded from head to toe with these waves, and literally within a few minutes, its temperature begins to rise. If the patient is able, and willing, to endure it—and here the doctor-patient relationship is extremely important—the temperature is kept at 105°F. for between one and one-and-a-half hours: the temperature at which cancer cells, but not normal cells, are damaged. Naturally during this treatment the body loses potassium, and this must be balanced by a diet which is rich in potassium, for instance bananas, rice, or potatoes.

"M. von Ardenne, Lampert and others have shown that cancer cells are very sensitive to heat. At a temperature of around 105°F. the malignant cells in the body can be adversely damaged. On the other hand, healthy cells are not damaged until a temperature of 109.5°F. is reached. Fever and hyperthermia therefore not only improve the potency of defense, but also weaken cancer cells to such an extent that they can be destroyed more quickly by the defense mechanisms—while healthy cells go unharmed.

"There are many other means of inducing passive fever, such as simply by giving the patient a hot bath and afterwards surrounding the body with hot water bottles and blankets. In this way the fever may be maintained for five or even six hours.

"Passive fever treatment is usually repeated twice a week, sometimes for months, until the desired results are achieved. During this time, it is important that pyretotherapy is sympathetically but firmly administered, its value carefully explained, and whenever possible, the patients taught to regularly keep their own temperature chart."

As for the substantial effects of induced fever, Issels states that:

"In such febrile conditions, active defense cells, neutrophilic granulocytes, are mobilized in the bone marrow and released into the blood. There is a marked increase in the number of leucocytes; the 'active defense phase' has been reached which can be seen in the blood count. These defense cells produce bactericidal substances and also proteolytic and detoxicating enzymes. They are able to 'swallow up' toxins, microbes and fragments of cells, storing them until they are dissolved in a process known as phagocytosis.

"The production of specific antibodies, or 'defense enzymes,' by 'immunocytes' (lymphocytes, lymph cells) is also greatly increased. Even a single feverish attack of a few hours' duration may, in some circumstances, cause antibody titres in the blood to increase ten times. In addition, febrile reactions stimulate the mobilization and elimination of unwanted inert deposits in the mesenchymal stores. They clear toxicants remaining after acute and congenital infections, for instance congenital TB or syphilis. The elimination and regeneration of damaged tissue may be speeded up. Alkalosis is simultaneously converted into a relative acidosis, so that the internal environment of the body undergoes a fundamental change. In short, during general febrile reactions, the natural resistance and recuperative powers of the organism are brought to a high pitch. A further benefit is that, if a patient is being treated by intermittent massive-dose chemotherapy, the drug dosage can be reduced by a third, sometimes even by a half, if it is administered at the peak of pyretotherapy. The curative effect is almost the same but there is a reduction in the harmful side-effects associated with chemotherapy.

"Whole body therapists know that the 'delicate' child, the one who goes down with one pediatric infection after another, will, later in life, be less susceptible to chronic disease. And doctors believing in biological methods of treatment will always aim to promote and assist this most powerful curative reaction by, for instance, using hot mustard packs. These are particularly indicated when cutaneous eruptions 'don't want to come out,' when they 'turn inwards,' when the body's own febrile reaction is not powerful enough to overcome the infection without artificial stimulation."

2. *Haemotogenic Oxidation Therapy, H.O.T.* This was developed by the Swiss worker Wehrli, and has been increasingly used since the early 1960s as part of modern medicine's arsenal against cancer.

"Unlike many other treatments, H.O.T. is essentially simple, and has the added advantage of being painless. A quantity of blood, which, depending on the patient's state, can range from 100 to 200 millilitres, is drawn off. Under suitable laboratory conditions, oxygen is then bubbled through it. This produces an effervescent effect and the foamed blood, previously usually blackish in color, is now generally changed to a distinctive red. At this stage it is irradiated by ultra-violet rays for between five and ten minutes. Finally, it is left to settle for up to an hour. Then it is returned to the patient by drip.

"In treating blood in this manner, oxygen is transformed into ozone. The result is that the oxygenated blood derives the same benefits as it would from ozone therapy. The blood itself is sterilized, normalized, regenerated and reactivated. Defense cells regain their aggressive capacity. Returned to the host, these cells can once more attack microbes and cancer-promoting viruses which are characterized by an anaerobic metabolism—making them unable to survive in the actively oxidized environment that H.O.T. creates. At the same time, malignant cells are attacked, and alien and alienated proteins and other unwanted compounds in the blood are chemically altered during H.O.T., so that they can be recognized as such and eliminated.

"H.O.T. is a regular weekly treatment which can go on for two or three months. There is no fixed time-scale; it depends on a number of factors, such as the condition of the patient at the onset of treatment, the progress and type of tumor. Needless to say, close clinical observation is necessary if a patient is anemic; blood from a donor must be used and treated in this manner before being drip-fed to the patient."

3. *Auto-Hormone Therapy.* This concerns the passing of ultra-short waves through the brain and its hormone-producing glands, to break up the typical autonomic freeze of the cancer patient. Repeated at clinically indicated intervals, it can normalize the autonomic control functions and thereby eliminate one of the most important causal factors of the disease.

"The autonomic, vegetative, centres of the brain, especially the thalamic and hypothalamic regions, respond to the irritative effect of the ultra-short waves by altering the body's metabolic reactions. There is an increase in hormone production. This, in addition to its immediate physiological result, will have a feedback effect within all the regulatory organs. Thus, this double-pronged attack not only initiates short-term normalization of neuro-hormonic activity, but it also has a 'training' effect whereby, in the course of time, the hormone-producing organs will begin again to spontaneously fulfil their biological tasks without the need for further ultra-shortwave treatment.

"Tumors which have hitherto shown themselves resistant to X-ray therapy can be made more susceptible by a preceding course of ultra-short waves; these will also allow for a reduction in the amount of X-rays needed, and this can only help to remove some of the unpleasant side-effects that so often accompany radiation.

"Rehydration and a high fluid intake assist these treatments by eliminating the products of oncolysis and metabolic residues and improve liver and kidney function."

4. *Substitution Therapy* includes all the measures aimed at restoring organic malfunction, by:

> *a.* the substitutive stimulation of detoxicating and defensive systems, by liver and mesenchymal extracts, and so forth;
> *b.* the regeneration of extremely stressed organs, by organ-specific RNA and DNA preparations;
> *c.* the normalization of metabolic malfunctions resulting from enzymatic defects, by regular application of specific drugs, as well as vitamins and minerals;
> *d.* the administration of proteolytic enzymes to replace the missing nonspecific dissolving activity.

}&* *&{

Again, while the basic therapy regime may appear complicated, in practice it is not. It is also reproducible. Further, the more effective the general measures, the less there is a need for substitution therapy.

5. *Neural Therapy.* Issels explains first that "the 'focus' is a chronic, abnormal, local change in the connective tissue, capable of producing the varied distant effects beyond its immediate surroundings, and therefore in constant conflict with local and general defense (Pischinger and Kellner). By this definition, even a fully-healed scar may sometimes act as a focus, spreading disease to distant parts of the body."

Dr. Issels concentrates, however, on what he considers to be the most lethal of these foci, namely, infected teeth and tonsils, indicating that "the removal of devitalized teeth and chronically diseased tonsils is one of the better-known aspects of my work. .... I *do not* recommend that healthy tonsils and teeth be removed ... but I believe that if they are diseased, they cause the body's natural resistance to be lowered, thus acting as an important contributory factor to tumor development. In these cases, I insist on their removal.

" . . . The beneficial results of tonsillectomy with cancer patients were first brought to my attention in 1953, and by chance. A tonsillectomy was performed on an incurable cancer patient in my clinic who had severe rheumatic pains and a long history of tonsillar disease. The operation was done to relieve the woman's pain, but it was remarkably successful in other ways as well: general toxic symptoms disappeared, and, most important of all, her pathologically rapid pulse rate was reduced. Many cancer patients have a high pulse rate, reaching 140 and even 160, and this always leads to a poor prognosis, but in the case of this woman, it was almost normalized. Soon her tumor began to regress, and ultimately she recovered from her cancer.

"This unexpected but welcome result encouraged me to arrange for tonsillectomies on two further patients with tonsillar ailments, who also had therapy-resistant cardiovascular disorders and toxic symptoms. In these cases as well, following surgery, cardiovascular and many other symptoms virtually disappeared. A positive 're-tuning' of natural defense and a certain inhibition of tumor growth was also observed. This improved situation naturally allowed more time for active immunotherapy to work.

"These early successes encouraged me to persevere with tonsillectomies. Before making them virtually obligatory in my clinic, forty percent of those who died there, did so from heart attacks. Afterwards the figure dropped to five percent. This, I contend, is incontrovertible proof that tonsillogenic toxins find their way into the bloodstream and eventually can cause, for instance, a fatal myocardial disease. This is one reason why more people die from heart disease than from any other.

"In addition, my experience shows a direct connection between dental and tonsillar foci and many of the illnesses responsible for early debilitation and untimely invalidizing."

Issels says that, as long as the body's own defense system is in good working order, "the extent of the disease-provoking activity of a focus in distant parts of the body depends on whether the body is able to oppose the focus with its own defense mechanism. As long as the focal situation is kept under control by the local defense mechanism, no focus-induced remote effects will arise. On the other hand, distant effects will arise when the body's resistance has more or less broken down: control of head foci will then gradually collapse, and there will be a consequential gradual increase in generalized focogenic intoxication. This will cause an inevitable deterioration of the body's defense power with a concomitant promotion of malignant growth.

" . . . The diagnosis and treatment of dental foci remains generally unsatisfactory. A survey conducted at my clinic found that, on admission, ninety-eight percent of the adult cancer patients had between two and ten dead teeth, each one a dangerous toxin producing 'factory.' Very often we are confronted with X-ray negative dead teeth, root remnants, and residual ostitis which had not been diagnosed and therefore had not been removed.

"Only total, thorough dental treatment will really succeed in giving the body's defense a chance. In addition to X-ray diagnosis, it is therefore necessary to use other diagnostic aids, such as infra-red techniques and tests, to estimate tooth vitality and periosteal resistance, and other electrometric methods."

Dr. Issels has studied this problem most intensively, and, in his challenging book *Cancer: A Second Opinion,* he discusses in impressive detail the scientific and medical data surrounding this problem, which led to his conclusions.

" . . . Ferdinand Huneke, the founder of neural therapy, whose remarkable contribution in this regard we shall look at in detail later, discovered over forty years ago that injection of a local anaesthetic near a primary focus may immediately remove any symptoms of distant disease induced by the focus. This effect—the second-phenomenon—usually takes place only a few seconds after the anaesthetic injection, and lasts for hours, days, or even for a lifetime. Naturally the improvement occurs only in those regions influenced by the injected focus. Nevertheless, the measure has therefore a remarkable diagnostic value as well."

Issel considers that the toxic activity of odontogenic foci may be even "more perilous for the organism than their neural effects.

" . . . The identity and chemical structure of certain of the biogenic amines were mainly clarified in the 1950's by Schug-Koesters, Hiller, Gaebelein and others of the University of Munich. Following similar findings in America, the metabolic and exchange processes in solid dental structures were further investigated by the German researcher Spreter von Kreudenstein. He showed the drugs injected intravenously were, four to five hours later, discernible within the intradental capillary ducts or even devitalized teeth, and in a concentration only slightly lower than in the blood.

"That endodental exchange may also take place in the opposite direction has been reported by Artelstone (USA) and Djerassi (Bulgaria). If radio-iodine, I-131, is deposited in an evacuated pulp cavity which is then sealed off with a filling, the iodine will appear in the thyroid some twenty hours later, as can be demonstrated by taking a scintograph of the thyroid region. Similarly, dyes can be washed out of a sealed pulp cavity.

"All these findings prove conclusively that within solid dental structures, there may proceed an unimpeded substantial interchange in either direction. Consequently, odontogenic toxins, wherever they may have been produced, are able to diffuse and circulate within the organism.

". . . The close connection between teeth and tonsils was proven when it was observed that Indian ink injected into a sealed dental cavity appeared as spots on the tonsillar surface in about twenty to thirty minutes. These experiments showed that pathogenic substances from the jaw region, including toxins from devitalized teeth, are conducted to the lymphatic tonsillar ring, there to be detoxicated and excreted. Besides their 'natural' physiological load, the tonsils are thus additionally exposed to continuous attack by odontogenous toxins provoked by the devitalization of teeth.

". . . As already mentioned, before I began paying special attention to the tonsils, I lost many incurable patients, *not* as a result of cancer, but through acute cardiocirculatory failure. After introducing tonsillectomy, such deaths became much rarer.

"Toxic circulatory death, however, is only one of the many dangers constantly threatening the life of the chronically sick. Phlebitis, thrombosis, embolism, pneumonia, pleurisy, and cystitis all too often complicate the course of treatment. In my experience, these, too, became noticeably rarer with the introduction of routine tonsillectomy.

"Another observation, one I believe very important for cancer treatment, is that often following tonsillectomy, in a large proportion of patients, I have found that the tongue, not coated before the tonsillectomy, later has a marked yellowish, brownish, or blackish coating. Experience shows that the canalizing activity of the intestinal mucous membranes is indicated by the surface condition or coating of the tongue; a change in this coating suggests that a previously blocked 'gut filter' has been opened, leading to the conclusion that tonsillar foci also disturb the detoxicating and excretory activity of the gut. Restitution of this function is of crucial importance in the treatment of cancer because the largest proportion of the necrogenous toxins which develop during tumor solution is excreted by this route.

"The widespread opinion that degeneratively destroyed tonsils may still be of importance for cancer patients as detoxicating and excretory organs and must therefore be preserved at all cost has, in my experience, been quite clearly refuted. Anyone, having seen the degenerative destruction in the tonsillar tissue of cancer patients, will be convinced that, on the contrary, these tonsils have contributed in potentiating the virulence of the tumor milieu and the defense deficiency.

"Tonsillectomy must be followed by desensitization with vaccines obtained from dental and tonsillar foci. Neural treatment of the tonsillar bed concludes this treatment.

". . . Nevertheless, my own unhappy experience shows that with cancer patients, foci treatment has generally been left to a very late stage. In the vast majority of the patients I have treated, it was quite clear that foci treatment should have been carried out years before—and certainly long before the manifestation of the tumors.

"That this was not done is a sad reminder that far too many doctors and dentists fail to recognize a fundamental truism; untreated foci can be linked to the development of cancer."

6. *Immunotherapy in Progressive Metastatic Cancer—a Fifteen-Year Survival Follow-Up.* This paper by Dr. Issels, published in the *Clinical Trials Journal* (London) 1970, 7, No. 3, 357-66, is a precise and comprehensive approach to the science of immunology—and an important record of treatment of several hundred patients. The simple, underlying principles that he used follow in abridged form:

a. Disorder occurs in the mesenchymal system regulating and controlling the growth and distribution of normal cells and the lysis of abnormal cells.

b. The tumor milieu is the result of secondary damage to organs and organ systems.

His combined cancer therapy, therefore, consists of the basic treatment of the body to prevent the development of abnormal cells and the use of other therapeutic procedures that attack the tumor itself. His calculated, carefully evaluated combination therapy to eliminate the original tumor may include surgery, irradiation, chemotherapy, enzyme therapy with lytic enzymes—such as asparaginase—and immunotherapy by both active immunization with mycoplasma vaccine (Gerlach) and passive immunization with antibodies prepared from cancer cells.

But it must again be emphasized that Issels uses the traditional medical modes circumspectly and, at that point of crisis in the pathology where it is an imperative, as a life-saving necessity. However, whenever such action is invoked, his stern caveat is that it must be complemented by immediate, accompanying measures that stimulate and reinforce the body's own immunological defense system.

Dr. Issels has used the Gerlach mycoplasma vaccine in what he calls "active immunization." As for "passive immunization," he has this to say: "Passive immunization is effected with standard preparations such as Centanit, Sarkogen, and Lymphogran, which induce formation of specific antibodies. Centanit is used in cases of all types of carcinoma, Sarkogen for all types of sarcoma. A special indication for Lymphogran is Hodgkin's disease (lymphogranulomatosis).

"By this basic treatment of a cancer patient (the host), it is possible to increase the effect of tumor-specific immunotherapeutic agents. This therapy improves the results of prior conventional treatment because it eliminates the otherwise unaffected tumor milieu and, therefore, the tendency for relapses or metastatic growth formation.

"Our observations and experience in cases unsuccessfully treated, including the use of immuno-biological drugs, may be explained in that the principles of comprehensive treatment of the whole cancer-affected organism have not been observed."

The cellular immune system, according to Dr. Issels "has a homeostatic control function or immune surveillance. It is this system that differentiates between 'self' and 'nonself' and destroys alien or outlaw cells including cancer cells." In fact, all of these specific measures can be optimized to restore the body's ailing immune system when integrated within the framework of the basic concept of whole-body treatment—Ganzheitstherapie.

THE SEVEN DEADLY SINS

Besides offering profound food for thought to every concerned human being, Dr. Josef Issels, in a striking challenge to the medical and scientific community, formulated a critique of certain "transgressions" of the practicing physician, which affect the medical, physiological, and psychological factors at work in the pathological condition. He dramatically calls his treatise "The Seven Deadly Sins of Cancer." (The emotional and psychological influences that are present in the clinical situation are elaborated at greater length later in this book.)

"1. The 'charitable' white lie, in which the doctor keeps the diagnosis of cancer from his patient, is without doubt the most deadly of all these 'sins.' Withholding the truth, apart from being ethically dubious, also means that a patient cannot become involved in the essential two-way partnership with his physicians that allows curative measures to achieve the maximum effect.

"2. Equally wrong is the 'sin' encompassed in the oft-heard arguments of many doctors that whole-body therapy, either as a pre- or post-treatment to other methods, is not necessary. To reinforce their case they argue further that, in the case of surgery, the operation has been radical, that the 'accepted' way of 'curing' cancer has been achieved, and that there is no need for any other treatment. Similar arguments are applied to radiotherapy. The patient and his relatives are left in a state of induced euphoria which is too-often shattered when the disease returns.

"3. The third deadly 'sin' is ignorance of the role that whole-body therapy as a follow-up treatment can play. Coupled with this is the further misapprehension about the very meaning of follow-up treatment. The popular idea of follow-up treatment after surgery is to order a course of radiotherapy. But, at best, this is not more than a tumor-specific measure which does not have any part in treating the actual cause of the cancer. Yet, to succeed, any follow-up treatment must attack the source and the actual cause of the cancer to avoid metastases and secondaries recurring. That is the avowed aim of whole-body therapy—and happily there are many cases who can testify to its success. This therapy is the only means available of returning the abnormal metabolic milieu to normal so that the host can recognize and destroy cancer cells already existing or in the process of formation. Further, this method allows for an actual cure of the disease by removing the host's predisposition to produce tumors.

"4. The fourth deadly 'sin' is the widely-held belief that proper follow-up treatment does exist within the framework of conventional medicine. In practice this turns out to be routine 'check-ups,' in themselves necessary because over fifty percent of all those who have survived surgery and radiotherapy have, in fact, a high chance of contracting secondaries. The 'follow-ups' are designed in the hope that such recurrences can be discovered at an early stage. It is true that metastases may be discovered during such a check-up. But it is equally true that the check-up has not PREVENTED the secondaries appearing. And, by the time they are found, the patient is often deemed as beyond further treatment. The tragedy of these check-ups is that they lull the patient, and sometimes his physician, into a false state of well-being. Worst of all, the patient too often believes the check-up is actually some kind of preventive treatment. It is nothing of the kind.

"5. The fifth deadly 'sin' is the belief that a few weeks' holiday is beneficial following surgical or radiological treatment. It is certainly pleasant to have such a rest after a spell in the hospital. But the time should be applied to the far more urgent and important matter of undergoing positive whole-body aftercare. Those days and weeks following an operation or irradiation are, as we have seen, crucial for a patient's long-term survival. This is NOT the time to lie on a beach or putter about in the sun. This IS the time to strengthen a patient's bodily defense. Too often, a period of blissful convalescence is followed by the discovery that the cancer has returned, and that the patient is about to be consigned to the category of incurables.

"6. The sixth deadly 'sin' is performed by those doctors who urge patients who have undergone conventional treatment to go on special diets designed to fatten them. Now, it is common knowledge that overeating is harmful even for healthy people. It is doubly wrong then to pump food into cancer patients in the belief that it will 'build them up to go out into the world strong and healthy.' Numerous experiments have shown that such feeding, far from increasing bodily resistance, lowers it—and so contributes to recurrences. Further proof of this can be seen in the cancer statistics for the two World Wars. During the war years the numbers dropped significantly; one reason for this was the fact that cancer patients, like everybody else, were kept on reduced rations. My own clinical observations show that a pronounced weight increase is a triggering factor in the development of metastases.

"7. The seventh deadly 'sin' is to recommend whole-body therapy as a follow-up and then fail to see that this is carried out properly, and that a patient has all the benefits accruing from such a treatment. The problem is one of education; a realization that it is not enough to pick and choose from a carefully-tailored program. The whole regime must be followed through. For instance, it is virtually useless to lay down dietary rules—and then neglect to deal with foci. All the measures within whole-body therapy are framed to interlock and complement each other. Partial treatment is not enough.

"By removing these 'sins,' a major step would have been undertaken in coping with that most important of all problems—that of the so-called 'incurable' cancer patient."

2

Misdirection and Detours:
The Origin of Ganzheitstherapie

Medical manuscripts dealing with cancer manifestation and treatment go back to the ancient Chinese and Sumerians—three thousand years before the birth of Christ. Certain of the concepts and components of Issels's Ganzheitstherapie clearly started to surface in the fifth century B.C. with the advent of Hippocrates, the founder of modern medicine.

Hippocrates hesitated to use surgery, giving his prime emphasis to the elimination of toxins and the purification of the blood, a natural food diet, herbs, and drugs—representing indeed, some of the elements of the holistic approach. His "whole person" view encouraged observance of the natural laws through abstinence from anything that was harmful not only to the body, but to the "soul and spirit." His path to healing is best remembered by the much-quoted dictum: "Let food be your medicine, and let medicine be your food."

In the second century B.C., Asclepiades, a Greek physician, preferred methods that are today recognized as the "natural hygiene" system. This was characterized by a natural foods diet, exercise, and rest. Clarus Galen (A.D. 131-200), the founder of experimental physiology and pathology, was in the same ball park, considering cancer a disease of the entire organism.

Then came the towering giant Paracelsus, dominating medicine in the sixteenth century. He recognized the body's natural healing powers, and contributed much to the doctrine of totality in medical treatment. He it was, too, who first opened the door on psychosomatic medicine, elaborating the important role played by the mind and the spirit in illness. Paracelsus's remarkable intuitive powers led to his propounding his startling analogue to Jung's precept of "the wounded physician," in his perceptive instruction: "Let the highest motive in medicine be love."

Each was on the track of truth. With the brightest minds in medicine pointing to the essential quality of wholeness in the approach to healing, where did we lose the way? Where did we deviate from the mainstream, when the most advanced thinkers over three millennia had already set the course, clearly pointing out the road? Why did modern medical science regress to a Precambrian frame of mind—reverting to the minutiae—losing sight of the universal dimensions by deciding that cancer was a localized disease problem?

Rudolf Virchow, perhaps the outstanding figure in pathology in the nineteenth century, enjoys the dubious distinction of having thrown medicine off the track. He theorized and presented convincing evidence to prove that all morbid processes occur in the cell. This egg hatched beautifully, but not as Virchow had anticipated. He, himself, believed in the whole-body concept in medicine, and intended his work simply to contribute to what was already known—to be integrated into the existing body of knowledge. Instead, the members of the institution of medicine seized Virchow's postulate, convincing themselves, irretrievably, that they could now locate the disease in the cell—ergo, cancer could now be viewed as a problem of local origin. The symptom—the tumor—was now declared to be the disease itself. Unwittingly, Virchow's work in the area of cellular pathology changed the face and course of medical history in education, in research and—not least—in the treatment of the patient.

This was not exactly surprising in an age that was soon ushering in supermicroscopes, miniature transistorized spectaculars, and exciting gadgetry and instrumentation, which cast its fatal spell—as the credulous public in the medical marketplace daily waited with bated breath the anticipated pronouncement that God had just been produced in the laboratory.

The origins of the disease process were lost. Everything that had been learned before went out the window, was now forgotten, including—especially—the priceless inheritance from three thousand years of the finest medical minds in history, namely, that cancer was a disease of the entire organism, and that the restoration of the body's innate resistance through its immunological defense system was the heart of the problem. Obsessed with the mechanisms, the conventional mind in full ecstatic bloom easily approached a state of blissful idiocy. Eyes bulging with fanatic zeal, doctors enthusiastically boned up on the Merck Index, honed their scalpels, and charged into their radiation rooms, intent on blasting symptoms to Mars and Jupiter.

Over the years, science and technology had deposited a beautiful Christmas package, a veritable gold mine, on the doorstep of modern medicine—the accumulation of three millennia of concepts, principles, and methods—a master road map on the path to good health and the treatment of disease, every inch of the road having been painfully detailed by all the venerables in the history of the healing arts. All jettisoned, just when twentieth-century technology, undreamed of by Hippocrates, Paracelsus—or Virchow, for that matter—made its appearance on the scene. Instead of serving as a springboard to carry medical science forward, it carried it farther and farther away from the mainstream.

How far away was simply but tragically stated at the Tenth International Cancer Congress where six thousand famous cancer research workers met in Houston, Texas, in 1970. Many of the world's foremost scientists and doctors, one after another, categorically reiterated that to continue along present lines of research and treatment would bring us from our present dire state of "crisis, to catastrophe."

It becomes clear that, throughout history, the underlying principle in medical practice was in the constitutional treatment of the patient, although the accent of the changing times differed with respect to components. For example, over the ages, one or another therapeutic agent or method was given a more conspicuous place. During one period, plants, herbs, and their derivatives—like the hellebore, sedum, and garlic—were dominant; at another time, powerful drugs like arsenic and mercury were administered. Though hard to credit, the records of those "dark ages" abound with stories of cures. Above all, the direction was maintained, despite some bumbling and stumbling along the way.

Pioneer Josef Issels would be the last person to challenge the laurels so painfully won by the nobility in medical history. He is among the first to acknowledge the valiant contributions of those trailblazers who marked the path so well. His work with Ganzheitstherapie is not a claim to their grand idea, but rather a tribute to their struggle, and to the victory. Where others feared to tread, Issels has dared to follow the leaders over a hazardous personal path, risking name and fortune. His has not been a rejection of traditional practices, but actually a process of adding, improving, refining and complementing, in a dedicated and selfless effort to achieve a harmony of the practice of clinical medicine with the natural laws of the universe.

Issels can be faulted by orthodox wisdom only because he refused to turn back from the path already marked, as did many of today's valiants whom we shall discuss in the pages of this book. He took what was available, and, in addition, applied any or all of these superb weapons in a struggle against ignorance, disease, and death.

3

Mistletoe in Cancer Treatment

Hauntingly, as if to tantalize the growing awareness in man, there rises, out of the seemingly primeval mists, a pungent nostalgia that pursues his emerging intellect with the nagging persistence of an old joke, whose details are well remembered but whose punch line forever eludes recall.

Such a game of hide-and-seek insinuates itself upon the heels of Middle Ages mysticism and old Germanic legend, venturing with a sacrilegious audacity into the restive environs of obstinate orthodoxy in the European scientific and medical community.

This irreverent intrusion stems annoyingly from rather humble origins, the root cause for complaint being a half-parasitic "animal-plant" with astonishing healing properties, which is held to be a hangover from an earlier period of earth's evolution. Belonging to the botanical family of Loranthaceae, it is sometimes referred to as *Viscum album,* but is more familiarly known as mistletoe.

Tales of its therapeutic magic come from the Edda, a collection of old Germanic myths and legends, which is replete with compelling tales about this mysterious plant: of good and evil, right and wrong, redemption of guilt, and of evolutionary trends and tendencies. The Druids, priests of the early Germanic tribes, used to cut this holy plant with a golden sickle. Even in our own times, we enjoy a happy legacy from this ancient past: in accordance with old Teutonic custom, the romantic may still exercise his privilege of kissing a woman standing under a sprig of mistletoe.

Right up to modern times, mistletoe has been recognized and used as a remedy for many diseases, including epilepsy, sterility, high blood pressure, and depression. Rudolf Steiner was the first to discover its extraordinary qualities in cancer. As far back as 1917, Steiner gave his first instructions for the therapeutic use of mistletoe; and in 1920, he initiated physicians in mistletoe therapy. In close working conjunction with pharmacologists, he gave instructions to transform mistletoe into an effective cancer remedy that was called Iscador.

Spiritual-Scientific Medicine, or Anthroposophical Medicine, as Rudolf

Steiner came to call his system of healing, was in complete harmony with his philosophical teachings of the natural and universal laws, and their manifesting phenomena. It trespassed heavily, in those days, upon the stage and scenery of traditional medical practice, which was comfortably bedded down in a glittering surgical arsenal of scalpels and knives, and in the chemistry of drugs.

Unfortunately for the entrenched medical community, Steiner was not just another garden variety of intruding intellect, but a rare genius at dissembling the dogmatism of conventional knowledge. Although he carried superlative credentials as a scientist in his own right, and was an eminent philosopher and educator to boot, insult was added to injury by the fact that Steiner was without any medical background. Yet he dared to challenge modern medicine on its own terms; even so, he did not discount the necessity—within precisely defined limits—for the use of surgery, having deep knowledge of nature acquired through spiritual training.

It is a basic principle of Anthroposophical Medicine that the physical organism cannot be considered as a separate entity, but must, in divine union, as it were, work hand in hand with the human mind and spirit. Prima facie, this open-ended, multifaceted thesis presented unbending medical doctrine and practice with its gravest challenge, no less threatening than that posed by Dr. Josef Issels, whose whole-body concept had certain things in common with Anthroposophical Medicine.

The success of Iscador and its complementary regimen can be attributed to the diamond quality of Rudolf Steiner's grand design, beginning with spiritual insights (the "science" of Anthroposophy), which were then engineered into sound medical procedures. In other words, an Austrian clairvoyant—the least likely candidate for membership in the "club"—had obeyed all the rules. First, he developed a sound conceptual base. Then he proceeded to establish incontestable pharmacological support, attracting in the process a brilliant professional staff. Last but not least, he dared to move his game-play into the crucible situation: the brilliantly lit stage of clinical testing and practice.

Mind-boggling indeed was the fact that Steiner, an outsider, carrying the incongruous trappings of an esoteric philosophy, had penetrated orthodox medicine's inner sanctum by transmuting his premises into iron-hard therapeutic procedures for successfully treating the disease of our times—cancer—by introducing new possibilities in this area of traditional medicine.

Dr. Alvan R. Feinstein, Professor of Medicine at Yale University, one of today's bright, courageous minds, expands on this in broader terms, echoing Anthroposophy. He says that the presumed "scientific evaluation" of drugs ignores the vital human factors that make the "science" strongly suspect and seriously challenge the validity of its "evaluation." The use of control groups, the random division of test groups—including those receiving only placebos—and the trial procedures that are designed as the scientific basis for assessment of a drug being tested, "do not contain provision for evaluating the complex crucial issues that distinguish a person from a *dog,* or a field of *wheat.* . . . We have not worked out adequate methods for analyzing the distinctively human issues that characterize the treatment of people."

Virtually all "human" information is considered to be "soft data," and as such is deliberately omitted from scientific evaluation. Dr. Feinstein contends that the so-called "hard data" that remain are "no more valid indexes of the realities of human medical therapy, than the 'body counts' in Vietnam were valid indexes of progress in human warfare."

His conclusion is that the real answer to effective treatment is with the full-time practicing doctors who are actually using the medications in the clinical situation, and who know the patient inside out as a complete human being. The golden key, once the medicaments are understood, lies in that subtle, indefinable area of humanics, not mechanistics. It will not be found in a dog or a field of wheat. Let us see what results are being achieved by full-time practicing doctors who use Iscador in a total treatment approach.

Throughout the world today there are more than a thousand medical doctors in more than twenty countries who are members of the Anthroposophical Society, subscribing to the whole philosophical system, and to spiritually oriented medicine, with Iscador playing the central role in the treatment of cancer patients. There are, in addition, many more thousands of physicians, outside of Anthroposophical Medicine, who also subscribe to, and administer, Iscador in the treatment of malignancies, and in the postoperative care of their patients. These practitioners have not exactly been turned on by some itinerant spellbinder, but have been completely convinced and committed by hard-core proof.

In a survey carried out in 1973 by Dr. G. Kienle in collaboration with the Society for Cancer Research in Stuttgart, among 912 practitioners using Iscador, seventy percent observed "marked" to "impressive" improvements in the disease, and ninety percent reported a noticeable improvement in the patients' general condition under treatment. More than ninety percent of the doctors stated that Iscador also had "marked" to "excellent" effect on pain due to cancer, and ninety percent of those who commented on the value of Iscador considered it crucial to success in the treatment process. The physicians participating in this survey, had a total medical experience encompassing more than a hundred thousand clinical patients.

In another study presented under the auspices of the Austrian Surgeons' Congress in May 1972, Dr. M. Lindemann, who had started a

comparative trial with postoperative treatment of lung cancer patients
at the lung sanatorium "Baumgartner Hohe" in Vienna, reported that
the results of a two-year trial run had already been so impressive that
there could be no doubt about their being positive over the longer term,
and this conclusion came from rock-hard conservative medical men.
Professor Dr. G. Salzer had operated on seventy-eight patients with lung
cancer, about half of whom were given postoperative Iscador therapy.
The other half of this patient group had been referred to the hospital by
doctors who were not interested in follow-up therapy, so they in fact
constituted the control group. Patients were classified according to the
stage of their cancer, and all surgical reports were assessed by the same
pathologist. The distribution of stages was the same in both groups. After
this two-year period of observation, eighty-one percent of patients treated
with Iscador were still living, compared with twenty-nine percent of those
who had not been given follow-up treatment.

In lung cancer patients, metastatic pleural-carcinosis is one of the
most common complications of a spreading malignancy. It often leads to
exudate formation ranging from severe dyspnea to life-threatening cardio-
respiratory insufficiency. Over the years, many methods have been
employed to inhibit exudation and seal the pleura, with limited degrees
of success, cytostatis averaging from 11-19%. Tube-thoracotomy and
talcum methods have shown an 80-90% success rate, and Wobe-Mugos
enzyme therapy 47-81%.

In a study published in the medical journal, *"Praxis und Klinik der
Pneumologie"* (32, Jahrgang, Heft 11, Nov. 1978, Seite 683-748), fifty
cases of carcinomatous pleural effusions that were given *topical treatment
with Iscador* were examined. In 92% of the patients the exudate disappeared after an average of 3.3 applications within eighteen days. The
journal indicated that "Pleural reaction to Iscador is minimal: almost no
pain reported; subfebrile increase in temperature is common; extreme
increase in temperature is rare; no cases of pleural shock." And—of
crucial importance—*Iscador therapy can be administered in ambulatory
patients or during house calls.*

To the oncologist who works with lung cancer and who knows the
grim statistics (five-year survival rate: 9 out of 100), such an assist
as Iscador when the patient's condition is complicated by pleural effusions,
with its convenience in administration, could be life-saving.

Considering the morbid threat posed by lung cancer throughout the
world today, these results are encouraging, to say the least. In the U.S.,
lung cancer is the number-one killer among the male population, the
death rate having increased more than twenty-five times in forty-five years.
The condition usually is inoperable by the time of its detection, with
poor response to chemotherapy—only ten percent having any chance to
be saved.

In the area of gynecological malignancies, Professor Dr. W. Bickenbach, Director of the First Gynecological Unit of the Munich University Hospital, with Professors Ries and Breitner, conducted a study that was designed to evaluate the efficacy of follow-up therapy for the prevention of recurrences. Iscador therapy was administered after the primary treatment normally employed at the hospital, which consisted of combined radium and X-ray therapy only. Between 1956 and 1961, eighty-one cervical cancer patients were given three years follow-up therapy with Iscador. In this group, the mortality was about forty percent less than among controls.

}⊱ ⊰{

The Lukas-Klinik, which is a forty-four-bed hospital in the village of Arlesheim, Switzerland, under the direction of Dr. Rita Leroi, is the heart and principal focus of a worldwide center of healing based on the principles of Anthroposophical Medicine—an extension of the art of healing through spiritual knowledge.

While steadfastly providing enviable leadership, Dr. Leroi never fails to recall that the great innovator of the Lukas-Klinik was her late husband, Dr. Alexandre Leroi. As founder and prime motivator, his talents for organization and prodigious efforts in research were highly acclaimed by associates and co-workers alike for over thirty years, during which time his sterling work as a leader in the medical movement bore fruit through the development and perfection of Iscador. His pinnacle achievement was in the continual refinement of Iscador as a miracle healing agent so that, today, extensive application by thousands of physicians in a total cancer regime represents the fruit of his lifelong hard work as a physician and researcher in the treatment of cancer.

The Lukas-Klinik uses Iscador as its primary medicament, Iscador being the oldest and most differentiated internal remedy for the treatment of cancer patients, having been in actual clinical use for more than forty years. Its success has been proven over many years of testing in public and private hospitals. It has no toxic side effects.

The Lukas-Klinik stands in a natural fairyland of breathtaking beauty amongst the hills and valleys lying between the Northern Jura and the Rhine, five miles from the university town of Basel. It is an ideal environment for the inspired work it is doing in treating the critically ill cancer patients, many of whom arrive at the clinic in terminal condition.

Patients at the clinic are under the medical care of a group of ten physicians. But the total clinical staff is a happy, harmonious, and totally committed group—a dedicated League of Nations, with—at last count—129 members from 23 different countries. Biannually, a medical

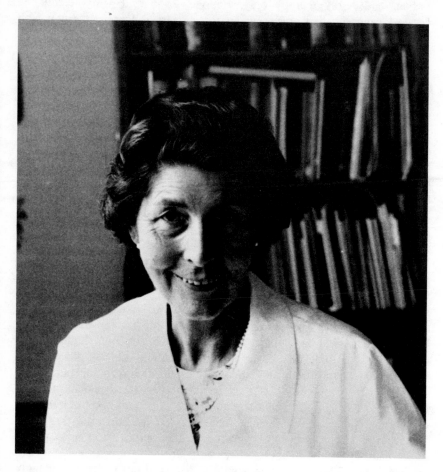

DR. RITA LEROI

seminar is conducted over a period of three months at the Lukas-Klinik, where medical students and doctors from all over the world are introduced to medicine based on spiritual science and where practical training can be acquired.

Particular attention is paid at the Lukas-Klinik to the early detection of possible cancer symptoms. Besides other methods of early diagnosis, the Kaelin Filterpaper method and the Copper-crystallization method of Pfeiffer for testing the blood are used. These tests give the clinician a general idea of the state of the individual organs and functions, and make possible the better detection of a predisposition toward malignancy, long before pathological changes manifest. Using Iscador as a prophylaxis, effective measures can then be taken to intercept this precancerous state. Instructional booklets and experienced professional guidance are available to interested physicians.

On admission, each patient undergoes a thorough general examination of his physical and psychological condition, with complete case history and background material, after which the physician in charge works out the individual therapy. The effects of this are observed during daily visits, and the treatment is always carefully adjusted to the needs of the day.

The Lukas-Klinik is well equipped for general examinations, and for control investigations in the treatment of patients in every stage of illness. There are laboratories for hematological and biochemical investigation, X-ray equipment, and facilities for endoscopical examination. Massage and hydrotherapy are employed, and special rooms equipped for artistic therapy play an important role in improving the patients' mental attitudes. Specialists from Basel University and other hospitals are consulted on surgical and gynecological problems, and in difficult cases of internal disease.

Used as a prophylaxis, immediately after surgery and/or irradiation, Iscador has demonstrated that mortality in the various groups can be reduced by thirty to fifty percent, as compared with that of untreated groups. In cases of inoperable or recurring tumors (where metastases are often present), a radical decrease in the rate of growth, or complete stoppage of growth, has been observed, often accompanied by a regression of the malignancy.

The hospital team of physicians and nurses is, of course, intimately involved and concerned with the physical condition of the patients, but a vital part of the total treatment program is to help the patient achieve the right mental attitude toward his illness, and to take a positive approach to life. Artistic therapy has proven especially beneficial as a part of the psychotherapeutic modality.

Selection of the very particular mistletoe preparation according to the host tree on which it grows, e.g., pine, oak, apple, to be used with each patient, is based on the sex of the patient and the site of the tumor. It has been experimentally proven that even the constellations at the time of picking the mistletoe have an extraordinary influence on the quality of the plant. Anyone who has read *The Secret Life of Plants,* with all of its implications, would hardly doubt this possibility.

For genital carcinomata in women, for example, including breast cancer, the preparation used is Iscador Mali cum Argento (M c A$_g$, mistletoe from the apple tree, with traces of silver salt added). This is given by subcutaneous injection, in courses of various concentrations that are called "strengths." Every course of injections starts with one of the higher dilutions and gradually goes to the lower strengths (i.e., higher concentrations). A course consists of fourteen injections, one given twice or three times a week. Every detail of Iscador therapy, and its very precise administration, is explicitly explained in instructional booklets and manuals that represent the accumulation of forty years of clinical experience.

Dr. Rita Leroi, in explaining the adjuvant methods used in conjunction with Iscador, states: "In our clinic, in addition to Iscador, we give supportive therapy especially for the liver, the kidneys, the circulation and the digestive functions. These additional remedies are prepared from natural substances, mostly in homeopathic dilution, which we use according to the symptoms and the type of patient. We also use different medicinal baths with herbs and oil-dispersions, and we make use of hyperthermia and massage. Art therapy is a new form of treatment which is done in our clinic, be it eurythmy to harmonize the patient's general attitude, or painting and modelling to awaken his latent creative forces."

As part of a continuing series designed to assist the medical practitioner in his work, the following instructive reports have thus far been published under the overall title "Progress in Iscador Therapy of Malignant Tumors":

1. Brain and Skin
2. Gynecology
3. Tumors of the Digestive Tract
4. Breast Cancer
5. Kidneys and Urinary Tract
6. Leukemia

In a further revealing study of the impressive results achieved with Iscador by Dr. Alexandre Leroi and Dr. Bernard Wohrmann, ten case histories of selected patients are cited. These patients either had developed a recurrence or metastases after primary surgery or irradiation, or still had the primary tumor. The majority of these patients came to the Lukas-Klinik for treatment because the carcinoma was too far advanced for treatment by the usual methods. All of these patients were treated with Iscador, with no toxic side effects. The ten case histories include three gynecological cases, one carcinoma of the bladder, a sarcoma of the nose, one of the tonsil, a carcinoma of the thyroid, a hypernephroma, a radiation carcinoma of the skin, and a malignant melanoma.

To underline the virtually terminal nature of their condition when these patients arrived at the Lukas-Klinik—which is quite common —and the results achieved, four case histories, out of the above ten, are described in detail below. The startling results of successful therapy in this group, where virtually total remissions occurred in so-called "hopeless" and "inoperable" cases, are not unusual in Iscador therapy:

Case No. 1. C. H., born 1914, female factory worker. Clin. diagn.: Ovarian tumor. Path. anat. diagn.: Papillary adenocarcinoma of corpus uteri, papillary cystic ca. of left ovary with metastases in right ovary (Dr. Pendl, Vienna). Nov. 1955: Genital bleeding. Feb. 1956: Abdominal total hysterectomy and removal of adnexa: Ovarian tumor, the size of a small child's head, with partial cystic degeneration, adherent to rectum and sigmoid colon, so that total removal was not possible. In Douglas's pouch retroperiton, metastatic nodes up to the size of cherries; these are left. Patient refuses X-ray therapy. Feb. 1956: started ISCADOR THERAPY. March 1956: Gynecological examination: Solid infiltration in left parametrium. July 1956: Fully able to work. Iscador injections are given without interruption. Dec. 1956: Gyn. exam: No path. resistance palpable. In the years that followed, general condition remained good. Patient has to do heavy physical labor. 1964: Subjectively and objectively, nothing to indicate tumor. Period of observation: 9 years.

Case No. 2. B. A., born 1934, schoolgirl. Clin. diagn.: Ovarian tumor. Path. anat. diagn.: Polymorpho-cellular malignant tumor (teratoblastoma), with infiltration of appendix (Prof. Roulet, Basle). Feb. 1949: Tumor the size of a child's head, extending to the navel and filling the whole of the pelvic inlet (Univ. Hospital for Women, Basle). Exploratory Laparotomy: Removal not possible, biopsy. X-ray therapy with 600 r, increasing cachexia, hgb 56%, weight 32 kg. (70½ lbs.). June 1949: Started ISCADOR THERAPY. Tumor still extending to umbilicus. Aug. 1951: Tumor no longer palpable, weight gain 8 kg. (17½ lbs.), symptom-free. 1961: Symptom-free. Iscador therapy discontinued. April 1963: Examination reveals tumor in the area of the right anterior hip bone, suspected recurrence. Iscador injections resumed in 1964. Able to work. Period of observation: 15 years.

Case No. 3. A. T., born 1898, housewife. Clin. diagn.: Ca. of the bladder, inoperable. Path. anat. diagn.: Ca. of the bladder (Prof. Roulet, Basle). Confirmed by Prof. Werthemann, Basle; Prof. W. Fischer, Jena. Sept. 1947: Cystoscopy (IInd Surgical Unit, Burgerspital, Basle). Oct. 1947: Sectio alta: tumor inoperable, already adherent to the ramus of the pubis, with extensive infiltration of the wall of the bladder. X-ray therapy has to be discontinued after a few sessions because of haemorrhagic cystitis and rapid deterioration of the general condition. Nov. 1947: Started ISCADOR THERAPY. Violent pains in hypogastrium, lumbar pain, tenesmus on micturition. Pollakisuria. March 1948: Weight gain of 7 kg. (15½ lbs.), less pain. Patient is again able to work. Iscador therapy continues without interruption. Feb. 1949: Cystoscopy: Tumor has disappeared, only bare suspicion of malignant infiltration, granular cystitis. In the years that follow, cystoscopies are regularly done at the IInd Surgical Unit of the University Hospital, Basle. Occasionally mild bladder symptoms, but patient remains able to work throughout. March 1958: Last cytoscopy: No signs of malignant tumor. 1964: Patient feels well and is symptom-free. Period of observation: 18 years.

Case No. 4. F. K., born 1914, motor mechanic. Clin. diagn.: Malignant melanoma of the skin, with metastases in the inguinal lymph glands (Prof. Zollinger, St. Gallen). March 1956: Tumor on the R. shin, growing to walnut size within a year. April 1956: Excision of the tumor and removal of inguinal nodes. Patient refuses X-ray therapy. Started ISCADOR THERAPY, but only has regular treatment for six months. March 1958: After several months without treatment, there is one recurrence in the scar on the leg and one in the inguinal flexure. May 1958: Dissemination of about 80 skin nodules up to pea-size on the leg and in the groin. Intensive Iscador therapy. Sept. 1958: Skin secondaries have regressed considerably. Nov. 1958: No pathological findings. Depigmented areas where the metastases have been. Patient entirely symptom-free and fully able to work. 1964: Nothing to indicate further recurrences or metastases. Period of observation: 8 years.

In the standard administration of chemotherapeutic agents, now numbering something around forty being used in the United States alone (singly or in combination), side effects—such as loss of hair, nausea, loss of appetite, depression, and sometimes a frighteningly low white blood cell count—all present a morbid horror picture, quite apart from the depressing fact that—in the process—not just cancer cells, but normal, healthy cells are also being destroyed throughout the entire body. As if this were not enough for a sick patient to contemplate, there is, in almost all cases, a suppression of, and often grave damage to, the body's first line of defense—its immunological resources system.

In direct contrast, Iscador is the only cytostatic agent known that violates none of the laws of nature; rather, like a good soldier operating on a number of life-threatening fronts, it hastens to the rescue of the embattled body, and, insofar as the formidable worldwide array of permissible drugs is concerned, Iscador is one of the few *nontoxic* medicaments available today for the treatment of malignancies, although it is not permitted for use in the United States.

In spite of (perhaps because of) its nontoxic effects, mistletoe has been found to be one of the most effective agents known against all forms of cancer. The German research worker Vester discovered that some protein fractions of *Viscum album* "in vitro" (artificial environment outside of the living organism), and "in vivo" (within the living organism) have better activity against malignant cell growth than the strongest cytostatics, such as endoxan and other drugs, which are presently used in the treatment of cancer. Another group of workers (Selwary, Vester, Mai, and Schwarz) also isolated a number of sugar and protein-containing fractions with marked carcinostatic activity. These are the first protein fractions ever found to have demonstrable anticancer activity, more powerful than that of the usual anticancer agents. More recently, pharmaceutical studies with mistletoe indicate that the protein fractions are acting on the nucleic acid cellular control mechanism. It may indeed be these very fractions that assist the body's defense system by providing the trigger for the form-giving, reversal activities that are initiated against the wild, unregenerate proliferation of the cancer cell.

But, in healing, just to achieve destruction of the tumor would still be purely symptomatic therapy. The important goal is to put the entire organism into good order, creating a harmonious, balanced whole. It has been proven in animal experiments, and also in the clinical situation, that Iscador is the *only cancer remedy* that has the double property of of simultaneous tumor inhibition, and, at the same time, the activation, support, and rejuvenation of the immunological defense system, i.e., of the antibodies and blood cells that attack the tumor as a foreign body in the organism. How gratifying for the devoted physician, who must every day stand at that dark door with his patient, often without further choice—or even alternative—dreading the decisions! For him, Iscador can bring new hope, due to its profound healing capabilities:

1. *Increased Phagocytic Activity.* (Phagocytes are cells that envelop and digest other cells, microorganisms, or other foreign bodies in the bloodstream and tissues.)

2. *Activation of Leukopoiesis* (the formation and development of leucocytes, or white blood corpuscles).

3. *Stimulation of the Thymus,* a ductless gland that plays an important role in the body's resistance to disease; and also stimulation of the spleen, which acts as a blood purifier and blood-storage organ.

4. *Rise in Temperature.* (Usually the temperature in the cancer patient is low, and this rise in temperature has a beneficial effect. Better circulation also results.)

5. *Normalization of Electrophoresis.*

6. *Increased Erythro-Leukopoiesis.*

7. *Results in Higher Serum Iron Levels.*

8. *Lower Serum Copper Levels.* (The reverse is observed in progredient cases.)

Healing Substances Present:

1. *Protein components,* which in animal and cell-culture experiments have been found to have the strongest tumor-inhibiting effects yet known.
2. *Purified Protein Fractions* with marked carcinostatic activity (Selawry, Vester, Mai, and Schwarz).
3. *Polysaccharides and Fat Substances* that are efficacious against the tumor, and a stimulating effect on neutrophils (Mathé, Schneider, Amiel, Cotton, Schwarzenberg, *et al.*).
4. *Viscotoxin,* a polypeptide with necrotizing properties; also, sugars, resins, alcohol, choline, and acetylcholine (Winterfield, Rink, and Bijl).
5. *Free Amino Acids* in a specific configuration (Vester and Niehaus).

The activation of the defensive functions of the organism as a whole, and the consequent inhibition of tumor development, is evident from the following clinical observations of many thousands of patients:

1. relief of pain
2. improvement of general condition of well-being
3. return of appetite and weight gain
4. deeper and more restful sleep
5. lessening of tiredness and depression, with return of activity and enterprise
6. increased elimination of stool, urine, and sweat
7. slowing down or cessation of tumor growth
8. occasional regression of tumors
9. reduced incidence of secondary growths and metastases
10. no toxic side effects, even if Iscador is given intensively for many years.

In summary, what can we say has actually taken place in the healing process initiated by Iscardor therapy?

Viscum album, or mistletoe, the brainchild of Austria's great clairvoyant, Rudolf Steiner, has, within the parameters of Anthroposophical Medicine, "persuaded" the malignant condition to return to the domain of the laws governing the whole organism. Acting within the framework of total therapy, as postulated by spiritual-scientific medicine, Iscador employs the body's innate intelligence, using its physical and spiritual resources, to *reverse the process* of the cancerous cells by leading them back again to being normal cells. Thus the organism is restored to its original state of biological integrity.

It is no exaggeration to say that this constitutes a major revolution in today's world of medicine. It opposes the almost unanimous medical hypothesis and dogma, which categorically rejects the possibility of biological reversal of the malignant condition—of the taming of the wild and proliferative cell nature. Orthodox medicine makes its position implicit by its massive assault on the *symptoms*; by its commitment and addiction to the unholy trinity of surgery, irradiation, and devastatingly poisonous drugs. To doctors practicing drug medicine, mistletoe therapy completely refutes medical scientific doctrine in this respect.

In one astonishing series of observations in which clinical results were precisely confirmed by closely supervised laboratory tests, it was found that, in cases of cancer of the bladder and rectum in man, regression of the tumor occurred under Iscador therapy. When this happened, the usual stages of tumor development, i.e., chronic proliferative inflammation, polyps, papillomata, and finally infiltration of underlying tissues, *were all gone through in reverse*—proof positive that a healing pattern had been initiated in the organism, and continued in reverse order until the complete recovery stage.

This bears good witness to the prescience and wisdom of Portmann, a famous Swiss zoologist: "It is not the stones that create the edifice. The invisible entity at work *creates its own bricks*. The organism differentiates itself into systems; *cell formation is a later stage.*"

The overall proof—loud and clear—declares that there is *no such thing as complete autonomy of the tumor*. The very fact that the body's defense system goes to work and acts to *reverse the irreversible*, belies the prevailing premise.

The tumor cannot secede from its "society"—the body. As a discordant member of that society (symptomatic of a deeper malignant process), it is shown the way back through activation and strengthening of the basic defense systems and processes of the entire organism. Once again, the body assumes leadership, and restores order by controlling and regulating the differentiation process in cell formation—which has been running formless and wild. The tumor (and the entire malignant condition) goes through a reform and rehabilitation period, as the body slowly rebuilds to its original healthy state—in perfect balance and harmony.

In the "Gospel" of Spiritual-Scientific Medicine, interpreting the metamorphosis that has taken place, the "wayward cell" (the prodigal son) has been brought back into the family fold. The errant cell (the son), by the gentle persuasion of divine love, gives up its self-willed, ego-directed ambition, which has harnessed it to the sense world, and which has caused its "fall": regression to a primitive stage of evolution, i.e., a fermentative state for its life's energy.

In the "resurrection" and the "ascension," the body is restored to the higher consciousness of its original healthy state, and once again energy is generated by the normal process of oxidation instead of fermentation.

Thus the wayward cell has, in the process of reversion, made a full confession of its guilt, and, in effect (by cellular emancipation, as it were), been absolved from all sin. The "disease" has run its course: through the cycle of ignorance and delusion; through aimless wandering and regression; from sin to absolution.

God's "Church," the Temple of the Soul, is now rebuilt. Within the framework of Rudolf Steiner's spiritual science, and of Anthroposophical Medicine, the prophecy and the law have been fulfilled.

4

Zadig, the One-Eyed Man

To everything there is a season, and a time for everything under the sun. We come now to a point and place where it is fitting to discuss the incisive—if not always constructive—role played by the governmental and/or privately endowed control bodies that operate in the medical amphitheater, and their impact on certain original and creative research efforts, particularly nontraditional methods. The agencies referred to often exert a radical, sometimes irresistible subliminal influence, which can obstruct an ongoing, evolving process.

At the outset, let us say that it is not any part of our purpose to enter into a polemic against the Establishment. However, with respect to one particular organization, the American Cancer Society, we are impelled to make our point in that area where this Society straddles—like a monolith—the nerve center of our primary interest and particular concern—the so-called unorthodox cancer therapies, in which area the Society looms as the most influential organ of public propaganda in the United States.

We preface our remarks with an expression of thanks and appreciation to the many government agencies and private organizations, and individuals without number, whose help and counsel made it possible to accomplish our work. Very special plaudits and thanks are due the Food and Drug Administration, whose staff were most generous in assisting with much-needed research material. Their cooperation was extended unconditionally, although they knew that ours was a highly controversial project. Thanks, also, to the National Cancer Institute, and—truly, not least (for they helped with so much)—to the American Cancer Society.

We beg all others who assisted in many diverse and important ways, to know and believe that by our works they may be known.

If it smacks of ingratitude to take the American Cancer Society to task now, it is because we consider that a point of honor takes precedence over the protocol of debatable manners. Our observations concern that area that is critically consequential to our work, in which area the

33

American Cancer Society exerts its most profound influence, impinging on the past, present, and future. Those names on the Honor Roll that bear defending are the unsung heroes of this battlefield—the "Unknown Soldiers" of this war—and the point of honor concerns our responsibility to reach for the torch flung from their failing hands.

The American Cancer Society, Inc., is a private, independent corporation that has, over the years (among its other diverse programs and objectives), become a self-designated watchdog for the U.S. government over what it chooses to call "unproven methods" of cancer treatment. It touches base with the National Cancer Institute, the government giant in the field of research and education, joining hands in promoting many programs of common interest.

The Society is very active in the general public domain, and with the medical profession in the field of education—publishing pamphlets and brochures, holding lectures and group discussions, presenting film showings and exhibits. Its own medical organ, *Ca—A Cancer Journal for Clinicians,* has a circulation of over 350,000 and is distributed to physicians, medical students, and medical libraries throughout the country.

It has built its strength by means of a volunteer citizens organization, which numbers approximately 2,300,000 Americans, with 58 Chartered Divisions, 2,792 local units (in every state in the country), and more than 68,445 community leaders who direct the Society's programs on the county level. Its "Committee on Unproven Methods of Cancer Management" is the central coordinating force for directing its work in this area—and, as stated in their literature, "is actively involved in strengthening and encouraging the passage of state legislation to control the use of worthless cancer remedies and tests."

The officers of this corporation and the medical doctors and scientists who form the pool of expertise in the ACS carry a grave responsibility. The consequences of error or misinformation can affect—in the United States alone—370,000 Americans who die each year of cancer, and more than 55,000,000 Americans now living who will contract the disease during their lifetimes. Assuming ethical, principled motivation, the last thing such an organization should be guilty of is complacency, or categorical rejection of any therapeutic agent or method that holds out promise of benefit.

Yet, regrettably, the American Cancer Society has developed its own form of catechism whereby they identify and proscribe the "heretic," virtually excommunicating him from the medical congregation. It has coined—and continues to use—the following stock paragraph in its literature, which is tantamount to categorical rejection of the "unorthodox" remedy under scrutiny:

After careful study of the literature and other information available to it, the American Cancer Society does not have evidence that treatment with Iscador [or whatever the remedy under review may be] results in positive objective benefit in the treatment of cancer in human beings.

This is the ultimate in dismissal notices, and carries the kiss of death in medical circles. Using this pat statement, the Society has done away with Iscador, for one; with the "Gerson Method," for another; with CH-23, an important therapeutic agent used by Dr. Josef Issels; with the use of KC-555 by Dr. Morvyth McQueen-Williams; and with Dr. William F. Koch's antitoxins. All of these involved men of medicine and science suffered public humiliation and ostracism in one way or another, and carried the mark and stigma of the outcast. Some of these pioneers and their medical agents and methods are documented in the pages of this book.

We do not take issue with the American Cancer Society—or with any supervisory agency or organization that acts unselfishly in the common interest. Charlatans and frauds do exist. But, noting the confirmed success of Issels, Gerson and others, we raise the question of whether, in many crucial instances, the baby is not being disposed of with the bath water.

The lone, independent pioneer in research is—not surprisingly—a maverick, often endowed with superlative academic credentials, but working outside of the flock. This is not always from choice, but sometimes from grim necessity. As one example, Dr. Max Gerson (who conducted his practice in New York City) was hailed by Albert Schweitzer, his intimate friend, as the "Man of the Century." He established a fully documented record of remissions and cures of hopeless terminal cancer patients, unbelievable to the medical community; yet he was so ostracized and oppressed that his hospital privileges were revoked. He was compelled to use his own home—with its austere accommodations—as his clinic and hospital. Some laboratories even refused to examine his tissue specimens.

It becomes obvious that the nonconformist is not welcome on the medical scene. Drug and pharmaceutical companies, manufacturers of medical equipment and instrumentation, and important research laboratories that depend upon government and private grants for their lifelines, abhor and isolate such a man. Although often depicted as a rough-riding outlaw by the regular news media (who are quick to pick up the trail), our typical martyr is the least likely candidate for the FBI's list of most-wanted criminals.

Such authoritarian tactics lay the grounds for easy suspicion that the American Cancer Society is less than objective in its pronouncements.

Although it numbers four Nobel Prize winners among its grant recipients, as well as other notables in medicine and science, a close examination of the parameters of research projects that are uniformly approved, discloses that they follow conventional lines, falling conveniently into a comfortable and happy wedlock with medical orthodoxy.

The Society, in its literature, declares its commitment to the bankrupt concept that "cancer begins as a localized disease." It follows through by stating that we continue to have "new and better cancer treatments"— which turn out to be the same Unholy Trinity in the same old costumes: "New methods of *surgery* . . . (which) . . . have enabled surgeons to perform thousands more life-saving operations each year. . . . New supervolt *radiation* equipment to . . . eradicate tumors . . . and *chemotherapy.*" (Our italics.) Nothing has changed but refinements in the quality and quantity of technological overkill. Science is still treating man as a dog and a field of wheat.

It becomes altogether too clear that those following the house rules dictated by traditional medicine are the recipients of appropriate rewards in the form of research grants. Although some modest gains have been registered in such research, the returns on this investment of billions of dollars have been grievously disappointing. On October 15, 1975, a CBS documentary, "The American Way of Cancer," stated that "in the last twenty-five years, the cancer mortality rate has increased 20 percent." At the Tenth International Cancer Congress in 1970, six thousand famous cancer researchers met in Houston. Many of the world's foremost scientists and doctors, one after another, categorically reiterated that to continue along present lines of research and treatment would bring us from our present dire state of "crisis to catastrophe." If the object of the exercise is to get people well, and if orthodox medical research and practice has proven barren of result, then one is tempted to ask, "What is orthodox and what is nonorthodox?"

It is less than an open secret among the initiate that cancer congresses and conventions, conferences and seminars—worldwide—are dominated in the wings by the entrenched bureaucracy—governmental and private— by the major drug and chemical industries, and by entrenched research laboratories—comfortably supported over the years through the largess of government grants and subsidies and special interest private support.

The portals of the open secret are widened a little more by conventional medical wisdom, which knows how all too often; the papers and reports generated are sterile in conception and inconsequential in their applicability to practical cancer therapy—at the patient's bedside. Yet these are the groups and the individuals who are given the bulk of the hundreds of millions in cancer research funds every year.

One example—definitely *not* the recipient of any assistance, which he desperately needs and wants—is Dr. Albert Szent-Gyorgy, M.D.,

Ph.D., a Nobel Prize Laureate in 1937 in Medicine, for isolating Vitamin C (among his other impressive achievements). Today, at eighty-three, mentally and physically vigorous and alert, he is afloat without a paddle, trying to champion an exciting new theory on cancer cause and therapy. Although his laurels in chemistry and medicine amply qualify him on the one hand for, surely, a modest subsidy, his decided reputation as a scientific rebel, on the other, leaves him with empty pockets.

He was compelled long ago to release his last assistant, a chemist, from his own Marine Biological Laboratory at Woods Hole, Massachusetts, on Cape Cod, for lack of funds. Dr. Szent-Gyorgy, aging but brilliant man of science, is puttering around in circles for lack of financial support, reminding one of the proverbial hoop—which has no end to it; while endless millions are spent lavishly on scientific flyspecks that compose the discordant music of a forever unfinished symphony.

When the proof required for the submission to the Food and Drug Administration (of an application for an important new drug) is a mind-boggling tens of thousands of pages of documentation (in 1968, 77,200 pages of data were necessary to license an anesthetic), and approximates, on an average, an expenditure of one to ten million dollars for requisite animal experiments—as it does in America today—it becomes even less noble to castigate so severely the humble innovator in our midst.

Without a power base, nothing much can improve in this direction for the lone rider. Under these conditions, the mores of traditional free enterprise, and the much-touted rewards for the bold and venturesome, have come to a dead end. The democratic process in this dimension remains tragically defeated.

In the large sense, all of the whips and scorns cannot be laid just at the doorstep of the American Cancer Society, because it is not the main, or only, organization that can and does influence the flow of money. However, with a budget of approximately $2,000,000 a week, it does have the capability of playing a more constructive role.

In moving to a conclusion, we cannot help recalling the tale of "Zadig, the One-Eyed Man," from Voltaire's *Candide*. In ancient Babylon, Zadig, a man of innate goodness, was to be married to a beautiful and talented lady, Semira. One day, while walking along the bank of a river, they were set upon by a gang of cutthroats led by a spurned suitor of Semira. Zadig valiantly fought them off, but suffered an arrow wound under his left eye, which developed into an abscess.

This was cause for grave concern, so the great doctor Hermes was sent for from Memphis, arriving with a considerable retinue. He visited the distraught invalid and declared summarily that he would lose his eye. He even predicted the day and the hour that this would occur.

"Had it been the right eye," he said, "I could have cured it, but wounds of the left eye are incurable."

Two days later, the abscess burst of its own accord, and Zadig made a complete recovery. Hermes wrote a book in which he *proved* that Zadig ought not to have recovered. Zadig did not read it.

Under the cold, impersonal light of overwhelming scientific proof of the efficacy of Iscador and of other therapies described in this work, conscience alone would dictate some concession by the American Cancer Society to exercise objectivity and competent discrimination in their examination and appraisal process. Classifying the not-so-rare, though poor genius (and his works) as charlatan and fraud is unbecoming to an agency with such grave lifesaving duties and responsibilities. The resulting blanket ostracism may easily result (as it has in the past) in the loss of important anticancer tools to our sick society.

A strong dose of open-mindedness, and decent, substantive encouragement and help will bear superior witness to truth and integrity. There is even the distinct possibility that such an attitude, implemented by constructive action, could contribute something of value to the healing arts—perhaps even to posterity and long life.

Surely a departure from the present static policy, with its self-defeating formula, would be regarded as a greater fulfillment of the public trust than the rather dubious honor of one day having to write a treatise on why abscesses of the left eye should not be cured.

5

Chinese Music

"The history of medicine reveals that reformers who bring new ideas into the general thinking and practice of physicians, have a difficult time. . . . Each new idea has been fought bitterly, and most of the reformers did not live to see the realization of their ideas."

These were the prophetic words uttered by Dr. Max Gerson in the preface to his classic work, *A Cancer Therapy*. He passed away on March 8, 1959, not long after its publication date.

His ideas and his proven methods, to this day, have not been seriously looked at by any one of the privately endowed medical research institutions or governmental research agencies, despite the incontestable mountain of hard scientific evidence that is available in officially documented medical and governmental records.

Apart from five "investigations," such as they were, made by the New York County Medical Society, detailed evaluations—if they were conducted at all—remain to this day a carefully guarded secret. The sum total about Dr. Gerson published anywhere by the officiating medical community, appears in three brief pages, a very chancy sketch, by the American Cancer Society in its tome *Unproven Methods of Cancer Management*.

In this somewhat battered fragment of Gerson's regime, the following is mentioned:

> Gerson's method of treatment for cancer was essentially dietary and was based on:
> (1) detoxification of the whole body;
> (2) providing essential contents of the potassium group; and
> (3) adding oxiding enzymes continuously . . . in the form of green leaf juice and fresh calf's liver juice. This creates a near normal condition of the oxidizing system of the body, to which malignant cells with the fermentation system cannot adapt.

It would seem that, if the interested professional medical doctor would have a thoughtful look at this all-too-brief, fractionated extract of Dr. Max Gerson's comprehensive therapeutic program, the underlying truths of the concepts impregnating these few words could surely not escape him. The precepts clamor the soundness of the underlying doctrine, directed at helping the organism in a natural way, and encouraging it toward a renewal of its innate vital activities. Grim fact: Nobody was listening.

The ACS article continues: " . . . To the layman . . . it makes sense because it views the problem in the 'concept of totality,' placing emphasis on the deteriorated metabolism as a whole, with the liver as the central organ."

Is it implied here that this is an absurdity to which only a layman would subscribe? Is the concept of *"totality"* a fraud, something to poke fun at? Is the liver *not* actually the "central organ" of the body? Do malignant cells *not* perish when the cancer metabolism is changed from the *fermentation system*—in which the malignant cell *lives and thrives*— to a normal *oxidizing system*—in which it *dies?*

Not quite content with having reduced to nit size a monumental idea whose time had come, the American Cancer Society hardly gains any points by its cavalier opening statement to this same article:

> After careful review of the literature and other available information, the American Cancer Society does not have evidence that treatment of cancer in humans by the Gerson method results in any objective benefit.

From a letter written by the director of an Eastern cancer research center comes the following comment on Dr. Gerson's book *A Cancer Therapy*: "It is a serious, careful and honest record of observation and analysis, and, as such, will make its contribution to the advance of knowledge so sorely needed by all of us. I hope that clinical men who are connected with the National Cancer Institute and the American Cancer Society will be given the opportunity of reading it."

Even the most cursory investigation would have disclosed that the files of the New York County Medical Society were replete with case histories and related data from five different investigations they had conducted of Dr. Gerson's treatment methods, as would, also, a reading of his medical classic *A Cancer Therapy,* which was available in 1958— three years prior to the first published date of the article by the American Cancer Society—and still appearing in the pages of their 1971 (latest) edition, thirteen years after Gerson's book first appeared! Again, no one seemed to be listening.

Not generally known is the fact that tumor cells live on fermentation and not on the normal oxidation metabolism. Dr. Gerson observed that "they do not have a normal exchange with the blood and the serum, and grow and spread uncontrolled. Studying these, I felt there must be a way to prevent fermentation which is vital for the life of the cancer cell. That is the object upon which we could base further tests and explorations. . . . You have to realize that cancer cells live essentially on fermentation, but potassium and oxidizing enzymes introduce oxidation; *the high point of the treatment comes when the potassium and the oxidizing enzymes go into the cancer mass. And that is the point at which we kill the cancer cells, because we take away the condition of fermentation which they need to continue to live.*

"But now, we have a mass of dead cells which must be eliminated, or they can poison the body, and kill the patient; and this is where my *detoxification* program comes in, because it helps the body to throw out the dead cells. I lost a few of my patients before I learned this sad lesson. They were getting better and better, but suddenly they died. I was shocked. I couldn't believe it. What was I doing wrong, I asked myself? Then I realized the problem. And do you know what first gave me the hint? One day, with a lady patient, we had to completely repaint the room because the toxins which came out of her lungs and skin were so strong that they peeled off all the paint from the walls and ceiling! So I realized what must be happening.

"Because of my strong attack with my therapy, with fruit and vegetable juices, the liver juice, the potassium solution and the iodine, the cancer cells were dying very quickly, and these dead cells were like poisons building up in the patient's body, because they were not coming fast enough out; so, somehow, I had to get rid of them more quickly. I remembered about Dr. A. A. Meyer in Göttingen, and some experiments he did with Prof. Heubner. He gave caffeine solution into the rectum of animals and observed that the bile ducts were opened up, and more bile could flow. I felt that this was very important, and I worked out the idea of coffee enemas, which was successful beyond my dreams. I was relieved of my heavy worry. I found it even necessary to order *alarm clocks in every patient's room* to wake them up for their enemas—even in the middle of the night—so that we could remove the poisons of the dead cancer cells.

"The healing of cancer in the latter part of my treatment can be considered as a *parenteral digestion.* After I recognized the healing of cancer to be a parenteral digestion (other than through the alimentary canal), the entire therapeutic endeavor was subordinated to this purpose. This means that after the cancer mass is killed, *the dead pieces must be dissolved.* If you are interested in such horrible things, I can show you a whole collection of such *eliminated dead pieces,* from the rectum, cervix, bladder, vagina, esophagus, tonsils, intestines, or wherever they found their way out from the bodies of my cancer patients.

"And maybe you won't believe me—because the medical doctors

don't believe me, either, but after a few coffee enemas most of my patients—even those who had been on high dosage of morphine—did not longer need any pain relief."

With billions being spent annually on cancer research, why has not modern medicine paid even token tribute to the priceless contributions from ancient civilizations—those of the Egyptians, the Greeks, the Islamic world, and of Babylon, many of whose most noted physicians believed in the healing value of diet, rest, sunbathing, and massage—with occasional natural herbs and medicines—or with the decent homage of a nod in the direction of great standard-bearers of holistic medicine like Hippocrates and Asclepiades, Paracelsus and Galen, Jennings, Tilden, and Trall, all of whom sanctified the natural approach? And, from ancient testimony, too—from Genesis; "And God said, 'Behold, I have given you every herb bearing seed, which is upon the face of the earth; and every tree in the which is the fruit of a tree yielding seed; to you it shall be for meat.' "

Gerson commented on the quality of wholeness: "As science is not yet developed to the point of knowing all the enzymes, vitamins and many biological functions of hormones and minerals, it is safer to use food *in the most natural form, combined and mixed by nature* and raised, if possible by an organic gardening process, thus obeying the *laws of nature.* This observation helped the human race for thousands of years before any science was developed. In this way we bring in all known vitamins and enzymes, both the discovered and the undiscovered ones, and—to quote Professor Kollath, especially the *unknown* 'life-stimulating substances,' given best as fresh as possible and not damaged by refining or preserving processes such as canned food. These contain all of the necessary substances in their *proper quantity, moisture and composition, and are regulated by instinct, hunger, taste, smell, sight and other factors.*"

So why not a few paltry doubloons for an intensive investigation into Ganzheitstherapie, the treatment of the "whole man"? Yes, and why not one pilot plant to the memory of Dr. Max Gerson, say, a "Max Gerson Treatment Center," where medical doctors and nutritionists could work hand in hand, either to prove out his claims and works, or—conversely—throw the lie back in his teeth? A unique center where men and women in white can work as the copartners of Nature, instead of doing her violence. A fitting and proper monument to a great soul, not the forgotten grave of an unknown soldier.

Why not one strong thrust in the direction where the light is showing, instead of into the darkness, with its so tragic waste of money and superb talents that today characterize so much of the effort of our greatest research scientists and laboratory technicians?

In July 1942, Albert Einstein alerted President Franklin D. Roosevelt to the terrifying probability that the Germans might well be working out the technical problems of an atomic bomb. At this prompting, Roosevelt activated a top-secret operation to be known as the Manhattan Project, headed by General Leslie Groves of the War Department. Its objective was to create a superexplosive by exploiting the nuclear fission process.

Some of the world's most famous physicists, engineers, and scientists—like Nobel Prize winner Enrico Fermi, Niels Bohr, and Seth Neddermeyer were involved, as was J. Robert Oppenheimer, who was director of Project "Y," which was to design the weapon. These, and many other top staff members, were enlisted in a network of research laboratories scattered throughout the country in this concerted effort.

It was at the University of Chicago's laboratory, on December 2, 1942, that a self-sustaining nuclear chain reaction was first achieved. The project's scientists and engineers then developed an experimental atomic bomb, which was detonated on July 14, 1945, near Almagordo, New Mexico, and, on two fateful days, August 6 and August 9, respectively, of that year, two atomic bombs of twenty kilotons each (the equivalent of twenty thousand tons of TNT) were dropped on Hiroshima and Nagasaki, ending the war.

The total cost of the Manhattan Project was two billion dollars. Success was attained in exactly twenty-six months—from start to finish—in what seemed, then, a problem fraught with insurmountable obstacles.

Estimates of the cost of medical expenses to a terminal cancer patient and his family run from $5,000 to as much as $100,000 during the course of the average illness. By any standard, a most conservative mean average today would be $12,000. Assuming this average of $12,000 per victim, with 370,000 Americans dying each year, the total cost in one year amounts to $4.4 billion. As for the mortality figures in two years, this would amount to 740,000 person (2 × 370,000 per year), or *more than the total of all the U.S. battlefield deaths (not counting injured) in all the wars ever fought in American history!*

Our cancer *research* bill in America alone, in any two-year period, easily runs the total cost of the Manhattan Project, which took about the same period (twenty-six months)—and which meant the winning of the war.

As for the war on cancer, a similar concerted effort could be mounted. The ground troops would be a handpicked consortium of the world's most brilliant men in the medical and related sciences—such as those who characterized our all-out atomic effort—unfettered by any preconceptions or peer commitments, or by dubious loyalties to hoary mores or dogma, or by the impinging arrogance or threatening motions of the status-burdened medical establishment with its idée fixe. Such frontiersmen would have to be given their heads—unconditionally—and, as the night follows the day, they would find their way to the light; and we would have *the answer to cancer in our time.* Their instructions would be simple, but explicit: *"Damn the torpedos, full speed ahead."* And, beyond any shadow of doubt, Dr. Gerson's work would then have its day in court.

The files on cancer today, if collected in any one spot, say, dead center in the Congo, would sink the African continent. One multimillion dollar research institute—as monotonously typical as a TV commercial—states in its brochure: "The goal of the institute is *to add to the store of knowledge* [our italics], of the fundamental nature of the diseases called cancer. . . ." (Note that the *plural* of "disease" is used!). "Overkill" is a mild term with which to designate the titanic mass of research material available on this subject. Properly sorted out, unified, and evaluated with the assistance of computers, there is enough here for cancer to be destroyed at least ten times over—give or take a few thousand tons.

As visualized, such an inspired team of the world's outstanding men in this field, devoted to the cure of cancer—in the cause of truth—would no longer prolong the agony, but would create the ecstasy.

In that great work *China in the Sixteenth Century: The Journals of Matthew Ricci: 1583-1610,* Father Ricci writes that the "leaders of the literary class observed a solemn day of sacrifice in honor of Confucius, if 'sacrifice' is the proper word! This particular celebration is attended with music. The priests who composed the orchestra, set about playing their various instruments, bronze bells, basin-shaped vessels, some made of stone, with skins over them like drums, stringed instruments like a lute, bone flutes, and organs played by blowing into them with the mouth rather than with bellows. They had other instruments also shaped like animals, holding reeds in their teeth, through which air was forced from the empty interior. At this rehearsal these curious affairs were all sounded at once, with a result that can readily be imagined, as it was nothing other than a lack of concord, a discord of discords. The Chinese themselves are aware of this. One of their sages said on a certain occasion that the art of music known to their ancestors had evaporated with the centuries, and left only the instruments."

Has medicine, too, gone the way of Chinese music?

"THE NAIL OF A WRECKED SHIP . . ."

Hundreds of millions of dollars a year are being poured into a bottomless pit of predominantly microsize cancer studies. The National Cancer Institute alone, in an average year, will probably finance from five hundred to seven hundred major project areas, representing several thousand grants. The awesome maze starts at an impressive policy level, with the grand design paying commendable homage to the ultimate goal of cancer research, which is "to eliminate or prevent all human cancers."

But, as the hierarchical plan and program strategy unfold, practical goals and objectives are translated into nit-sized individual studies that represent a maze of redoubtable proportions. As one follows this series of serpentine trails farther and farther into the labyrinth, there comes a point at which it will prove next to impossible for the microbiologist, biochemist, pharmacologist, radiologist, or other laboratory research worker or scientist to maintain any meaningful integrity with home base— the human organism as a whole.

Traversing the maze is much like being carried helplessly along an infinite number of diverging paths on spiderlike conveyor belts, which— as they fan out farther and farther from the starting place—move closer and closer to microscopically narrower and more perplexing vortexes. A point of no return is reached, and the way back is hopelessly lost amid brooding caverns and recesses, dimly lit chambers, and flickering shadows. Compasses are of no avail, because contact with the magnetic pole—the living body—as a point of reference, has long since vanished. It has become so fragmented that, as in a giant jigsaw puzzle in which many of the pieces—and even the picture itself—have been lost, relevance to the parent host is now so obscure as to have reached the vanishing point.

Any credulous attempt now to relate the atomic-scale activity of an isolated and fractionated cell, a gene particle, or a microchemical or physiological change in the body—which may be a billionth or a trillionth part of what is taking place on the grand scale in this cohesive human universe—with any measurable activity of the parent organism as a whole, can no longer be called science, but the metaphysics of miracles.

As an illustration of the type of project area fairly characteristic of cancer research in general, a few are cited as follows:

> 1. Study factors and steps involved in expression of oncogenic viruses after IUDR exposure, including details of gene derepression, excision, repair, and break relinkage processes occurring during activation of viruses and oncogenes. Apply results to prevention of virus-induced Ca.
> 2. Determine nature of secondary event resulting in rapid tumor growth after prolonged irradiation of mouse bone tumors induced by a primary event caused by a single acute dose of irradiation. Use results to restrict progressive growth of nests of cells made preneoplastic by irradiation.
> 3. Correlate genetic segregation of endogenous oncogenic viruses with the susceptibility of the cells to tumor induction in vivo and the susceptibility of cells to transformation by chemicals and radiation in vitro.

From a research center other than NCI, we cite the following area of cellular study, which constitutes a primary thrust for this particular center:

The fundamental aberrations of cancer are concerned with cell division. Research interests in this laboratory are concerned with cell divisional controls, particularly of chromosome replication. In order to study DNA synthesis in single cells, we have developed an immunological technique which utilizes antibodies specific for a non-biological base analogue (5-bromodeoxyuridine), of a precursor (thymidine) which is incorporated into DNA. Thus, newly synthesized DNA can be recognized by antibody binding to the "abnormal" precursor. This immunological technique is also applicable to studies with the electron microscope. so that ultrastructural localization of newly replicated regions of the chromosome can be visualized. We are currently applying this immunological technique in an attempt to "map" replication regions on human chromosomes. It is found, for example, that if cells which are synchronously dividing are "pulsed" with bromodeoxyuridine at various periods of DNA synthesis, their chromosomes become "banded," a band possibly representing that segment of a chromosome that is being replicated at a specific time interval. It is hoped that this kind of method will permit analysis of differences in the way chromosomes from cancer cells replicate in comparison to normal cells.

In *Clinical Judgment,* Dr. Alvan R. Feinstein, Professor at the Yale University School of Medicine, says that "the basic intellectual problems of treatment, receive comparatively little attention in contemporary clinical research. The clinicians of modern academic medical centers have become increasingly concerned with *laboratory investigation* of pathogenesis of disease or *mechanisms of cellular biology.* The problems of *clinical therapy* are often dismissed as a mere application of the 'basic science' studied in the clinical investigator's laboratory" (our italics). In other words, much of the hyperactivity goes on in a vacuum of pure fundamental research without intimate relevance to, or concern for, clinical application. As a matter of fact, only a fraction of the thousands who are involved in laboratory research have had more than passing experience with the moment of truth—the real life-and-death struggles that take place at the bedsides of cancer patients. Humanics has again lost to the machines.

Because the "elimination or prevention of all human cancers" is the avowed object of the multimillion dollar research exercise, today's orthodox therapeutic approaches must be judged on the record; so let's have a look at the scorecard again, if we want to know how the game is going. On the record, we have seen that, despite all, *"in the past twenty-five years, the cancer mortality rate has increased twenty percent."* When we consider this abysmal showing, with an increasing mortality rate, and with cancer deaths now running close to one out of every three, candor compels the harsh judgment that present-day ongoing research activity as a whole is not any more likely to contribute to a solution of the cancer problem than the proverbial fifty monkeys placed in one room with fifty typewriters

—and given endless time—would produce the complete works of Shakespeare!

More than fifteen hundred years ago, a physician of the court of Byzantium, working with drugs, charms and amulets, prescribed the following treatment for epilepsy:

> Take the nail of a wrecked ship, make it into a bracelet and set therein a bone of a stag's heart taken from its body whilst still alive, and put it on the left arm; you will be astonished at the result.

Anyone for Ganzheitstherapie?

}⊱ ⊰{

The handful of projects cited in the foregoing represent only a fraction of thousands of similar research efforts funded by diverse institutes and government agencies. In the main, they are, at best, of highly dubious value and applicability. The specialists work in a morass of watertight compartments. They focus upon minutiae—smidgeonized, fractionated, and atomized—where the way back from the microcosmic to the total human being becomes hopelessly lost.

It is all too dreadfully remindful of a hoary cliché—the definition of a specialist: a man who gets to know more and more about less and less, until, finally, he knows practically everything about absolutely nothing. Gerson's wry comment: "It looks as if we will soon know everything, and understand nothing."

By its very nature, mired down in the Virchow syndrome of cellular theory and localization, the "system" compels the application of mechanistic procedures that violate the human equation. First, by fractionating, i.e., mistaking the parts for the whole—the trees for the forest. Then, as a further extension of the error—into the minute—the introduction of narrow-focus systems, machines, and instrumentation. Thus the trend is away from humanics, from the dynamic unifying principles of the universe, and into the development of mechanized modalities, the structuring of formulas, and the calculation of dosages, series, and courses. Measurements are introduced, printouts elaborated, visual and auditory monitoring devices installed in such profusion that the fate of the patient is—ultimately—reduced to a *mathematical equation*—with a baleful *Star Wars* green-eyed monster in charge.

Dr. Ralph Crawshaw, on the subject of "Humanism in Medicine," presented a brilliant paper at the annual meeting of the Oregon Medical Association on September 19, 1975. His opening statement: "The preoccupation with a medical profession that appears more mechanical and less human grows each day. Our ears are bent, our minds filled, perhaps even our hearts weighted, with the burgeoning catalogue of iatrogenic problems. For me, I have had enough, a surfeit of these problems, moral and mechanical, which indicate that physicians, like it or not, are becoming less human under the sway of a Frankenstein technology and a Faustian government."

It becomes increasingly clear under these conditions that the following statement made about automation—though terrifying in its implications—gains formidable credence: "Automation does not really eliminate the chances for human error. It only moves that possibility to a higher level, so that, when a mistake is made, *it is a colossal one!*"

The newly spawned monster in medicine called iatrogenics—which might alternately be called the science of "negative healing"—constitutes abundant proof of ascending error in medicine. This is not surprising under the circumstances and conditions of mechanistic super-sophistication in medical technology today.

Dorland's Medical Dictionary defines iatrogenics as "resulting from the activity of physicians." In the *American Heritage Dictionary of the English Language,* the definition reads: "Induced in a patient by a physician's words or actions." Today, it is an accepted branch of medical science, an area for serious study, where the physician must be prepared to treat problems that he himself creates, through inadvertent overdose, poor or inadequate monitoring techniques, or the wrong diagnosis. Admittedly, twenty percent of the cases being treated by physicians today are caused by their own ineptness—medical error. Iatrogenics composes an entirely new curriculum that is now part of medical education and training. Are we, then, rapidly approaching that point at which it will be quite unfunny to say that the cure is worse than the disease?

The *CMA Journal* of March 6, 1976, states that "in Western societies about twenty percent of the disorders of hospitalized patients are iatrogenic." Some examples cited:

> 1. A young girl had a routine chest radiograph. It showed a soft-tissue lesion at the apex of the right lung. She was treated for several months for tuberculosis, but she recovered *naturally* because the radiographic shadow was that of a lock of hair lying over her right clavicle.
>
> 2. . . . a woman who had taken, in a period of some months, 27 different drugs, all prescribed by two physicians, neither of whom knew she was attending the other, was admitted to a hospital for gastrointestinal investigation. Three of the medications were for the treatment of diarrhea and another three were for the treatment of abdominal pain (and at least two of the latter—propantheline bromide and codeine—were contributing to the constipation). She had also been taking two drugs for hypertension; one of these contained reserpine, which in turn had been aggravating her underlying depression, for which she was taking three different mood-altering drugs,

one of which was probably also aggravating her constipation. *We discontinued administration of all medications and she got better.* [*Italics added*].

The treatment of non-disease, it is clear, can turn it into disease.

There is unanimous agreement among the experts that, almost without exception, the administration of any drug—even something as mild as aspirin—will result in a certain number of casualties, no matter how small the number. As for the application of stronger drugs, the percentages go higher. The medical position taken is that the end justifies the means, and it is hoped that, in the big picture, the favorable activity of the medication will outweigh, in the majority of cases, its potential for damage.

Looking at the picture statistically, then, does it come as any surprise that medical casualties litter the landscape, to the tune of twenty percent of those treated? And that malpractice suits (i.e., those actually brought into open court), have increased to about five percent of the patients treated? Or that premiums for physicians' malpractice insurance are so high as to be almost prohibitive today—with many insurance companies refusing altogether to handle this type of insurance?

The trite phrase "side effects" is nowadays glibly bandied about by so-called sophisticates. As in a movie where only "the other guy gets killed," they talk themselves out of being involved. Are we all victims of a psychotic syndrome, believing with some absolutely mad psychiatrist that, if we consciously project or verbalize our problems, they will all magically disappear?

Death and disability are hardly side effects that will go away easily, though they may come trippingly on the tongue. For example, those "side effects" precipitated by a U.S. Air Force B-29 flying over Hiroshima, Japan, at 8:15 A.M., on August 6, 1945; and again, three days later, on August 9 over Nagasaki. Two atom bombs, each with the force of twenty thousand tons of TNT, exploded in the clear blue skies on those fateful days. Seventy-five thousand human beings were incinerated in Hiroshima, and thirty-five thousand in Nagasaki, with tens of thousands frightfully injured, many carrying the scars, the pain, and the suffering to this day, with the long-term effects of radiation exposure affecting countless future generations. And so—the graveyard humor, goes—the new "improved" types, like those with hydrogen nuclear warheads of six megatons (equal to six million tons of TNT)—(and some even a bit more sophisticated), can remove the four Japanese islands altogether, and, for good measure, the city of Vladivostok, USSR, which inconveniently juts south in the direction of the Japanese archipelago!

And so it goes, with stronger and stronger drugs, with medically administered irradiation, and other therapeutic inputs every day—all of which seem to work on the very simple, if frightening, premise that the human body can withstand anything. After all, isn't the body just one vast chemical factory anyway? So let's try injecting it with this, or blasting it with that, and see what happens? Who knows, if the patient is lucky, it may work? Although, on the other hand, if the second, third, or fortieth generation winds up with flippers for hands, then we'll know we've made a mistake!

Today, oversized monsters keep children infinitely enthralled and deliriously happy at our TV tubes and in the movie theaters. But the giant-sized threat to humanity, as the ultimate result of our abuse of nature, her creatures and her laws, may less likely be of the King Kong variety. Rats, for example, used to shriek loudly, once or twice, then turn belly up, after a few nips of lethal warfarin—a deadly anticoagulant rodenticide. Now, having established resistance, they have settled on this delightful concoction as their dessert, devouring it like strawberry shortcake, and clamoring for more. One can almost expect threats and imprecations from the rat union if, in the future, their portions are not up to expectation. Yes, for the rodent today, warfarin has become his cup of tea, his pièce de résistance.

And then there are the microorganisms and viruses—smaller by far than the ant or head louse—those invisible creatures of that never-never world of electron microscopes where tiny mites (needing 30,000 to 40,000 magnifications to be seen) are learning to fraternize with our most deadly germ-killers. New strains of pneumococcus, for example, can withstand anything in our medical pharmacopoeia today. According to *U.S. News & World Report,* measles and gonorrhea are increasing substantially, with gonorrhea considered by some officials as "out of control." One strain of gonorrhea, which first reached the U.S. from the Philippines, "is completely resistant to penicillin and is threatening to spread. Syphilis is also now starting to increase . . . and new pockets of tuberculosis have been discovered." As for influenza vaccinations, these are usually for one strain only, and are rarely effective against other types! The basic reason and problem in all this? The emergence of new, highly resistant strains.

Frenzy and panic are often generated—such as that which resulted in the crash program initiated by President Ford in the fall of 1976, when 140 million Americans were inoculated—then, suddenly, everything stopped. A medical doctor, writing in *Good Housekeeping* in October 1976, said about the swine flu vaccine, "Because it contains only *killed* viruses, there is no possible way the vaccine itself can cause infection." Shortly after this pronouncement, 23 deaths occurred—alleged to have been caused by the vaccine. Another 494 persons who received shots were paralyzed by Guillain-Barre disease. The program was then halted.

So our giant-sized monsters may turn out not to be the real danger after all. Who can tell which one of the hundreds of drugs or medicaments presently being brewed in laboratories all over the globe will one day mutate a strain that will inherit the earth? It seems pretty apparent that we have met the enemy—and they are *us*.

THE IMPAIRED PHYSICIAN

The pressures of our modern industrial society, with their disastrous impact on the well-being of our citizens, have compounded the difficulties for the medical practitioner in coping with its resultant health and disease problems, proving too much for many. It is not surprising therefore that the physician, out of sheer instinct for survival, may seek escape from his oppressive dilemmas by retreating to the machines—or, else, to something much, much worse. The refuge found in sophisticated equipmentation affords at least a modicum of security—particularly against the terrifying threat of malpractice suits, and—on the record—it provides prima facie evidence that the doctor did, in fact, take such measures with his patients as were necessary and compatible with approved professional standards and procedures. Yet it does provoke us to a natural question: Are we in fact living out now—on earth—a *Planet of the Apes* scenario, in which our captors are not apes, but computers?

In postwar Japan, the language problems were so formidable that Japanese employees working as interpreters infested every single office of the U.S. Occupation Forces. Interpreters by the thousands were deployed throughout the organization at every echelon—from the lowest levels of labor services to the War Crimes Tribunal, to the hearing rooms of the Allied Council, and even in the office of the Supreme Commander for the Allied Powers, General Douglas MacArthur himself. It was often remarked that "the real occupation is by the interpreters." And is it so, too, with medicine and its machines?

In the lighter banter that sometimes protrudes to relieve the otherwise somber topics of doctors' intercourse, a physician was once overheard to remark ruefully: "Fifty percent of the things we are doing are right; and fifty percent of them are wrong. The trouble is, we don't know which is which!"

We dare to venture here that, if medicine does not know which is which, "Why not"—as the magistrate said in the German court to Gerson's accusers, when he summarily dismissed their case—"let Dr. Gerson do it?"

Although more than likely to be classified as damning with faint praise, it is nevertheless fitting that we pause a moment to pay tribute to the thousands of dedicated physicians who must fairly be counted among the ranks of the wounded physician. Testimony in this regard is distressingly provided by certain vital statistics that give us some clues relative to the devotion and involvement of many members of the medical community, which affect their lives and their deaths, and that give clear evidence of the severe stress to which they are exposed in their daily work.

The suicide rate among doctors tells a grim story, which bespeaks deep emotional involvement with their sick and dying patients. As Dr. Stanley Gitlow of the Mount Sinai School of Medicine commented, "Suicides are two and one-half times more common in the ranks of physicians than the general population average. This tragic waste of professional life means that 'one medical school graduating class of 100 students is needed each year to replace physicians who commit suicide.' "

As for alcoholism among medical doctors, this is observed twice as frequently as narcotics addiction. According to a survey by the American Medical Association, "One to two percent of the physicians are markedly affected by drug dependence. . . . Seven to eight percent are now, or will become alcoholics. . . . Alcoholism seems to be the most frequently encountered illness, constituting at least half of the sick physician pathology. . . . Some observers would place it as high as two-thirds. If we were to settle on 60 percent, then the aggregate number of doctors disabled by their alcoholism, drug dependence, or mental illness, would approximate 17,000, or from 5-6 percent of the total physician population."

All this is grim reminder of the inordinate psychological trauma experienced by the practitioner today. His physical energies and emotional resources are strained to the breaking point by the unceasing burden of the sick, the halt, and the lame.

The AMA has only belatedly become significantly involved in this appalling problem, the more frightening because (with some minor exceptions) such machinery as exists for detecting the presence of an impaired or sick physician is of such a low-key and passive nature that Gilbert Cant, writing in *Good Housekeeping* in January 1976, said, "In every state except Florida . . . men and women who have once obtained a license to practice medicine, may continue to treat patients long after they have become totally unfit to do so. . . . The medical machinery to protect patients against this threat is as grotesquely cumbersome as a Rube Goldberg design for a spaceship."

With the percentage of impaired physicians as high as one out of every twenty practicing, the quality of care delivered to the patient—whether in routine illness, or in chronic or advanced disease—is suspect. Operating within a collegial infrastructure, the hospital administration—literally—is terrified of possible malpractice suits should a physician's incapacity be suspected by the public. The physician's peers, also, hesitate to become involved in such decidedly sensitive and unpleasant situations, besides themselves often being frightened by seeing their own reflection in a brother physician's condition!

It is beyond the scope of this book to venture, in depth, into the general quality level of patient treatment, but it is impossible to abstain from an observation that, besides the tragic loss of much-needed professional personnel, a definite hazard exists because of the lower quality of health care given the general public. Surely, a primary concern of the government, and of controlling and involved institutions, should be in the revision of qualifying standards and criteria for admission of students into the medical universities. Interviewing and testing procedures and techniques need refining and strengthening to emphasize and appraise the psychological elements present in the family, social, and emotional background of the applicants, which would allow a meaningful evaluation of those indicators that measure the stable quality of an applicant's probable responses when precipitated into the stressful environment he faces upon graduation.

It is not as if we were here dealing with just achievement levels, and a general IQ, such as might be more tenable in professions like engineering, business administration, or law. The practicing physician is in a class by himself, because he is confronted in his daily working milieu with oppressive necessities that involve him without surcease in grave life-and-death decisions.

6

"We Got It All"

It becomes clear that, even under the best of circumstances, if the physician succeeds with one or more of the traditional approaches in "controlling" or "curing" the malignant condition, should he not complement his successful first thrust by employing nature's primary means—food—to regenerate the tissues and organs, and thus restore the body's basic healing mechanism?

Orthodox medical practice uses the "attack" means—aggressive assault—in cancer, i.e., surgery, irradiation, and chemotherapy (drugs). These may in some cases temporarily surmount the immediate threat—the crisis situation—but these measures, in the light of long-term results, remain in terminal cancer a hazardous undertaking and, in the main, not a final resolution of the malignant condition. The search-and-destroy effort may relieve and palliate, but, in a fundamental sense, it cannot repair or restore.

CHEMOTHERAPY

Take chemotherapy, for example, which today occupies the greatest attention of the medical research world. Chemotherapy is engineered for specificity, i.e., to attack a particular type of cancer cell and/or tumor site. It is designed to reach particular cells and cancer foci in the body, and to alter their organization and physiological activity in such a way as to bring about their destruction. Routinely, depending upon the drug, it is usually administered either intravenously and/or orally, most often in a combination of three or four drugs. They act as a general pervasive agent and permeate the living cellular structures of the body via the blood and lymph streams (just as the cancer cells do), damaging and destroying the healthy cells along with cancer cells.

Because these drugs have such generalized destructive action, they must be labeled as highly toxic to the body. No healthy cell in the body can escape the drug's action, having the same exposure as the tumor cell.

It is well, therefore, to have a look at the *desired actions* of these drugs first. These drugs:

1. block the cell's normal metabolic processes
2. inhibit the utilization of nucleic acids and proteins, causing the death of the cells
3. interfere all the way along the line with the chain involved in DNA synthesis
4. alter the hormonal balance of the patient
5. arrest cell division
6. block the production of certain amino acids necessary for cell survival.

It is readily seen that the healthy cells may be doomed to suffer the same fate as the cancer cells, and that the action of the drug is destructive in nature to the entire body. It is true that the malignant growth may be reduced, but the underlying causes remain, and consequently the probability of recurrence.

Most antitumor drugs also depress the cellular immune system of the patient, and thereby increase the probability of depressing some systems that restrain tumor growth. A point of no return is often reached with advanced cases.

Side effects such as nausea, vomiting, diarrhea, baldness, uterine bleeding, depression of the normal content of the bone marrow, infection and bleeding tendencies, skin rashes, pigmentation of the skin, edema, and hoarseness are among some of the reactions. They prove aggravating, distressing, and depressing to the patient. The suffering of some of the patients is indescribable, and must become a part of the physician's conscience, in which he shares their wounds.

The selection of one drug, or a combination of drugs, by the chemotherapy specialist is immediately directed at the tumor site and the cancer cells in general. But his first and perhaps most frightening confrontation is with an array in the medical supermarket arsenal of about forty drugs (at last count) that are recognized for use in the malignant condition. More often than not, he will choose a combination of three or four, rather than a single drug. Life-saving and life-risking decisions are inherently involved all the way along the line in any chemotherapeutic regime. However, there is very little, so far, in this uncertain kingdom of medical hit-and-miss, that has yet been reduced to empirical absolutes—and very little that is likely to be, in view of the bone-cracking, perplexing differences between patients, and their individual afflictions.

Authoritative opinion, as echoed by one specialist in the field, Dr. Victor Richards, agrees that "the outstanding shortcoming of chemotherapy is the failure of the drugs to destroy the cancer cells specifically without simultaneously damaging the host . . . for it is oftentimes impossible for the drug to kill the cancer cell without *simultaneously damaging all the normal cells of the host."*

Every chemotherapist has had patients die from the effects of drugs. In the *New York Journal of Medicine* of March 1, 1971, we learn of a study that admits to a death rate of ten percent—not from the cancer, but from the chemotherapy. In fact, chemotherapy suppresses the body's natural, immunological defenses against cancer, thereby helping the disease to metastasize, or spread.

Dr. Hans A. Nieper of Germany, world-famous cancer specialist and research scientist, has declared that it is in the nature of the beast, chemotherapy, to provoke an assault upon the body that results in "considerable additional suffering of the patient, or in a regression or remission *paid for with a final iatrogenic collapse of the endogenous condition."* In plain words, Dr. Nieper is saying that, although chemotherapy may initially cause a reduction in tumor size, or even accomplish a remission, it is usually of a temporary character; *ultimately the chemotherapy causes total collapse of the body's innate capabilities to recover.*

Nevertheless, despite its hazards and pitfalls, chemotherapy has burgeoned today into the forefront of cancer research and treatment, on an ascending, almost logarithmic scale. But the most morbid implications of all, in orthodox therapy, are that modern medicine is still hopelessly married to its interpretation of Virchow's cellular theory, and, by extension, to its ultimate fatal commitment to the *symptom as being the disease!* As the serpent lies sleeping in the egg, so does this concept carry within it the seeds of its own destruction, because the therapeutic modalities springing from its impoverished soil remain barren of true healing capability.

With the minor exception of a few types of malignancies such as childhood leukemia, Hodgkin's disease, cervical cancer, and some others that show good response when treated with modern-day methods—but that account for only six percent of the recorded cancer deaths—the cooked statistics channeling out to the general public are confusing in the extreme, and are used as a drunken man uses lamp posts: "more for support than illumination." What *is* illuminated, however, is the bankruptcy of such an all-out attack. If it is to be used at all, surely it must not fail to include, as an intimate, viable partner, a strong dietary regime?

The contention is made that, by reducing or removing the tumor growth, the body is given relief from the immediate pressures of cancer masses, which are infiltrating the tissues and organs and blocking vital functions, poisoning, disrupting and destroying the body's physiological systems. This theory is tenable as far as it goes. There is no doubt that, in some cases, the *immediate* desired result is accomplished. But, in the main, these are emergency measures providing symptomatic relief, too often temporary in nature. The application of palliative measures in such crisis treatment, dealing (presumably) with the underlying causes—*without knowing* what fine metastatic threads may be radiating throughout the body; *without knowing* what cancer cells are circulating in the blood or lymph systems, or have settled into other tissues and organs, which are approachable neither by the surgeon's most superlative skill, nor by the specialist's most ingenious combinations of drugs and radiation therapy —will defy the most valiant heroics.

In the last extremity—terminal cancer—when it is five minutes before midnight, we are dealing with a dying patient. With the body's resources seriously depleted, and with many organs and functions limping badly—some completely prostrate—despite the most intrepid measures of orthodoxy, there is rarely any possibility of a remission.

Long-term statistics provide macabre evidence that there has been no diminution in the overall death rate of cancer patients, quite the reverse: "In the past twenty-five years alone the cancer mortality rate has increased twenty percent," as indicated in a CBS documentary.

Given the body's straitened condition, how, then, can a turnaround be expected? How can exhausted, sick, and dying cells be renewed? How are tissues to be regenerated, the organs rejuvenated, the functional mechanisms reestablished—in other words, the metabolism, and the body's whole immunological defense system, returned to normal—if not with nutritional therapy? Is there any truth, after all, in the oft-quoted assertion "You are what you eat"? Dr. Max Gerson thought so, and he successfully practiced the art and science of healing, using a logically conceived, clinically tested, and—as we shall see—extremely effective dietary regimen.

Cells certainly cannot derive true sustenance from synthetic chemicals manufactured in pharmaceutical laboratories, and certainly not from the more lethal types used in chemotherapy. Potent drugs such as cyclophosphamide, nitrogen mustard, 5-Fluorouracil, and Thio-TEPA do not by sheer force of strength miraculously purify the bloodstream and wash the tissues clear of cancer cells. *Nor* does the scalpel by divine fiat accrue omnipotence by some feat of surgical legerdemain as it cuts cruelly through whole cellular worlds, parting flesh from flesh. *Nor* does irradiation unfold a magic umbrella that spreads an all-pervasive power of healing. All of these means, prima facie, are attack-and-destroy expedients. None of them is even remotely conceived or intended to accomplish the task of restoration in a fundamental physiological sense. Do not then the theory and the practice suffer from a fatal flaw? Let's face it: there is simply no feat of legerdemain in the lexicon of traditional medicine that can pull a rabbit out of a hat and reverse the ongoing malignant process without the introduction of a rejuvenating dietary regime. The mortality statistics are tragic proof of that.

Dr. Gerson's nutritional program is completely discussed later in this book. However, it is pertinent here to note that he discovered—the hard way—that, even within his tightly controlled and highly reinforced total therapeutic regime, certain hormones—and even certain food factors, also —acted as virulent carcinogens in his terminal patients.

In the case of his women patients who had had their ovaries removed (a not uncommon procedure in premenopausal women with advanced or disseminated breast cancer), he observed that the tumors started immediately to regrow upon the administration of hormones in the form of ovarian substance. The tumors also regrew when he gave these patients fats in their diet. This latter was a general phenomenon observed also in his other patients. He learned through painful experience that even so much as the addition of the yolk of one egg had a carcinogenic effect, and acted to retrigger the malignant process. Once, leaning heavily upon the work of Professor Huggins about successful results achieved with hormone therapy, Gerson decided to use it with some of his patients. The consequences were catastrophic. As Gerson reports it:

> The most dramatic setback occurred when I added to the therapy the opposite *sex hormones,* so highly recommended at that time by Professor Charles Huggins. These hormones were first applied in five cases which could not recover fast enough. In the first three to four months, I observed a pronounced improvement. Therefore, I administered these hormones to an additional 25 patients.
> *All of these patients were already free of cancer symptoms,* but they still felt weak. Most of these cases had received previous X-ray treatment of long duration. The outcome of this hormone treatment was *disastrous.* I lost 25 of my best cases. After a remarkable improvement within three to five months, they died within three to four weeks. Only five of them could be saved. I feel that the specific sex hormones, even small doses, stimulate the liver and consume the painstakingly re-accumulated reserves of the liver.

Dr. Gerson took this so very personally that severe depression resulted. He was moved to give up at this point, but friends and patients prevailed to have him put this tragedy behind him, and to continue with his work.

Happily, at about this same time, Gerson discovered a giant balancing truth: that iodine (which he usually prescribed in the form of lugol solution) was a potent inhibitor of tumor growth. In consort with his Ganzheitstherapie, the lugol apparently acted to reinforce the immune factor, and to establish a new resistance front against the disease.

Can it be more clear, then, even from the nature of the overall healing activity, that any therapeutic program demands superior nutrition, as an issue of life and death? Not just any good food, but the *correct* food, in type, quantity, and quality—and in the right combinations. Dr. Gerson, with long years of research and experience in food technology, in his towering work *A Cancer Therapy* happily shares with the medical practitioner his entire food and medication regime.

For medical doctors to ignore completely the life-threatening consequences of a faulty diet—especially in our grossly poisoned environment—is to negate any possible gains they may be achieving with their indecisive methods. Given the patient's devitalized condition, how critical it becomes to provide the body with life-sustaining nutrients! But, more than that even, *to avoid abuse of the body with either oppressive and possibly carcinogenic medicaments, OR food factors!* The caveat of Hippocrates illuminated the pure heart of this precept. He said, *"primum non nocere,"*—first, do no harm.

From start to finish, according to Dr. Gerson, the primary objective must be twofold: on the one hand, to eliminate the cancer foci by placing them under continuous siege and assault with certain prescribed therapeutic measures, and at the same time to administer a potent, reinforcing nutritional therapy. This double-barreled combination will undermine the malignant condition, and simultaneously rouse the body from its poisoned stupor, so that its own native intelligence mechanism is reenergized to take over the job of reorganizing, rebuilding, and reinforcing its physiological defense systems, ultimately restoring the body to its natural health, strength, and vigor. Gerson continued to reiterate, however, that "diet alone cannot cure cancer. Medication also is necessary."

Insofar as the basic philosophical premise of this book is concerned, it should be clear that the accent must be upon therapies that work with nature and with her laws—with an absolute minimum of medications. In principle, the application of potent drugs, of irradiation, and of surgery, is admissible only in a crisis situation, as, for example, when the blockage of a vital organ or function threatens life. Otherwise, the potent healing activity inherent in the integrated Gerson therapeutic program will do more to overcome the pathology than orthodox methods.

Common sense alone should tell us that the habituating use of drugs and medicaments on a virtually permanent basis is unnatural, creates addiction, and must in due course destroy the body's native ability to maintain an integrated defense system. A drug is an alien agent, and when it is introduced into the human body it acts as a stimulus, triggering assorted responses, which we call "reactions" or "side effects." Instead of allowing the body to work out its own solutions to the underlying disease cause, the drug alters and/or inhibits the natural metabolic processes, misdirecting and disrupting the organization of the communication and defense system. Paracelsus von Hohenheim, about four hundred years ago, called this self-healing power "the physician within," without which even the most practiced medical doctor could not perform his healing.

The knowledge of the ages, genetically engineered, and the instinctual responses hidden deep in the innermost recesses of the cellular intelligence, is short-circuited by these artificial stimulants. Attention is diverted from the real miscreant, because the body is now compelled to deal with the more immediate threat—*the new drug!*

In severe chronic disease and in terminal cancer, energy resources are at a dismally low ebb. As a result of the oppressive orthodox therapeutic regime, the organs and functions become *disoriented,* and their normal power of discrimination and appropriate response seriously weakened. In other words, the defense systems have been breached and eroded by the pathology underlying the systemic condition, which continues to grow worse under the remorseless pressure of a harsh and unabating therapeutic assault. In truth, *a whole new and synthetic internal environment has been created!* The body's previously integrated system is now on the brink of disaster, tottering along on crutches, using artificial supports, such as drugs and medications, intravenous feedings, powerful pain killers, oxygen tents, and other assorted paraphernalia and methodology—all of the disquieting adjunctive aids, fittings, appliances, and trusses from the arsenals of medicine. It is fair to say that, somewhere along the line, the oppressed organism—frightened, disoriented, and disconcerted—has been placed under such unendurable stress that it has reached a state of *madness—and in this madness has actually built an accommodation to the illness!* The familiar landmarks are gone, and the path obscured beyond recognition. The road map, with its strange and bewildering signposts, has become a giant maze that puzzles the will, and will—inevitably—lead to that "undiscovered country from whose bourn no traveler returns."

The body can act correctly to restore good health only if it is provided with the necessary tools, the essential ingredients. The introduction of alien materials in the form of destructive and addictive drugs and medications—the traumatic invasions of its subtle but profound privacies by surgery or other intervention—*will not restore anything,* least of all the body's own healing capabilities. So-called reactions and side effects are nothing more than the body's valiant efforts to defend itself against this gross violation of its sanctity by rejecting the alien incursions. The harsh assaults with radiation and drugs—yes, and surgery, too—are highly traumatic, and sometimes fatal intrusions of the body's sacrosanct cavities, too often unnecessary, and rarely curative.

The use of attack means in cancer therapy has severe limitations. They may help the terminal cancer patient survive a short battle, but rarely the war.

Overwhelming the forces of chronic disease and cancer is not unlike total war. In battle, there is the initial assault phase, then the establishment of defensible positions to hold the ground won, following which the foot soldier, with air and ground support cover, moves out to overtake and destroy the enemy. In medical metaphor, surgery, radiation, and chemotherapy can be likened to such an assault on the enemy's forward positions, for the establishment and maintenance of the beachheads. The temporary digging-in and holding action may be compared to the maintenance dosage (keeping the valuable ground won), until the arrival of reinforcements. But over and beyond these first battles, if the war is to be won at all, the troops must advance farther into enemy territory and wipe them out, forcing nothing short of unconditional surrender.

In the illustration given, confronting the enemy on the decisive level means the use of nutritional troops, carrying all the weaponry and armaments for "invading" the body's enemy strongholds—the alien, cellular infrastructures that hold the body captive. The enemy troops in their preliminary forays and early thrusts have now reached the point where a subversive Trojan Horse action has completely undermined the inner defense system. They have commandeered the heights (tissues and organs), seized the depots and storage facilities (reserves), and captured the transportation and communication systems (blood and lymph). At this point, only a dietary regime can repel the invading armies, recapture all positions, and once again establish a defense bulwark along the entire perimeter, so that a new great wall of invincibility, the body's renewed immunological defense system, now faces any future invading force.

Is it not clear that, over the long term, chronic, life-threatening disease requires incisive dietary treatment as an inseparable part of Ganzheitstherapie?

To give you just an inkling of the hairsplitting considerations on which a human life may hang, let us have a look at the dilemma of the chemotherapist: Which drug or drugs should he use? In what amounts? How long should the series be in one so-called "course"? How many courses? How closely must the patient be watched, and with what specific monitoring procedures, to be sure that the selected drugs are proving helpful, and not damaging? What countermeasures must be instituted immediately in the event of serious, sometimes catastrophic developments, like a sharp drop in the white blood cell count, sudden bleeding or infection, functional failures, or other frightening—even though expectable —reactions? And when the danger signals flash, should the dosages be reduced, the combinations changed, or the therapy completely abandoned? And in this last eventuality, are there any longer any alternatives, or is the patient now—*hopeless?*

Perhaps one of the most morbid doubts of the physician with a heart hangs on the harrowing thought: "Are the *observable* symptoms really telling the whole story with respect to the efficacy of the therapy; or are the available testing and monitoring techniques, at best, providing only fragmentary bits and pieces, not truly adequate to cope with the life-and-death crisis?"

There are uncounted cases in medical history where patients have been given a clean bill of health following a thoroughgoing physical examination—only to fall victim to cancer shortly thereafter. These beg the fact that there may be underlying pathological deterioration, empirically undetectable, but, nonetheless, in any etiology, as crucial to the matter as all the observable clinical phenomena for which the patient is being treated. Dr. Max Gerson reported, "I have seen a number of cancer patients who had been examined in excellent cancer prevention clinics only a few months earlier, in whom nothing pathological or suspicious had been found."

Likewise, there are instances where a physician receives a patient with a puzzling malaise and is quite unable to put his finger on the trouble, yet is deeply disturbed by the patient's condition, sometimes, even, with forebodings of an incipient malignant basis. Yet his best diagnostic efforts prove unavailing to resolve the dilemma. Dr. Michael B. Shimkin states, in *Science and Cancer,* that "difficulties in diagnosis will increase as patients bring smaller and earlier lesions to the attention of the physicians, and as physicians confront the pathologist with progressively earlier stages of cancer"! Under such conditions, the physician, in short, is compelled to send the troubled patient home with nothing more valiant than a placebo, and an injunction, in effect, to "Come back when it gets worse"!

To Gerson, such a case, puzzling and gnawing to the average practitioner, would have been "a piece of cake." His simple injunction to the distraught physician would have been: "Attack the condition with a strong nutritional therapy—let the 'inner physician' do the healing. I have given you all you need in my cancer therapy book to heal the patient. Do you want to know something?" he would have added with a glint of the elf in his eye. *"A cancer metabolism starts where the body is no longer able to produce a healing inflammation.* This can help you with your diagnosis. Dr. Kempner proved that slices of tissue, taken from malignant rat tumors or human cancer tissues, are killed fast in an inflammation exudate because the fermentation metabolism of the cancer cell cannot be maintained in those surroundings.

"Look also at the work of Dr. J. Alibert, a famous French surgeon at the Hospital of St. Louis in Paris, who experimented upon himself and a few volunteers. He took cancerous material from a female breast tumor, broke it into small particles, and finally made an emulsion with which he injected himself and three of his students. A severe feverish inflammation appeared, and lasted a few days, but there was no further reaction. He repeated the experiment, with the same result. You can see from this why the whole weight of my therapy is to reinforce the body's own physiological healing mechanisms with those very oxidizing enzymes which will create a normal oxidation metabolism in which cancer cells cannot live. They must die because their life depends upon a fermentation process that cannot survive the total assault of my restoration treatment.

"Cancer patients have different types of allergic reactions. . . . The patient may have enough power for an allergic *reaction,* but not enough for an 'allergic *inflammation'*—which is the decisive part of the body's 'weapon of healing power.' . . . An allergic reaction may be thought of as a diminished enzymatic reaction (Lichtwitz), and allergic inflammation to be an increased enzymatic reaction (von Bergmann).

"I, myself, have used cantharidin plasters with my patients to test their inflammatory response. Cancer patients could not produce such a response, but I noted that as my treatment regime continued, the inflammatory mechanism—which is, after all, part of the immunity system—returned, proving that my patients were getting better. I think I will repeat myself: A cancer metabolism starts where the body is no longer able to produce a healing inflammation. So, if you are asking me my suggestions, I have to say two things. One, as a preventive measure, and to assist with the diagnosis, why not test the patient who is showing puzzling symptoms, to see if his body can produce an inflammation? Two, if the inflammation reaction is weak or nonexistent, then we must definitely suspect the possibility of a malignant condition, even if there is no sign of it yet, and we must begin an aggressive preventive routine with strong nutritional treatment, as I say in my book. As part of the continuing monitoring process of the patient's condition, we can use the cantharidin plaster or some other similar agent, to measure the return of the inflammation response to the metabolism."

Gerson would surely have smiled broadly at this point, in his open, confident fashion: "Is that so difficult to understand?"

SURGERY

Surgery, too, represents a radical assault upon the body. In surgery, the tumor may be extirpated—as far as can be seen—but, like the tip of the iceberg, especially in the presence of metastases (often undetected and undetectable), invisible metastatic threads may have woven themselves throughout the physiological structures, blocking the therapist's (and the surgeon's) best efforts. Tragically, autopsies too often provide the only "proof" of "success" in this direction, i.e., direct observation of the cadaver, and of the reduction or elimination of the *visible tumor.* So the symptoms were palliated but the disease remained, and continued its inevitable ongoing process. The painful cliché, "The operation (or chemotherapy) was a success, but the patient died," remains appropriate.

In a remarkable study covering intensive postmortems of eleven thousand deceased persons, Berg and Lundberg found that in 44.1% of the cases a malignant condition was discovered, "whereas only 26.3%

of these persons were previously considered as suffering from cancer. In hypothetical allover micro-dissection," they indicated, "perhaps 80-90% of the deceased would have been cancer carriers."

Jane E. Brody, Science Reporter for *The New York Times,* writes: "When a surgeon tells the patient and his family, 'We got it all,' he may really mean, 'We got all the cancer we could *see.'* Microscopic . colonies of cancer may have escaped his scalpel, and for this reason, anywhere from 10 to 80 percent of patients from whom the surgeon thought he removed 'all' the cancer, will experience a recurrence of the disease."

Cancer has many faces, according to classifications by orthodox medicine. There are, they say, a hundred viruses and a thousand chemicals capable of causing it. According to orthodox theory, also, there are many different kinds of cancer. The American Cancer Society rushes in where angels fear to tread and says, right out, that "cancer is a *large group* of diseases"! The National Institute of Health seems to agree, saying in its turn that "cancer is a *group* of diseases," omitting the word "large," whereas the National Cancer Institute regards cancer "not as one disease but a *family* of diseases, having certain common characteristics." According to Dr. Michael B. Shimkin, of the Department of Health, Education, and Welfare, "At the present time, cancers are classified by their appearance under the microscope, and by the site of the body from which they arise. By such criteria of appearance (morphology) and localization, devised by pathologists during the past century, at least 100 different cancers are identified." And so it goes. . . .

It is apparent that the evasive cancer cell wears many disguises; and, if one goes searching for the rascal with instruments that make a loud bang, or sporting a light as broad of beam as a lighthouse beacon, the culprit may still evade all efforts to be caught—as we have already seen in the eleven thousand autopsy cases, where approximately eighteen percent remained undetected.

It is expecting overmuch to believe that the surgeon—any more than the radiotherapist or chemotherapist—will succeed in discovering and routing this wily cell from all of his hiding places. Under such anomalous conditions, surgical intervention must be viewed with utmost caution, even alarm, particularly when other less violent means are available, with less pain and suffering.

Reasonable doubt also intervenes, permitting serious question whether the highest motives of altruism underlie the necessities proposed by the surgeon. In February 1976, Washington's UPI correspondent reported that a House committee, after completing a survey of *surgery* in ninety-five hospitals, estimated that *"Americans spent $3.92 billion for operations they did not need, and found that almost half of the postoperative complications and 35 percent of the deaths studied were preventable."*

One authoritative hospital committee, which was created to curb the removal of normal appendixes, gallbladders, uteri and the like, reported that about a quarter of the surgical operations reviewed were unnecessary.

Discretion, therefore, becomes the better part of valor, and it becomes very much in order to question the desirability of surgical intervention at any time, particularly when reasonable alternatives are possible and available.

RADIATION THERAPY

Radiation therapy, too, destroys the healthy along with the malignant cells, and may have gross side effects that may damage specific organs, the gut or the spinal cord, and suppress the immune response of the body. In excessive doses, irradiation itself can cause cancer. The body's high sensitivity demands the greatest care in the weighing of factors involved, and requires the highest level of competence by the radiotherapist. It has been found that *"a single X-ray film of the abdomen of a pregnant woman produced significant increases in the incidence of cancer, including leukemia, in the child."*

Modern techniques and sophisticated equipment, such as telecobalt units and linear and cyclic accelerators, allow the high energy radiations to be focused on a specific site, sometimes with an infinitely small locus. Here, too, however, healthy cells in the surrounding area (or intermingled with the tissues' malignant cells), will suffer damage along with the cancer cells. Nor can irradiation, in most cases, cope with a generalized malignant condition, because it is virtually impossible, and highly undesirable, to attempt to irradiate the entire body.

Although irradiation is being employed with the adjunctive modalities of surgery and/or chemotherapy, even the medical community will freely concede that results of this cooperative front have been less than overwhelming. In what is called adjuvant or concomitant therapy, a controlled test study was conducted by the NIH to determine the efficacy of administering drugs in conjunction with breast surgery. Twenty-three major American institutions participated, with eight hundred and twenty-six patients being followed—all of whom had had radical mastectomies. Dr. Victor Richards, Chief of Surgery, Children's Hospital, San Francisco, in his book *The Wayward Cell,* reports that "this study demonstrated that in all categories, neither thio-TEPA nor 5-FU, the two drugs of choice administered at the time of surgery, or shortly after surgery, in a maximum dose compatible with the patient's safety, reduced either the recurrence of the tumor or enhanced the 5-year survival rate. The present therapeutic results obtained in adjuvant chemotherapy have been unsuccessful. . . ."

Does not all this make out the strongest case for whole-man therapy? For Ganzheitstherapie? For addressing ourselves to the restoration of the body's own healing powers—a totally integrated entity—through incisive nutrition? Should we not begin to take note of the endowment from that creative force that engineered, through countless eons of trial and error, the evolution of instincts; that evolved the incomparable intelligence stored in every cell of the human computer and soul; and that, through genetic magic, permits the organism, under natural conditions, to cognize and sort out, from an infinite nutritional availability, those rich unadulterated elements most needful for its healthy maintenance?

Can it be more than gross conceit to imagine that, with a few fragments of experiential data, sorted out by a handful of humans (against the vast backdrop of countless ages), the healing practitioner of today can challenge the instinctual wisdom locked within the secret bosom of this incredible human machine—where, Dr. Shimkin writes, one tiny "mammalian cell contains an estimated 100,000 different enzymes to perform up to 2,000 chemical reactions"?

Invisible to the naked eye, this tiny cell, approximately one-thousandth of a millimeter in size—of which there are approximately twenty-seven trillion in the average body—operates a bewildering number of chemical factories, all running full-tilt at one and the same time!

Let us contemplate for just a moment the far reaches of the human mind, which carries, in its microcosmic structuring at the cellular level, worlds within worlds. It has been calculated that, were we able to construct a computer that would cover the whole face of the earth, it would still not equal the capacity of one human brain! This soft, spongy mass of gray matter, containing something over ten billion cells, and weighing about three pounds, carries the image and imprint of the infinite universe.

Nature simply abhors rape, and will not succumb without violent retribution. She will yield her superlative secrets only to the gentle ministrations of man—in consonance with the quality of his character, his will, and his soul. Her innermost treasures will not be so easily available to the marauder, the miser, or the felon. Or to those of little faith. It is simply not in the natural order of things that there should be disharmony or imbalance in the universal grand design.

Is it possible, also, that those biological phenomena that remain subliminal—beyond empirical observation—perhaps from ages-old wisdom, carry the messages of the greatest significance? Is it not begging the question to believe that an ordinary mortal with a few years of university education can knock on nature's door and be instantly rewarded with the solution to timeless mysteries, like sickness and health, affecting the most awe-inspiring creature in our universe—Man?

Over the ages, raw data on a cosmic scale has been feeding into man's cellular genetic "memory banks." Would the most dilettantish computer specialist dare to venture where angels fear to tread—into this endless labyrinth—without a programming guide, indispensable to instruct the computer on what to do in order to solve the problem? Second, *from the very start,* according to computer science (as, for instance, a million years ago—in the human example!), he must instruct the computer on what to do with the information. So far as we know, the Creator has not yet sent this guide to His publisher.

D. H. Lacy, Jr., in his treatise on computers, says, "Without a program, the computer is an impressively elaborate and frighteningly expensive contraption *which cannot tell one number from another. . . .* One false bit of logic could be catastrophic [because] *the mistake might be learned only when disaster struck."*

Does it not then make more sense to let the body's native intelligence systems take the lead in the healing process?

In attempting reasonable brevity, we have not even begun here to evaluate the endless considerations upon which the introduction of radical surgical intervention, or other therapeutic measures, hangs balanced by a thread.

Each cancer patient represents to the physician a distinct and delicate mechanism, an individual calling for sensitive diagnostic interpretation and decisions, with—normally—psychological implications inherent in the overall problem. The nature of the malignancy, its type and degree of severity, physical accessibility (i.e., whether outwardly visible and/or palpable, or deeply imbedded in the recesses of tissues and organs), whether metastasized—and if so, to what extent?—all of these considerations present a forbidding, boulder-strewn moonscape to the truly compassionate—the wounded physician—where rough terrain calls for a crucial series of speculations. In the case of the terminal patient, compared with Russian roulette, the hit-and-miss character of today's modalities remains a nightmare.

Statistical proof is not wanting of the long odds present in this situation. Fundamental failure of the system is evidenced by the deteriorating melodrama of cancer mortality statistics: 370,000 victims dead each year in the United States alone—and this figure is growing annually; 55 million Americans alive today who are doomed to develop cancer during their lifetimes. Certain types of malignancies such as childhood leukemia, Hodgkin's disease, cervical cancer, and a few others have shown good response when treated by modern-day methods, but these account for only six percent of all cancer deaths recorded, whereas the remaining ninety-four percent are in those areas where no significant progress has been made.

Despite incredible advances in medical instrumentation, surgical technology, and exotic new chemotherapeutic drugs, a CBS documentary, "The American Way of Cancer," broadcast on October 15, 1975, stated that *"in the last twenty-five years, the cancer mortality rate has increased over twenty percent."*

We have come now to the end of the road in our somewhat abbreviated discussion of the essentials of the three primary modes used by medical orthodoxy in the treatment of cancer. And we have dealt also with the thrusts now being made to combine therapies, but, up to the present time, no controlled clinical studies are available that prove that this form of partnership has resulted in any advantage.

Is the evidence then not overwhelming that *all* of the traditional modalities have severe limitations—having their genesis, from the start, in the failure of the concept? Surgery, chemotherapy, and irradiation, all brutalize to a lesser or greater degree the sacred integrity of the body.

In all this, little has been said about the human equation, which seems to lie in a deep freeze in most medical literature. So little emerges from the operating rooms, the irradiation rooms, and the drug treatments to convey the dreadful pain and suffering, the anguish of the patient, and of his family and friends—yes, and of the staff around him. What hidden trauma, what indescribable torment—of a soul desperately needing—wanting—to shed a tear—to somehow reveal to his dear ones that he, too, *knows!*

And they do! In the majority of cases, surprisingly, the terminal patient not only knows that death is impending, but is prepared for it. Dr. Elisabeth Kübler-Ross is an eminent woman psychiatrist who specializes in helping dying patients, many of them children, to pass over the threshold. She tells a touching story—one out of hundreds—of Liz, a twelve-year-old with a malignancy, who seemed to linger on and on—almost deliberately, it seemed. Liz was not afraid to die; as a matter of fact she was prepared for it—as was her family. "So," as Dr. Kübler-Ross tells it, "one day I asked her straightforwardly, 'Liz, something prevents you from dying, what is it?' Liz's calm reply, 'I can't die because I can't go to heaven.' The child's ingrained belief was that 'Nobody goes to heaven unless you have loved God more than anybody else in the whole wide world.' 'And,' she confided in a whisper (as if to keep God from overhearing her), 'I really love my mommy and daddy more than anybody else in the whole wide world.' "

At this point, with great skill, Dr. Kübler-Ross employed what is known as "symbolic language" and was able to clarify a certain ambiguity in the psychological situation, so that Liz could realize God's loving and understanding nature. It set her mind completely at rest, and was the end of all conflict. As this sweet sick child fell back on her pillow with a deep sigh, her face was illuminated with a radiant, happy smile of relief and contentment. Two days later, she passed peacefully away.

The wounded physician accepts all responsibilities. He suffers with all his patients, who, in his heart, are already endeared as his own family. As for the cold-blooded physician, the martinet who shuns emotional involvement with the patient—under pretense that it allows him to perform more efficiently—he will one day, in that still, quiet space where the soul resides, face his own conscience, and then may he pronounce judgment on himself.

"In memoriam" to the suffering hearts, those uncounted human souls who have been inhumanly abused through man's inhumanity to man, we consider it importune to relate a moving but tragic tale from Dr. Virginia Livingston's book, *Cancer: A New Breakthrough.*

> I recalled reading a story in one of the books I had researched, about a woman, a patient who had sought out a new doctor after having had a *radical mastectomy, both ovaries removed, cobalt treatments, more lumps, more X-Ray treatment, more lumps on her neck, more radiation, male hormones, bone destruction, liver impairment, chemotherapy, more hormone treatment, and then the removal of her adrenal glands.*
>
> The doctor had described with compassion the examination of this patient:
>
> "We removed the covering sheet from her body. Experienced physicians that we are, we could only look at her with anguish and a sense of self-guilt that our profession had not rescued her from this dread disease but had mutilated her beyond recognition.
>
> "The dark-rimmed beautiful eyes, the hairy, coarse, yellow face, the angry, furrowed deep red of the rhinoceros skin of her neck and chest, the nodules and ulcerations overlying the old mastectomy scar, the swollen abdomen with the wide transverse scars, the scars across her back, the thin swollen legs, the tremendously distorted right arm, the bent and shrunken body—was this once a lovely bride, a loving mother, a tender wife, a friend, a good neighbor, a woman concerned for her community, her country, her world? A spiritual being clothed in flesh?
>
> "As I placed my arm across her shoulders in an involuntary gesture of compassion, she whispered, 'They said it would be better this time but I am no better; I am worse. There is no more help. I won't let my husband see me anymore nor sleep in the same room. I must spare him this agony. How much longer can I keep up? Doctor, shall I kill myself?' "

Part 2
Dr. Max Gerson

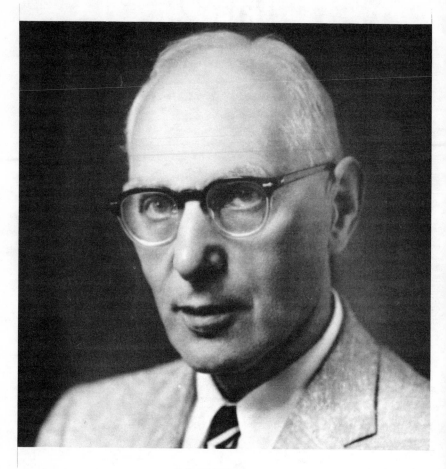

DR. MAX GERSON

7

Where Are the Monuments?

If Jesus of Nazareth were to appear today in the marketplace, healing the sick and raising the dead, he probably would be arrested for practicing medicine without a license. Past being prologue, it would be altogether reasonable to expect that—license or no—Christ would find himself in grave difficulties with the Establishment. His road to today's Calvary would be just as tortuous; the cross just as difficult to bear; and his crown of thorns just as painful.

Not so many years ago, there appeared in our midst a divinely inspired doctor with Christlike credentials. His name was Max Gerson. Albert Schweitzer said about him that he was "one man in a century. . . . A medical genius who walked amongst us; a medical Christ with healing powers."

The life and works of Dr. Max Gerson encompassed the entire spectrum of the healing arts, illuminating especially those dark and anguished corners that are usually given over to the solemn wringing of hands, and to tearful supplications in prayer.

The revelations that follow may quite easily move you to tears, perhaps to anger. Be that as it may, the story is true. The facts presented are fully documented. If it is a shock for you to learn that what you have been led to believe all your life is untrue, then prepare yourself for a shock. For example, if you have come to believe that cancer is an incurable disease, that, when you are terminal, you should resign yourself to die, then Dr. Gerson's unblemished record of curing fifty to eighty percent of terminal cancer patients may provide you with new food for thought.

We hope to prove to the objective reader, beyond any reasonable doubt—be he layman, scientist, or physician—that Dr. Gerson routinely cured patients for whom all hope had vanished. Not by that accidental miracle sometimes referred to as "spontaneous remission" (one out of one hundred thousand), but through the application of a medically sound, holistic therapeutic program, backed by fifty-two years of challenging experience in clinical medicine—in Germany, Austria, France, England,

and America—including a number of unbelievable "firsts," in which he more than once broke the medical "healing barrier." Ninety to ninety-five percent of his patients were terminal; i.e., either all recognized treatment had failed, or the patients were inoperable.

In his classic work *A Cancer Therapy,* Dr. Gerson addressed himself primarily to the medical doctor. He laid everything bare in its simplest terms so that his colleagues might go out and do likewise.

It is a great tragedy that no medical doctor thus far has chosen to do so, because Dr. Gerson achieved, with his treatment methods, a record of curing the vast majority of his patients, virtually all of whom had been labeled incurable—given up by their own physicians. Many came to his clinic on stretchers, a few comatose, some unable to speak or eat—in the very last stages of terminal cancer.

Once, when confronted with the hapless stream of the dying brought daily to his door, Gerson lamented: "On one side, the knife of the AMA was at my throat, and on my back I had only terminal cases. If I had not saved them, my clinic would have been a death house. Some of the cases were brought on stretchers. They could not walk. They could no longer eat. It was very, very difficult. I had to work out a treatment that could help these far advanced cases. I was forced into it."

8

The Sauerbruch Story

Let us begin then in Europe, in the spring of 1923. Listen now to the traveler who is telling the story.

I was sitting in a train traveling from Munich to Davos, where I had once again been invited. It had been an exhausting day and I tried to sleep, but in vain. I had probably drunk too much coffee. Grimly I leaned back and tried to read the medical journals I had with me.

After we had crossed into Switzerland, another traveler got into my compartment. The man seemed bored, and it was plain that he was looking for a chance to open conversation. He irritated me by shuffling his feet, twitching his legs, fidgeting with his clothes, and by his general restlessness. Before long, he made his opening move.

"Are you going to Davos, too?"

"Yes," I growled.

After a very short silence, he tried again. "Are you a patient?"

"No."

He peered across to try and read the titles of the periodicals that I had thrown down beside me on the seat.

"So you are a doctor going to Davos?"

"No, I am not."

"Thank God for that. Doctors are fools. All but one."

We rattled on through the night. I was desperately tired. I could not read, my eyes were aching, yet in spite of myself, I was curious concerning this exception. It was not difficult to set him off again. As I stared at him, he asked, "What can you see on my face?"

"Burns," I suggested.

"Burns!" he cried. "These aren't burns. They are the scars of skin tuberculosis, and I was cured of it by this doctor."

"What!" I exclaimed, though with some restraint. Skin tuberculosis, lupus, an unsightly disease for which there was no known cure. I decided that my fellow traveler was just bragging. "There's no cure for lupus."

"There used to be no cure," he replied, "but one has been found. I have been cured."

Before he realized what was happening, I was unfastening his jacket and shirt, for we were alone in the compartment and some distance from the next station. And on his chest I saw large areas of

75

perfectly healed lupus. I asked him to tell me his story. (From his accent, I judged him to be Russian.)

The disease, he said, had developed in his home country; he had gone from doctor to doctor. Being well-to-do, he had been able to afford treatment abroad and had visited various German hospitals— in vain. Feeling more and more like a medieval leper, he had been on the brink of suicide, when he was told that there was a doctor named Gerson in Bielefeld who claimed to be able to cure lupus. He decided to go to him. Why not? The effects of the disease on his face were such that he would soon be forced to retire from the world. People shrank from him, and few hotels would admit him.

As soon as Dr. Gerson saw him, he exclaimed, "Ha! Lupus, lupus vulgaris."

"Can you help me?"

"Of course I can help you"—and he did.

I asked him how he had done so.

"By diet."

In the whole range of medical literature, there was no reference to the treatment of lupus by diet.

"When I was cured," he continued, "I went to all the famous doctors who had told me there was no cure, and they all laughed at me. Doctors!"

"Did you ever go to Sauerbruch?" I asked.

"It wouldn't have been any use. He's in Munich, and, anyway, he always quarrels with everybody, shouts and bellows at them. He wouldn't listen."

I told him that I knew Sauerbruch and that I could guarantee that Sauerbruch would see him. And then he told me why he was going to Switzerland. He was hoping to acquire a building for the treatment of lupus patients free of charge. It was to be a gesture of gratitude for his release from this dreaded scourge. But he knew that he would need the support of some prominent man, for Dr. Gerson's name was practically unknown.

"Do not forget to call on Sauerbruch" were my parting words to him. "I shall see that you are received by him."

About a fortnight later, the Russian was shown into my office, accompanied by a modest man with a highly intelligent face. Dr. Gerson himself, I guessed.

"So you were Sauerbruch yourself!"

Gerson declared that he had cured a number of patients by excluding salt from their diet entirely. My Russian visitor was one of them. And of his cure there could be no doubt, however amazing his claim might seem. I could see no apparent connection between treatment and cure, but that did not prevent me from beginning a series of experiments immediately.

I put my assistant, Dr. Hermannsdorfer, in charge of a wing of the clinic, which was fitted up as a lupus station. The patients were to be fed in accordance with Dr. Gerson's diet. Lupus patients were found. We securely barred doors and windows to prevent escape. A person, who, over a long period, is given food with no salt at all, suffers agony and will use any means to obtain salt or to escape from his situation.

Dr. Gerson returned to his practice and I promised to keep him informed of our progress.

Results were catastrophic. We kept the patients locked up for weeks. Not a grain of salt went into their food, but there was no trace of improvement. On the contrary, in each case the disease advanced according to rule. Dr. Hermannsdorfer and I were at a loss, thinking of the Russian who had been cured, and of humble Dr. Gerson in whom we had put complete faith.

We felt that we must drop the experiment. Sadly I wrote to Dr. Gerson, telling him of the failure of the experiment and our decision to close the lupus ward. I dictated the letter in the morning. That afternoon, a sister called me to an emergency case: a patient had severe postoperative hemorrhage. I hastened along corridors and down stairs and did what was necessary. Pensively I was strolling back along the corridor near the lupus ward when I saw a nurse, the fattest nurse in the building, carrying an enormous tray loaded with sausages, bowls of cream, and jugs of beer. It was four o'clock in the afternoon, hardly the time for such a feast in a hospital. In amazement, I stopped and asked her where on earth she was going with all that food. And then the whole story came out.

"I couldn't bear it any longer, Herr Beheimrat," she explained. "Those poor patients with skin TB. The stuff they are given—no one could eat it."

She was astonished when I dashed her tray to the ground. It was one of the occasions when I completely lost my temper. Every day at four o'clock when no one was around, she had been taking the patients a nice, appetizing, well-seasoned meal.

I sent off a telegram to Dr. Gerson, asking him not to open the letter I had written him. We were back at the beginning again, and from that moment we took extra precautions in guarding the lupus wing. In comparison, a prison would have been a holiday camp.

Soon Dr. Gerson was proved right. Nearly all our patients recovered; their sores almost disappeared under our very eyes. In this experiment involving four hundred and fifty patients, only four could not be cured by Dr. Gerson's saltless diet.

Dr. Gerson was the first man in medical history to cure lupus vulgaris, skin tuberculosis. How Gerson stumbled upon a nutritional regime as the key to a total therapeutic program that would lead him ultimately to the pinnacle of his career—the treatment and cure of malignancies—is still another stirring tale.

In his mid-twenties he suffered excruciating migraine headaches, which were so severe that he was hardly able to function; more than once he contemplated suicide. He would get violently ill at times for two or three days, when he would seclude himself in a darkened room, oppressed by a hideous nausea, retching and vomiting. When he asked his teachers— the medical doctors and professors—"What can I do?" they all shrugged their shoulders and said, "Read the book; there is nothing you can do. When you're fifty-five, you'll feel better."

The more he thought about the problem, the more he felt that the answer lay in the body's chemistry. Even when he was a little boy of seven he was already experimenting—in his mother's flower beds—adding chemicals and trace minerals to the soil here, and—with glass prisms—changing the incidence of the sun there, just to see what would happen. Usually the plants died—simply because he didn't know enough about them. But he did learn a lot—and he created some extraordinary varieties —like a green rose with red leaves! Even at this early age he already had that craving to experiment, to change things and see what would happen. So, since his professors couldn't help him, he decided to attempt this trial-and-error method on himself.

His first sally was with milk. He reasoned, "Since a baby can digest milk, surely my body must be able to handle milk."

He was wrong. Milk didn't work.

Pondering further upon the problem, he conjectured that our ancestors had lived on fruits and nuts and greens. He decided that, since the most available fruit in Germany was apples, he would start with apples.

So for a while he lived on nothing but apples—in every shape and form. He ate them raw; he grated and juiced and baked them; he even churned them into applesauce. And—he discovered—as long as he lived on apples in this way, he remained completely free of his headaches. With this experience as a base, he began to add other foods, because he knew that no one could long survive on just apples. And the minute a new food did not agree, he knew it, because Newton's law worked remorselessly. The reaction was quick and retributive: his migrane returned full force, usually in half an hour or so. Soon he discovered what additional foods he could and could not eat, with a basic apple regime. At this stage, the diet consisted for the most part of fruits and nuts, green salads, and some slowly cooked foods, without meat or salt. Gerson came to call what he had developed until now his "migraine diet." He was content. He had cured his migraine, and could now apply himself to his work with renewed confidence.

Then came that banner day that was to change the course of his life. Emil Schmidt appeared on the scene. He was a new patient complaining of unbearable migraine headaches. Dr. Gerson told him, "Look, as you know, the books say there is no cure for migraine, but I had migraine, and I'm taking this and this diet—and I reject all other foods. Why don't you try it—and come back in a few weeks?"

It was about a month later—early morning. Dr. Gerson was looking over some case histories, when he heard a commotion in his outer office— the sound of singing, amid uproarious laughter. Something, or someone was provoking high amusement among the patients in his waiting room. He opened the door and peered out—to confront a wild scene. A man stood in the middle of the room (obviously a lunatic) whirling like a

mad gypsy, and snapping his fingers like castanets, as he sang a popular
and slightly naughty ditty of the day. It was Emil—his migraine patient!
Dr. Gerson fixed him with a dour gaze, and said sternly, "Step into my
office."

Emil swallowed his embarrassment, following meekly, to the sound
of titters from the other patients.

Once inside, the man could not contain himself. Overcome with
emotion, Emil bent low over Gerson's desk and in a quite un-Germanic
flush of passion seized his hand and kissed it fervently. "Thank you, Dr.
Gerson, thank you!" he exclaimed. "I'm cured! I'm cured!"

A softer look crept into Dr. Gerson's eyes. *"Wunderbar! Wunderbar!"*
He was beginning to understand. And then, as full significance dawned,
his own mounting elation became so great that he could no longer repress
a burgeoning smile, which illuminated his entire countenance. He repeated,
in contagious joy, *"Wunderbar!* So you finally got rid of your migraine!"

"What are you talking about my migraine? I'm not talking about my
migraine!"

"You are not talking about your migraine? Then what are you talking
about?" Gerson was flabbergasted.

"Dr. Gerson, look! My lupus! My *lupus!* It's *gone!"* He was shouting
at the top of his voice.

"Your *what?"* Gerson exploded.

"My lupus! It's finished. I'm cured!"

Gerson snapped at him, "That's impossible! It was not lupus, because
lupus is incurable."

"No," said Emil firmly. "It *was* lupus!" A knowing smile appeared on
his face. "Look, I have here the laboratory reports," and he placed them
in front of Dr. Gerson. Gerson's deep blue eyes widened as he quickly
scanned the medical records. He was stunned. There could be no doubt!
It was incurable skin tuberculosis!

"Dr. Gerson," Emil suggested, "why don't you look closely at me?"
He pulled off his jacket, then his undershirt, and Dr. Gerson (just as
Dr. Sauerbruch was to do at a later date), stood up and leaned forward
over his desk. He stared transfixed, incredulous at the scars of the dread
disease, resembling syphilis, which had been eating away at the man's
eyelids, cheeks, nose, and chest. There could be no doubt: he was looking
at the unmistakable signs of completely healed skin tuberculosis.

Gerson laid his fingers over some of the scarred tissue on Emil's
back, moving them gently over the ridges and furrows. *"Ist gut! Ist gut!*
I'm very happy for you."

Deep in thought, Gerson sank back slowly into his chair. The words
of Professor Werner Kollath, which were to inspire his life, echoed again
and again through the chambers of his mind: "The incurable is curable."

Gerson did not remember when his patient departed, but, of a sudden it seemed, full realization shattered his quiet reverie like a thunderclap. Forgetting everything, he catapulted to his feet, and started jumping over the scattered chairs in his office, in a frenzy of joy. At the top of his lungs he sang a long-forgotten gay Bavarian drinking song from his college days.

Migraine and lupus, they had both been cured! What had happened was earthshaking in its implications: It didn't matter at all what the specific symptom or symptoms might be, which manifested, nor even the name of the disease. What *did* matter was to put the body right, to restore its own natural healing powers by proper nourishment, and by incidental—though temporary—medication, depending upon the condition of the patient. The nature of disease was systemic; the symptom was *not* the disease. If the body's own defense systems could be put back into sound working order, any disease could be routed. This was the supreme revelation, running directly contrary to what medical science held most dear: that you treat what you see—the symptoms.

Like Paul on the road to Damascus, Gerson had been struck with a lightning bolt. That very moment a horoscope was cast in the fire of his illumination, foretelling that Dr. Max Gerson would, one day, by a divinely inspired experiment—in which he joined two mice together, surgically—prove his theory that a healthy organism can resist and heal malignant cancer. The prophecy also carried an omen: that the implications of this ingenious experiment—tragically ignored up to the present time—would one day shake traditional medical practice to its foundations.

It was this experience with Emil Schmidt that eventually crystallized Gerson's determination to abandon his specialities, and to become a general practitioner. It marked the turning point in his medical career, and was destined to change the course of his life.

But his exhilaration also had some more pregnant roots at the moment. He savored the prospect of honor and fame for his contribution to medicine and science. He clearly remembered that Dr. Niels Ryberg Finsen had in 1903 received the Nobel Prize for his work in the treatment —but not cure—of lupus vulgaris. Yet here was an even greater achievement—the actual curing of this hitherto incurable disease. Should *he* not deserve at least equal recognition?

And so Gerson skipped among his chairs in high spirits. Great days lay ahead—of challenge and of accomplishment. Life was an exciting adventure—especially in the joy of giving hope to the condemned.

Before long, he found himself treating more and more patients for migraine and skin tuberculosis, and for all disorders and maladies that flesh is heir to. They came to him with heart and liver problems, gall-bladder and kidney malfunctions, arthritis and diabetes. And his results (as he worked continually to refine his earlier therapeutic methods) were uniformly more and more successful. He applied the same principles and practices that had succeeded so well for him with migraine and lupus—and they worked. His success brought him patients in droves, so that his fame spread in ever-widening circles. It soon appeared, however, that he had succeeded not wisely, but too well.

As his surviving daughter, Charlotte Gerson Straus, put it, "The next thing was not the Nobel Prize, but charges brought against him by the German Medical Association."

9

J'Accuse!

And the accusation? Gerson had transgressed his medical speciality; his shingle read, "Internal and Nerve Diseases," but, because lupus was a skin disease, he had no right to treat it!

German jurisprudence of his day allowed final decisions in such matters to be made by the presiding magistrate. The judge in this case listened attentively as three physicians, austere in dark conservative suits, presented the charges on behalf of the German Medical Association.

At the start of the proceedings, the judge reclined comfortably in his high-backed, black leather chair, prepared for a routine case. But before the spokesman was half through with his recitation of the bill of particulars, the judge had set his elbows firmly on the bench in front of him, listening intently to every word. He had removed his gold-rimmed bifocals, and with his right hand he held the earpiece in his mouth as he leaned forward.

The long-winded doctor enumerating the charges explained Gerson's violation of medical protocol, ethics, and practice, but completely ignored mention of the results Gerson had been achieving with his treatment.

As he droned on, however, he grew more and more aware of the fixed, disconcerting stare of the judge. He began to fidget and to lose something of his cool. Another of his colleagues developed a nervous tic, constantly loosening the starched collar that was chafing the back of his neck.

Finally, the medical spokesman summed it up: "Dr. Max Gerson is authorized to treat internal and nerve diseases, as it says in his papers, so he is in absolute violation of the law by this treatment of patients with skin tuberculosis."

The judge turned to Gerson, "And what is your answer to this accusation?"

Gerson looked up at the judge with his clear blue eyes, and with a show of asperity said, "It is true: I have been treating many patients with lupus—and I am curing them!"

The judge seemed almost too nonchalant as he turned to Gerson's accusers. "Somewhere I have read also that the defendant, Dr. Max Gerson, is having very good results with his treatment. Is this not true, gentlemen?"

The trio seemed flustered. "Yes, that is so, but it is not at all to the point of our charges, your honor."

The judge ignored his comment. "And now, kindly tell me, do *you* also cure this . . . what is it, lup . . . tuberculosis?"

"Well, no, it's incurable. It is a most difficult disease to manage, but we are making good progress with our research, which is going on at this moment; we expect soon the situation will be changed."

"Hm! Now, getting to the exact point, what is the punishment you are asking for Dr. Gerson with your charges?"

"Since it is against the medical code of practice for a doctor to treat anyone outside of his speciality, we request that the license of Dr. Gerson to practice medicine be revoked, because he has violated this code by treating patients with lupus."

The judge directed his next question to Dr. Gerson: "Do you have anything further to say in this matter?"

Gerson's reply was prompt and passionate: "Your honor, I'll be very proud to be punished for curing lupus patients!"

The judge, ever so carefully, wiped a speck of dust from his spectacles, and replaced them. "Gentlemen," he stated coolly, "it seems that, on the one hand—and please correct me if I am wrong—you are treating skin tuberculosis with not much success, but, on the other hand, Dr. Gerson is *curing* it. Do I understand this is the correct situation?"

The three medical doctors glanced at each other, and started mumbling and fumbling among themselves, trying to sort things out. Finally they looked up at the judge—and nodded their heads. "Yes, your honor, the answer to your question is yes, but—"

The judge interrupted, "Then surely, gentlemen, is it not also in the code of ethics, and in the spirit of good medical practice, that patients should receive the best possible treatment? As honorable members of your honorable profession, surely you will agree, no?" A thin smile curled his lips. It was clear he did not intend, or want, to have an answer. There was a cutting edge to his voice as he abruptly concluded: "Then why don't you let Dr. Gerson do it?" His gavel came down once, but hard. "Case dismissed!" and he stood up. They, too, had thus been curtly dismissed.

As the judge gathered his robes around him, he looked over his spectacles toward Gerson, and sent him a warm, congratulatory smile, then turned quietly and made his way toward his chambers in the rear of the courtroom.

10

The Lady from Bielefeld

As an eager mother plaintively beckons her baby to take his first step, encouraging him with loving words, with coaxing and clucking sounds, so it was with Gerson—and his beckoning angel—urging him ever onward toward the light, and to his destiny. In his journey of a thousand miles, each step was sometimes imperceptible, but its dramatic revelation formed the warp and woof of the exciting texture of his life.

In 1928, Dr. Max Gerson was practicing medicine in Bielefeld, Germany. One day, he received a puzzling phone call from a lady, whom we shall call Mrs. Henke, who lived on the outskirts of the city. She urgently begged his immediate attendance but refused to tell him over the telephone anything about her problem—and with good reason, as it turned out. When he arrived at her typical, middle-class German dwelling, he was confronted with a terminal cancer patient.

Mrs. Henke had undergone exploratory surgery at a well-known, nearby clinic, but, upon their discovering hopelessly metastasized cancer of the bile duct, they had simply sewed her up again, and sent her home. There was nothing they could do.

Dr. Gerson found her running a high fever, compounded by severe jaundice, unfortunate evidence of serious liver malfunction. Altogether every sign pointed to a typically hopeless condition.

Sadly he told her, "I'm sorry, but I can do nothing for you. I don't know how to treat cancer. I have not seen any results in such an advanced case as this, especially where there is no possibility of surgical help."

"Dr. Gerson," she pleaded, "I called you because I heard of your wonderful treatment of patients with tuberculosis and arthritis. Won't you please try to help me?"

Even at this time and place, with all of his experience, Gerson's mind was still conditioned by the years of rigid indoctrination and training of his tyrannical professors in the German medical schools. He still did not dare the impossible dream.

Instead, since he could not face Mrs. Henke squarely, he turned away clumsily to leave, saying "I'm sorry, but there is nothing I can do, I'm sorry. . . ."

Ever so gently, Mrs. Henke sought to restrain him. She reached out a pitifully wasted arm and laid it upon his strong hand. "Please, Dr. Gerson, before you go, do me one favor. On that table over there, there is a book, and in that book, you will be good enough to read to me aloud the chapter where I have placed my page marker."

Dr. Gerson was puzzled by her request, but how could he refuse a fellow human who was dying? He picked up the massive work—twelve hundred pages long—and, of all things, about folk medicine! Indicating the page was a thin brass marker decorated in blue enamel, with a figure of St. Francis, the healer, a white dove perched in his outstretched right hand.

Little did Gerson realize as he started to read that Mrs. Henke had already won this battle. The chapter, "The Healing of Cancer," contained extracts written five hundred years before the birth of Christ—from the writings of Hippocrates, regarded from classical times as the father of medicine. It was all there: Hippocrates' ideas on diet, on growing food with natural fertilizers, on the elimination of toxins from the body, on temperance, even his recipe for a special vegetable soup—which Gerson was to adopt and use through the years, for all his patients!

And Gerson kept on reading. In the deep recesses of his mind, a strange alchemy was taking place. What had been soft, fuzzy clouds of confusion melted in the bright sun of ancient Greek wisdom, as many things fell into place through these revealed truths: about the unity of nature and man; about the importance of maintaining that harmony and connection by living in close communion with all of the natural environment, and all of nature's creatures. And most vital of all, perhaps, emphasis on nutrition through a good but simple diet concentrating on fruits, nuts, grains, and green vegetables, as the basis of the healing process, best expressed by "The Great Physician," Hippocrates himself: "Let food be your medicine, and let medicine be your food."

When next Gerson looked up from his reading and consulted his silver pocket watch, he was startled to find that fifty minutes had elapsed since he had first entered the house. He jumped unceremoniously to his feet, remembering his other appointments, but holding fast to the book.

"Dear Mrs. Henke, I wish to thank you very much, but I'm afraid it's late, I must return to my office. Please allow me to keep this book until I get a copy for myself. I must have it."

There was a twinkle in her eye as she asked, "And what have you decided about my treatment?"

His response was a long wail of complaint: "Do you not know how difficult it is for me now with the medical association? Because of my treatment for tuberculosis, they are opposing me more and more, even the physicians. With any more problems, they will force me to give up my practice. I must think of my patients—more coming in every day— how can I risk any more trouble? *Lieber Gott,* if I start now with cancer, I will be finished!"

Mrs. Henke allowed this storm to pass over her, now that she felt quite in command of the situation. She turned to her sister, who had been standing by, and instructed, "Please, dear Freda, bring some writing paper and a pen." When these were brought, she started dictating, and Freda wrote: "I, Ida Henke, do hereby declare that, of my own free will and desire, I have insisted to Dr. Max Gerson that he should treat me by his methods in spite of his strongest objections to do so. I alone am completely responsible for this decision to have Dr. Gerson undertake my treatment. I release him from any consequences, no matter what the results may be." She signed the statement, and held it out to Dr. Gerson.

An inner voice whispered, "It must be possible, it would be a crime not to do it." Dr. Gerson gave a heavy sigh, and sat down. His look confirmed her victory. He removed his own pen from an inside pocket, took her note pad, and started writing. And, as he wrote, he talked: "Mrs. Henke, I am writing down here the treatment. It is almost the same which I worked out and used for patients with tuberculosis at the University Clinic in Munich with Professor Sauerbruch. I am prescribing for you a strict diet. You will please telephone me every day at eight-thirty in the morning, just before my regular office hours, to report your condition. I will visit you every Monday and Thursday." He finished writing, and handed her the instructions.

His parting admonition carried a tone of mock severity, accompanied by a warm smile: "Mrs. Henke, since I am going to now be hanged for a sheep instead of a lamb, I expect you strictly to stick to my orders. Otherwise," he threatened, "I will never return you your book!"

What happened after that was a miracle. In Gerson's words, "In six months, Mrs. Henke had fully recovered. She was up and around in good condition. Then she sent me a relative with inoperable stomach cancer— also cured. Then another stomach cancer—also against my will, also cured." As Gerson was to tell it in later years, "Had it not been for Mrs. Henke, I might still be practicing the treatment of disease instead of the restoration of health—which is the natural process. It is nature who teaches us totality—who teaches us not to lose the way by classifying man's diseases into little pieces, and treating isolated parts instead of the integrated whole."

His success with Mrs. Henke brought new light into the tunnel, but he was caught up in an ever-expanding practice, so there was little time for quiet, creative thought. He had stumbled upon the Rosetta stone, but it was not until he arrived in the United States that events moved him to consecrate his life to the treatment of cancer patients. In the interim, his guardian angel gave him no surcease, but continued to haunt him with the three cases in which he had succeeded. His innate modesty is revealed in his own self-examination: "I don't know how this happened, how I stumbled into that. If somebody had asked me about the theory, just what it was I was doing, I would have to answer, 'I don't really know myself!' I didn't know why they were cured. But, once it was in my head, and hands, and heart, I could no longer separate myself from the cancer problem."

11

Last Train from Berlin

In the fall of 1932, at the urgent prodding of Dr. Hermann Zondek, an internationally famous lung specialist, Dr. Gerson decided to settle down in Berlin, and to cooperate with him. All told, there were three Zondek brothers, all specialists in their respective fields.

As MacArthur said, "There is no substitute for victory." Dr. Max Gerson's continuing victories in clinical medicine brought his name constantly to the attention of the German people, chiefly through the popular media. Such a flood of acclaim could hardly be ignored or stemmed by even the most deliberate efforts of the German Medical Association and its hidebound inner clique. Gerson began to receive invitations to address small gatherings, and meetings of medical groups at clinics and hospitals. These, too, served to reveal the light that had been shining underneath the bushel.

His past collaboration with the renowned Dr. Ferdinand Sauerbruch, and now with Dr. Hermann Zondek, brought added prestige to Gerson's name, and helped to establish his own credentials in an ever-widening circle of his colleagues. These were not medical castoffs, or carpetbaggers hitching a free ride. Sauerbruch's name, especially, was a household word in the medical community. Among a host of other innovations that he had contributed to surgical instrumentation, methods and techniques, Sauerbruch invented the first pressure chamber, a device responsible for saving countless lives in thoracic surgery. Until the development of this ingenious piece of equipment, opening up a patient's chest cavity was tantamount to a sentence of death. After many hard trials and agonizing failures, Sauerbruch perfected the method that brought miraculous relief from this deadly threat. He was one of Europe's leading surgeons and consultants, world famous, ministering to the great and near great, to statesmen and to royalty, and to such unlikely contrasts as the elder Rothschild—the richest man in Switzerland—whom he charged mightily—though he had some difficulty in extracting his fee—and Ulyanov, a pauper student, later known as Lenin, whom he treated gratis.

In the face of Gerson's mounting publicity, patients kept goading their own doctors for results. Adding also to his spreading notoriety was a little-known story dating back a year or so, which—because of Gerson's characteristic modesty—had only just surfaced, having been stumbled upon by an enterprising newspaper reporter. Once the story was out, it made the rounds quickly.

It concerned Helene Schweitzer, the wife of the famous Albert Schweitzer, renowned theologian, accomplished musician, philosopher, humanitarian, and noted doctor in his own right, awarded the Nobel Peace Prize in 1952. Mrs. Schweitzer, just over fifty years of age at the time, had been suffering for some years from lung tuberculosis, with her condition gradually worsening. Despite his own imposing skills as a medical doctor, Dr. Schweitzer had been unable to curb the progress of his wife's disease. He had almost given up hope when—in the depths of the jungle, at his primitive clinic and hospital in Lambaréné, Gabon, French Equatorial Africa—stories reached him of Gerson's exceptional work with tuberculosis patients. He appealed to Gerson to intercede, sending his wife to Gerson for treatment.

Without fanfare, Gerson quietly applied himself to treating Mrs. Schweitzer, and, within a few short weeks, he had completely reversed her grave condition. She was out of danger and, three months later, well along the road to a full recovery.

This experience with Mrs. Schweitzer marked the beginning of an intimate, lifelong friendship between Max Gerson and the great missionary doctor. When Gerson passed away, on March 8, 1959, Dr. Schweitzer wrote Mrs. Gerson, "I was moved that you sent me a cable as if I belonged to the family. How I take part in the loss you suffer, you know; and that I mourn a friend whom I counted among my closest, you also know. I owe him such gratitude for all that he did for my wife. Without him, she would have died when our child was small. How gratefully she always thought of him! But in the hour when I received the news of his death, I also thought about what he has meant to the world.

"I see in him one of the most eminent geniuses in the history of medicine. He possessed something elemental. . . . His was the hard lot of searching and working as an uprooted emigrant to be challenged, and to stand as a fighter. We who knew and understood him, admired him for working his way out of discouragement again and again, and for undertaking to conquer the obstacles. . . . We who knew him, mourn him as a medical genius who walked among us. . . ."

Over the ensuing years, a strange quirk of fate brought Schweitzer's entire family to Gerson's door. The first was Mrs. Schweitzer; later his daughter Rhena, gravely afflicted with a strange ulcerating skin disease that covered her entire body; and, finally, the great doctor Schweitzer himself, almost totally incapacitated with diabetes. When they sought

Gerson's help, they were all in extremity, in crisis condition—yet all, with the help of divine providence, quickly improved and were restored to good health through Gerson's genius.

All this growing acclaim notwithstanding, Gerson's characteristic modesty remained reminiscent of the Biblical injunction contained in the Sermon on the Mount: "When thou doest thine alms, do not sound a trumpet before thee '. . . that thy alms may be in secret, and thy Father which seeth in secret himself shall reward thee openly." But before the reward, there was rancor, envy, and carping criticism—even gross calumny.

One rank bit of scandal-mongering making the rounds went something like this: "Did you hear? That Gerson is a fraud! His real secret is not his vegetable soup at all; it is his skill in retouching his X rays, just to prove he is curing people! Why doesn't he get a job in a picture studio!" And at the very exclusive professional clubs and private dining nooks, it was all too easy for the small, jealous minds to laugh away "that Gerson fellow" by such sick jokes as "Look, I, too, have no trouble to cure incurable tuberculosis patients, especially if they don't have tuberculosis in the first place!"

In order to impress the hard-case medical doctors with the validity of the results he was achieving with his lung tuberculosis cases, it was necessary, somehow, to establish incontrovertible proof—to banish all doubts. So Dr. Gerson decided that he would accept for treatment only those patients whose condition was certified by *three authorities* to be *uninfluenced by any normal or accepted therapy.* In other words, he was, in effect, carrying his standard to that sector of the battlefield where the fighting was thickest, and thundering his defiance in the teeth of the opposition, determined once and for all to break through the Chinese Wall of medical resistance.

With a reasonable defense perimeter thus established, Gerson now proceeded with his work. It did not surprise him or his few supporters that results continued predictably according to his past experience—in inverse ratio to the statistical probabilities that afflicted the physicians who were hung up on traditional methods. They were still looking for fish in the trees.

Interest in what Gerson was doing finally reached flood tide. Even among many professional groups the clamor grew louder. In addition to practicing physicians themselves, specialists in related disciplines such as radiology, biochemistry, biology, and pharmacology were asking questions, wondering where the truth lay amid the storm of rhetoric. This ferment culminated in an unprecedented invitation extended to Dr. Max Gerson to appear in Berlin, the center of learning, as the featured speaker at a specially organized nationwide congress of German medical groups, including even the German Medical Association. For this distinguished gathering of Germany's outstanding doctors and scientists, he was asked to give a demonstration of his methods of treatment. Surely his career seemed now headed for the stars.

In planning for this prestigious conference, Dr. Gerson decided on the extra precaution of having the top authority in Europe, Professor Felix Fleischner of Vienna, certify each and every X ray that he proposed to exhibit before this elite corps. Because some time was needed in the preparation, Gerson, in anticipation of the Berlin Medical Congress scheduled for May 12, decided to get an early start. With this in mind, he scheduled his trip to Vienna for April 1 in order to prepare his case records and X-ray photographs.

Suddenly, from the rubble of the dying Weimar Republic, the thunder and lightning of Hitler's Third Reich struck with the violence of a tropical hurricane, and overnight turned Gerson's life into a shambles. Adolf Hitler, an Army corporal, and many-times frustrated artist—given to paranoid brooding—but with a satanic genius for Machiavellian scheming, thrust himself into the leadership of the Nazi Party, and then became both chancellor and president of Germany—making himself absolute dictator in the process. His invading armies—the ruthless and one-time invincible Wehrmacht juggernaut—were unleashed in a campaign of conquest and annihilation that was to change the face of Europe, and of the world. In the process, Hitler's Third Reich, like a giant bulldozer, with a remorseless unconcern for the individual human, ground into dust all of Gerson's blossoming hopes and dreams.

Since the end of World War I, the economic and political situation in Germany had continued to deteriorate. Naked struggles for power among the wishy-washy middle-of-the-roaders, the liberal and extremist socialist-communist groups, and the reactionary industrial right, brought fresh crises daily into the lives of a people who had enjoyed no surcease from internecine stress and strife for two decades. Growing daily in numbers and in strength, the violent Nazis, with their unconscionable political arm, the National Socialist Party, kept gnawing at the vitals of the Weimar Republic. At this stage, only the most prescient observer might have anticipated the ferocity of the holocaust that the Führer, Adolf Hitler, with his mad dreams of an Aryan superrace, was spawning in the witch's cauldron of his Nazi movement.

Jews had just been dismissed from government service and the universities, and debarred from entering the professions. Dr. Gerson was not ignorant of the gathering storm, but he could not take his mind and heart away from the daily casualties of quite another struggle, which had never ended—the war against disease.

It was late in the evening of March 31, 1933, just prior to his planned departure for Vienna the next morning. Gerson was in his dressing gown, in the library of his home, quietly reviewing case histories, and selecting the X rays that he planned to bring to Professor Fleischner in Vienna for certification. The family had retired. All was quiet.

Suddenly the silence of his study was jarred by the ringing of the telephone. It had to be an emergency, because it was much too late for any social call. Unconsciously, Gerson sighed, as he reached for the phone. He recognized immediately the voice of an old friend. It was well controlled, but guarded, because it had become altogether too risky to express oneself clearly on the telephone.

"Look, Max, are you still planning as you had?"

"Yes, my plan is for tomorrow."

There was an imperative note of urgency in the caller's next instruction: "I suggest you don't wait until tomorrow, *go ahead now.*"

The implications were unmistakable. Gerson thanked his caller, and hung up. He ordered a cab before waking the family; then started dressing as quickly as he could, while they helped him pack a simple overnight suitcase. There was little time left to catch the late evening train for Vienna. Throwing only a couple of shirts, a few pairs of socks, and a pajama suit into his bag, Gerson scooped up his notes, and a large envelope containing the X rays. Some strained last-minute goodbyes, and he was in the taxi, headed for the terminal.

Outwardly calm, but with his heart thumping inside, Dr. Max Gerson stepped up to the window, purchased his ticket, and boarded the last train that day from Berlin.

The next day, April 1, 1933, was the infamous Boycott Day, which Hitler declared against the Jews.

12

April Fool!

When Hitler declared his special Boycott Day against the Jews, on April 1, 1933, he passed it off to the world as an April Fool's joke, which turned out to be as amusing as the collection of teeth at the bottom of the crematorium in Auschwitz.

All hell broke loose that day. It marked the beginning of a systematic program of mounting violence against the Jews; of a series of pogroms, the destruction and appropriation of property and personal effects, beatings, imprisonment, and torture. Then followed the infamous Nürnberg Laws of September 15, 1935, which deprived Jews of virtually all civil rights, and prohibited marriages between Jews and persons of German blood. The persecution escalated in fury, to see its ultimate horrifying culmination in extermination camps such as Belsen, Buchenwald, and Auschwitz, where from six to eight million Jews perished, the latter camp achieving a grim record for production-line murder, for twelve thousand pitiful victims a day perished there.

Dr. Max Gerson had boarded the train in Berlin at the last moment, and so was compelled to take the least desirable seat available—the one on the passageway, by the door. This might indeed have saved his life.

The train kept chugging along until the small hours of the morning, when faint rays of crimson began to tinge the morning sky in the east. Suddenly, without warning, the whistle shrieked long and hideously as the engineer violently applied the brakes, throwing the passengers headlong out of their seats, as he brought the train to a complaining, screeching halt.

The frightened passengers lifted the shutters of the windows to look out upon a wild scene. It resembled a battlefield—wtih SA troops running madly in all directions to the shouted commands—in guttural German— of their officers. The siding where they had stopped was a bedlam of racing motorcycles and truck transports being hastily assembled in a staked-out area.

A wave of apprehension shuddered through the train's occupants. Some who had just awakened erupted into questions: "What is it? What's happening, where are we?" A voice remarked, "Be quiet and keep calm, or you'll get in trouble. It's the SA."

There was a Czech on board who knew the area. "We are about two kilometers from the Czechoslovakian border, where they have the border control. We never stopped here before."

The door of the compartment was thrust violently open, and the figure of a young storm trooper filled the doorway—complete with smartly pressed brown shirt, soft overseas cap, and black leather boots—a boy, scarcely out of his teens. He paused briefly, taking in the frightened looks with impassive indifference.

"Passport control," he spit out; he took one step inside, and deliberately straddled the aisle. He turned to the first person on his left—Dr. Max Gerson. "All right, you there, where are you going?"

Though trembling within, Gerson managed a smile, and calmly replied, "To Vienna," and then, with a flash of intuition, added, "with my X rays."

"What X rays?"

Dr. Gerson now displayed a childlike innocence and enthusiasm, brightened by his innocent blue eyes. He reached down, pulled out one of the X rays from the envelope; then, as a gesture of respect, he stood up and started talking: "See, here?" he said, pointing to the photograph. "Do you see this light area here, like a white line running across the middle lobe of the right lung? This means that water is already filling up the lungs of this poor woman, and you can also see—here . . . and here . . . these round cavities—the black circles—in both lungs. They are actually holes in the lungs. This is a dying patient, in the last stages of tuberculosis. But Dr. Zondek and I, we have found a way to save them, and in two weeks we will demonstrate our method to the German Medical Congress in Berlin—to show the whole world the superiority of our German medical skills, which can cure the incurable. I am sure you have heard of the great Professor Fleischner in Vienna?" Gerson did not wait for a reply. "Well, I have an appointment with him today to discuss with him these X rays and my case histories so we can make a good demonstration to the conference in Berlin."

The storm trooper, seemingly curious, asked, "Where is your office?" His tone was noncommittal, but Gerson sensed his thoughts—which spurred his final inspiration, "In Berlin—Kurfürstendamm 112; it's very easy to find. Look, here is my name card with my telephone number. If you are anytime in Berlin, or any of your friends needs help, don't worry about anything, just come to my office, and I will give you every attention without question."

The young man carefully placed the name card inside his jacket. Pausing one agonizing second, he took a last, long, heavy-laden look at Gerson—then coolly passed on to the next man.

"Are you a Jew?" he barked. The man answered in a shaky voice, "Yes."

The storm trooper's voice was an angry shout. "What are you waiting for? Out! Out of the train!"

An old woman sobbed out, "What about my suitcase?"

"Forget the suitcase, you won't need it. Are you deaf? *Rauss! Schnell!* Out!"

One after the other, as he proceeded down the aisle, he picked out the Jews, and signaled behind him to one of his comrades to come forward. Unceremoniously, the Jews were thrown off the train, and herded into a miserable-looking group. Trembling in the bitter cold of the morning, they were assembled into a column of four, and loaded aboard the waiting trucks.

By the hand of divine providence, Gerson was spared. The dreaded question was never addressed to him, and he was allowed, with the remaining passengers, to proceed without further incident across Czechoslovakia, and into Austria.

But before the train resumed its journey, Gerson and the others inside were witness to a scene of human savagery and horror, which took place on the siding just in front of them. In the bedlam and panic of being pushed around, brutally manhandled, and herded like sheep, one young Jew was discovered with a gun, which the SA immediately seized. Hardly content with that, they then proceeded—methodically—to beat him with their clubs and fists into the ground. And when he fell, they kicked and trampled him to death—right under Gerson's eyes. This nightmarish scene was to haunt Gerson the rest of his life. For weeks after that, he could not go to bed at night without breaking into tears.

And so this was the grand April Fool's Day joke that Adolf Hitler played on Dr. Max Gerson, and on the Jewish people.

THE EXILE

It marked the beginning of Gerson's self-imposed exile in Austria. He remained in Vienna, where he lived for two years, and where he assembled his family again.

Driven from pillar to post, from one country to another, he was swept by his guardian angel from under the Sword of Damocles, always just a hairbreadth in front of the encroaching armies of Nazi barbarism. By God's grace, he and his family were spared the dread extermination camps of Dachau and Belsen, of Auschwitz and Buchenwald, where ten million Jews, Poles, and other innocents were labeled as *"Untermenschen,"* subhuman, and hauled in cattle cars to their grim destinations, to perish in the gas chambers and incinerators, and in the grim experimental laboratories, through the merciless depravity of man's inhumanity to man.

But now, even in Vienna, there was no peace. Hitler's ambitions had early included Anschluss with Austria. The fateful Nazi phalanx in Austria worked with satanic glee to undermine this democratic people. Their success in destroying the Weimar Republic in Germany provided them with a working blueprint for treason, sabotage, and revolution. The death of Austria, therefore, was not long in coming.

The lesson being written in blood, in the book of chronicles and tears, was clear. It had been written many times before in the history of other civilizations: Corruption, venality, and perversion spawn erosive criminal activity. Intrigue is its blood and bones, often nurtured by a sick liberality that equates laxness with compassion; fraud with tolerable human error; and debasing sensuality with freedom of choice. Shame disappears, and—as the night follows the day—gross dereliction in duties and responsibilities follows on the heels of moral transgression, playing readily into the hands of any well-organized antisocial movement or group, be it criminal syndicate or political revolutionary force. Cunning and deception—as elaborated by LeCompte duNuoy, the great political economist—flourish mightily in the ideal hothouse environment provided by a benign democratic system that has lost the vital essence necessary to its dynamic growth. Finally, the malignant process metastasizes—as it does in cancer—into the very vitals of the host organism. Symbiosis gives way to parasitism, the most debased level of creature survival.

So the malignant Nazi presence would not go away. Their violent agitation and shameless treachery undermined the social, economic, and political life of the nation, while, behind the curtain, creating a climate of paralyzing fear, was heard the shrieking voice of the mad circus master, Reichsführer Adolf Hitler.

Gerson could not fail to see the handwriting on the wall; he decided to leave Austria before it proved too late. So, in the spring of 1935, he and his family, bag and baggage, entrained for Paris.

Not long after that, Austria was engulfed in the Nazi darkness. Intrigue and corruption had continued unabated, reaching into the highest places, and involving even the Austrian Chancellor himself, Kurt von Schuschnigg. Under pressure from Hitler, he obediently resigned his office, and at the same time ordered the Austrian army *not* to resist the Germans. The plot thickened. From Germany, the Nazi minister Hermann Göring was conniving with certain official sources in Austria to have a telegram sent requesting German military aid. Failing that, they conspired for a false telegram to be sent by their German agent in Vienna, and, on March 12, 1938, Germany invaded Austria, an event that was followed the next day by outright annexation. Thus, this proud nation fell, and was sucked into Hitler's insidious vortex of power.

While he had been practicing in Austria, Gerson found that his reputation had preceded him. Many of the affluent were Americans who sought him out for the treatment of arthritis and other debilitating ailments. During this period, a Mr. Horace Finali, who had also visited him in Vienna—with the cooperation of some of Gerson's grateful American patients—set up a sanatorium for him in Paris. Here, when Gerson arrived, he was able to continue his work, and at the same time apply his now proven dietary treatments and methods to many childern with bone tuberculosis, who composed the patient group at this clinic.

All this was not quite as simple as it sounds, because Gerson had to learn French—which, to him, was a foreign language. At the same time, because he did not have a French medical certificate, he was compelled to have a French doctor working with him.

Mr. Finali had at the same time been funding a camp on the North Sea, where patients with a morbid array of chronic disease problems were being treated. Having observed Gerson at close range, and visibly impressed with the results, Mr. Finali persuaded the doctor and his wife, who were running the camp, to visit Dr. Gerson in Paris and to learn and apply his unique methods of treatment to their own patients.

When the couple arrived in Paris, the wife applied herself to learning the food regime, such as the daily menus, the juice cleansing and rebuilding program, salads, and the Hippocrates vegetable soup. In other words, the entire nutritional modality.

Her husband, the medical doctor, accompanied Dr. Gerson on his daily rounds, following which they would hold extended discussions, delving into Gerson's personal philosophy of health, his theories on healing, and their medical and scientific basis. Gerson took pains to explain that his prime focus was ever upon the restoration of the body's own immunological defense system, and that, while he occasionally used some of the milder drugs and medications, these should always be considered as a temporary therapeutic intervention only, designed to support the patient's enervated biological systems through the chronic or crisis stages of his disease. Eventually, the nutritional reinforcement program would transcend the pathological course of the disease by restoring the body's natural healing powers. And the proof of this theory? It worked!

In the face of his medical training, the results that the visiting doctor could personally observe firsthand, at the patients' bedsides, quite overwhelmed him. He had had abundant experience with such cases—but mostly with negative results. With Gerson, he had ample opportunity to examine the case records, to confirm diagnoses, and personally to examine the patients from day to day and observe their progress, improvement—and even total remission!

The open camaraderie between Gerson and the doctor proved a welcome relief from the heavy strain of the last few years. It brought a large measure of satisfaction to have, for once, an opportunity to expound his theories with a companionable, sympathetic associate; to explain how he had developed his system of treatment. These were relaxed, joyful moments, after the long day's work, taking him back to his days at the university. The discussions were especially satisfying over a cup of coffee, which—*verboten* to the patients—constituted one of Gerson's few vices!

Now and then, Gerson noted that the friendly doctor exhibited a naiveté that brought a broad smile to his face; it was so refreshing. The visitor was rather an uncomplicated soul, having come from a simple farm family in the south of France. Although a typical product of traditional medical schooling, he had retained a childlike quality, which endeared him to Gerson.

It therefore saddened Gerson when the time finally came for his colleague to leave. As they stood at the hospital gate, saying their good-byes, this truly simple soul gave utterance to an impelling thought—one that apparently had long preyed upon his mind and that was now vibrating at the top of his head. "Dr. Gerson," he said, "your work is wonderful, like a miracle, but, Dr. Gerson, if we cure all these people, what's going to become of us?"

And thus future events cast their shadows before them. Subconscious fears, such as threats to security, often lie just underneath the surface of the mind, and play their sometimes ugly role, even with the most well-intentioned. Many times, in the ensuing years—in America—doctors echoing the same theme were to approach Gerson, and beg him to "Please help my wife" (or "Help my sister" or "Mother"), "but don't tell anybody I was here, because, you see, Dr. Gerson, if we use your method, what's going to become of all our hospitals, of all our expensive radiation equipment, of the surgeons and cancer specialists—and the nurses that are trained in these fancy methods?"

During the year and a half Gerson spent in France, the political situation there, too, began to deteriorate. The close German presence and the corrosive influence of the Nazi doctrines were being felt everywhere, having their demoralizing effect upon the nation. Already, many were choosing sides, and it was inevitable that anti-Semitic feeling would gain ground. Gerson kept receiving anonymous letters, some of them threatening. The French Sûreté were hardly any exception, so, every so often, he would be called down by the Commissaire de Police to report. Although seemingly petty in nature, this constituted harassment, and adversely affected his busy practice, which kept him on a very tight working schedule.

Gerson was haunted by the traumatic experience in Germany in which he had witnessed the murder of the young Jew at the railroad siding. As the atmosphere of the entire continent became more and more oppressive, Gerson's built-in warning system began to sound a clear alarm. It left little to the imagination to envision what would happen if Hitler, deciding to fulfill his predictions as recorded in *Mein Kampf*, were to march with his armies to the west.

This time, in France, the mills of the gods did not grind quite so slowly. The chemistry of transition was hastened by events that followed the induction into the French army of the young doctor who had been practicing with him. Gerson's German medical license was not enough; it was necessary to find another French physician to join him in order for Gerson to continue. But it proved impossible to secure a replacement. Many were interested, but they were being harassed and threatened by their peers, who wanted nothing to do with Gerson.

Gerson's dilemma was an exact replay from *Hamlet*. Having borne the "whips and scorns of time, the oppressor's wrong, the proud man's contumely, and the insolence of office," Gerson now took his cue from the melancholy Dane, and, with the native hue of resolution, seized the initiative. He, too, was committed to truth, not just in medicine, but as his personal philosophy of life. Finding it impossible to continue his practice, he was compelled to close down the clinic, and in the fall of 1936, he moved to England with his family. Here he stayed only briefly, treating a few prominent businessmen, most of them referred to him by medical doctors in America.

Then one day, out of the blue, he received a call to come to America to treat a man bedridden with crippling arthritis. He learned that this was the scion of an important American family, who we shall call the Gordons. He commanded a worldwide business empire, with interests in airlines, shipping, banks, and chemical industries. Mr. Gordon had learned of Gerson through his cousin, an Austrian, who had been afflicted with the same arthritis problems as he was. Having heard that, under Gerson's treatment, his cousin had improved remarkably, Mr. Gordon ordered his attending physician to invite Gerson to America for consultation.

Gerson was overjoyed to undertake this mission. It seemed like the answer to his prayers, and a good omen for the future. The red carpet was rolled out for him all the way. His passage and retainer fee were paid for in advance, and, upon his arrival in New York, he found himself ensconced in a luxurious suite at the exclusive Mayfair House.

There were some preliminary telephone conversations with the attending doctor, during which Gerson learned that the patient was also being attended by a coterie of other medical experts. Unfamiliar with the American medical community, its protocol or mores, Gerson faced his first meeting with a certain amount of trepidation. What would they think of a German refugee doctor with some pretty radical ideas about treating disease?

The truth of it was that the grapevine had already done its ignoble best—which, properly interpreted, meant that it carried the engaging smell of a thoroughly rotten egg. Gerson, the stories went, was a runaway German Jew with some far-out ideas, whose methods smacked of alchemy and mysticism. He was hung up on foods as a cure for everything from corns to cancer, dispensing such strange nostrums as Hippocrates soup and carrot juice. As a completely unorthodox practitioner, he had become the prize whipping boy of the German medical establishment, which came panting always just a few yards behind him, in hot pursuit!

With this overripe gossip as the galloping herald of truth, the raucous sound of the welcoming trumpets was somewhat less than triumphal. It is not difficult to imagine, therefore, that the American doctors viewed Dr. Gerson's arrival with at least a few guffaws, if not outright laughter. "If we were to believe all his claims," one of them commented wryly, "surely he can also walk on water."

Greeting him upon his arrival at the Gordon mansion was the family doctor, accompanied by a specialist in arthritis, and one other consulting physician. The actual confrontation—for them—was anticlimactic. They were surprised to find Max Gerson soft-spoken and mild in manner, with an even temperament, and a quiet, likable reserve. He could easily have passed, by any standard, as a good example of a respectful and respected medical doctor. There was something droll, however, about his awkwardness in his spanking new English drape tweed suit, which reeked of London's Savile Row. It was not really Gerson's own taste, but had been purchased at the urgent prodding of the irrepressible Johanna, his eldest daughter. "It will be just the thing to impress the Americans!" she had insisted.

After some introductory formalities, following his entrance, Gerson was brought face-to-face with the patient, at his bedside—a sad, thin figure, joints deformed, arms stiff, his body gnawed with continual torments, which only pain-killing medications could relieve. Under the watchful eyes of the three medical doctors, Gerson's examination was slow, deliberate, and thorough. Finally he stepped away from the bed, and looked up. They caught his signal, and retired to a drawing room for consultation.

There was a look almost akin to smugness on their faces, which seemed to say, "See, we could have told you, nothing much can be done. After all, disabling arthritis is a disease that endures but never ends." But instead—with a feeble attempt at sounding cheerful—what the house doctor actually said was "Well, what do you think?"

Gerson's easy reply was "I find this a quite typical case of advanced arthritis. Everything is in order with the classical situation, and is just exactly as I expected, according to the case history which you sent to me in London. I would propose that we should use, in fundamental, the same treatment which I wrote in my letter. This method improved very much the condition of Mr. Gordon's cousin in Austria and has been used by me very successfully. I sometimes use a few simple medications which are necessary only in the beginning—but not for so long, to help with the reduction of inflammation and also some relief from the pain. This, I hope, we can discontinue early in the treatment, maybe in one month. To give some strength to the patient, it is necessary to have a good nutritional program. This is really the heart of my treatment." Gerson smiled, then continued. "Doctors always ask me what is my 'secret'." He laughed. "How can good food be such a big secret? In my opinion, diet must be the basis of all medical therapy, but it should not be a treatment by itself. I can write out easily for you all the details of the nutrition and medications by tomorrow morning."

A short silence followed Gerson's comments. He stood quietly by, waiting for their reaction. The specialist, feeling perhaps more personally challenged, spoke up first. He smiled plastically, and with the barest hint of irony said, "So you place a great deal of confidence on diet, Dr. Gerson—like carrot juice, salads, and vegetable soup—like you get cafeteria-style in the restaurant?"

"Well, it's something like that!" Gerson laughed, thinking it a little joke.

The specialist continued: "We admit we have no experience in treating such advanced patients with anything but the conventional drugs and agents which—I am sure you know—are recognized and approved by the most up-to-date medical practice. Since you have been called in as a consultant, we have of course a high regard for your views and your recommendations; that goes without saying. However, we still have our heavy responsibility for the results of our patient's treatment, so, naturally, we must tell you that we are, here, all in agreement with what is in acceptable usage today by the leading specialists in treating the chronic arthritic condition."

"Do you mean using the usual drugs and medications *only?*" Gerson sought to determine where the conversation was leading.

"Yes, naturally," the specialist replied.

"Gentlemen, please do not misunderstand my question, but I would like to ask you how long you have been treating Mr. Gordon for his condition."

"Since six years ago, when Mr. Gordon complained of continuing aches and pains in his arms and shoulders."

"Has there been any improvement since you began with your treatment?"

This time the family physician responded. He was candid and complete: "No, on the contrary, the arthritis has advanced further through the neck, back and shoulders, and more recently become aggravated in the arms and legs. Frankly, our patient has been slowly deteriorating. And, as you can see for yourself, he is now almost a complete invalid."

Gerson thought this over for a moment, then spoke: "I will not be so foolish as to make any promises in such a serious case. However, by my prognosis and my opinion, if you follow my treatment, Mr. Gordon will, in thirty days, be free from his severe pains. After four to six months, he will be able to leave his bed and to walk without trouble, and, maybe in a year, he should be functioning normally in everything, and carry on his regular duties."

Dead silence blanketed the room like a vast Newfoundland fog bank. Gerson's quiet confidence had carried disconcerting conviction. If he had dropped a live bomb, it could hardly have produced a more devastating effect.

At first, Gerson thought—from the silence—that they were not familiar with any cure for arthritis, and so were thinking up some further questions to ask about his therapy. He was soon disillusioned. They were not wrestling with questions, but with consternation.

He ventured innocently to inquire, "Would you like me to explain some more details about my treatment?"

The ball was now fairly in their court. Finally, the house doctor spoke. He was so deliberate, so careful, it seemed to have all been rehearsed.

"Dr. Gerson," he began, somewhat patronizingly, "you're new here, so perhaps a little explanation is in order—to be shared, shall we say, on a gentleman's basis with you—confidentially, of course." He paused to let this sink in. "This patient is the head of the R. W. Gordon family. They live here in this very elegant penthouse on Park Avenue, as you can see. They are multimillionaires. Their industrial and banking interests are spread all over the world. Don't you see, Dr. Gerson, this man is not going to die of arthritis. One doesn't cure people like that, one treats them! . . . So why don't we all agree to just continue with our present medications?"

Max Gerson's moment of truth had arrived—and now hung by a hair. He blinked foolishly like an owl, and gulped as if he had just swallowed a stone. In his nervousness, he fingered his lapels, as he tried to contend with this unexpected but terribly delicate development. A stranger in a strange land, he had just been handed—on a silver platter— a gilt-edged invitation to "join the club." The door had been thrown wide open by the three austere figures standing in front of him, waiting.

To Gerson, it was almost too staggering. America to him still meant the golden dream, still the land of opportunity, still the land where freedom rings—and where his shattered life might be patched up again. But the dismal song they were playing was from an old, familiar album. Was he doomed forever to the impossible dream?

Under the pressure of the situation, a flush rose to his cheeks. At the same time, the scene in the German court flashed through his brain, and he remembered the mockery of it all. But then—as he recalled the judge's warm congratulatory smile, following the dismissal of the sordid proceedings—something clicked in his mind. He had made his decision.

He was quite unaware that his jaw was now jutting forward an imperceptible fraction, his lips firmed in a straight line. Even the timbre of his voice was different as he spoke with a cool assurance. "Gentlemen, I thank you for your time. I appreciate the chance for my consultation. My way may seem to you somewhat . . . 'eccentric'?" He shrugged his shoulders. "But I am a simple doctor, and so I follow a simple way. Maybe you call it old-fashioned. How do you say it, 'When in Rome, do as the Romans do?' Who knows, maybe an old dog like me will one day learn some new tricks, but in this moment I cannot think of any different way to treat Mr. Gordon except in my old-fashioned way." Gerson was finished. He picked up his instrument case. "I think I cannot do anything more here. If you need me, I will be in the Mayfair Hotel for the week. I will be very happy to send you my detailed dietary and medical prescription for Mr. Gordon—if you wish it, of course."

They stood looking curiously at this strange human specimen. Gerson nodded briefly as he turned to each of the physicians and shook their hands. They were loose and cool. The house doctor escorted him to the door.

"By the way, Dr. Gerson," he said, "we appreciate that you will no doubt be very busy with your many personal matters. So it is not necessary to trouble yourself in sending us any further details. We have a quite clear idea of what we have to do. Of course, we will send you your fee—by mail." He smiled mechanically. "Don't bother to call us; we'll call you."

13

"Good Works"

"A city that is set on a hill cannot be hid. . . . Let your light so shine before men that they may see your good works. . . ."

From the time Max Gerson first hung out his shingle early in 1938, and until 1946, he was forced, because of a lack of funds and facilities, to treat on an ambulant outpatient basis only—even the very sick cancer patients. Despite this very severe handicap, the good news spread by word of mouth, and it was not long before he had more cancer patients than he could handle, virtually all terminal cases.

He was constantly improving and refining his methods, but essentially it was the same treatment that had been used by him in Germany, Austria, and France in the treatment of tuberculosis and other chronic disease cases.

Gerson found himself returning always to the laws of nature, the holistic universal framework. "In science, art, and philosophy," he wrote, "scholars have recognized the law of totality in their fields of research." In philosophy, he mentions Henry Drummond, who contemplated the continuity of the physical and spiritual world, the coherence of the physical inorganic world with the organic world of plants and animals. And, in physics, the approach was exemplified by Einstein's theory of relativity, and eventually the transformation theory, which included gravity, magnetism, and electricity within the same basic physical system, which Einstein called the "unified field view." In art, it was the work of Schaefer-Simmern, which took the explanation of art out of the narrow limitations of the old rational principles and demonstrated that art is a creative power inherent in our being, and developed according to the body's growth and the mental, emotional, and intellectual maturity. "The creative potentialities in men and women, in business and the professions," Schaefer-Simmern observed, "are always present as an entity with all the other powers of the body."

Gerson commented that "medical science has broken the totality of natural laws in the human body to little pieces. It has studied and restudied single processes and overestimated them. The symptoms of a

104

disease have become the main problem for research and clinical work. The medical theory of the old and middle ages to combine all parts in a body into a biological entity was pushed aside almost involuntarily, and finally became far removed from our thinking. How such thinking of totality will help us to find the cause of cancer can best be seen in practical examples—not animal experiments—in the nutritional field of peoples who do not get cancer, and, on the other hand, of those who succumb to cancer in ever-increasing numbers."

Although he had by this time built up the core of his therapy, he always considered it an open-ended, ongoing process. There was systematic growth in the search for perfection, and refinements in clinical treatment contributed more and more, as his experience was enriched through an expanding case load. Gerson had a very retentive mind in this respect, and kept detailed records, which assisted him greatly in quickly capitalizing upon, and incorporating into his therapy, advances and innovations that proved advantageous.

So, as Gerson's fruitful mind continued to apply itself to improvements in his methods, with measurable results, the press paid him more and more attention. It was inevitable. Something of his fame filtered through the grapevine route; some were referrals by the Gotham Hospital. And especially by word of mouth—one patient, friend, or family to another. There appeared to be a "cancer underground." Nurses at other hospitals could not bear the agony of simply waiting for hopeless patients to expire. Theirs was the most trying kind of nursing vigil: keeping a smile, a happy voice, that stiff upper lip, giving encouragement—when all knew that the doctor had already pronounced his verdict of "hopeless," as he shrugged his shoulders.

So these nurses, who had heard about Gerson and what he was accomplishing, would secretly whisper to the patient, or his family, that they knew of a refugee German doctor, Max Gerson, who was doing wonderful things for cancer patients—even curing them! "Why don't you see him?" they suggested.

Patients emerged from the woodwork, drawn like a magnet to the new healer, reminiscent of another who had once walked the shores of Galilee. More than one doctor was overheard to remark about Gerson: "His patients believe he's Jesus Christ!"

Gerson, himself, attributed his inspiration, insights, and success to divine intercession. He firmly believed that grace—through "holes in the net"—descended into the human equation, in varying degrees, and on different levels.

The wounded physician and his committed staff were the instruments, the channel, so to speak. And later, as often developed, the patient's families were drawn into this healing vortex. Subtle psychological and spiritual principles and elements, which constituted the frame of reference of the human and humane chemistries, were set in motion. From day to day Gerson could observe startling transformations. He never stopped repeating that love was the supreme catalyst involved.

As he analyzed it, the causes and dynamics of extreme trauma shattered the gross consciousness layers imposed by modern society's sordid conditioning. Repressed sensibilities and sensitivities, long lost or forgotten —which had been deadened by sense-polluted lives—surfaced, and began to breathe normally. Affection was rediscovered, and proved an uplifting experience. Altogether, a finer harmony and attunement of the physiological, psychological, and spiritual forces were at work. The chemistry of the old mix began to change. Negativity and gloom gave way to cheerfulness, good humor, and joy. An aura of revival could be felt, strongly pervading the entire process.

In this strangely illuminated environment, good things continued to happen. Families openly displayed affection and consideration for each other again. So often, this spilled over to all the other unfortunates in the clinic—there seemed now to be so much to give. Hope returned, and, for the first time—as the patients visibly improved—their families began excitedly asking, "When can we take Francisco—or John—or Rebecca home?"

On the viable side—the observable physical phenomena—the Gerson regime brought into play transforming electrical properties and energies, oxidizing enzymes, and other rehabilitating nutrients and detoxifying therapeutics that comprised the measurable physiological parameters characterizing this healing modality.

Dying patients brought in on stretchers were, after a week, around and walking, returning home after a month or so, with Gerson's strict outline of the combined dietary regimen they were to follow. Even in this brief period of stay at his clinic, reduction in palpable tumors was observable, and many patients, as it turned out, went into complete remission and ultimately cure. When news began to leak out that even medical doctors were quietly bringing patients to Gerson—sometimes members of their own family—it stirred apprehensive ferment in the bastions of the mighty.

Through a stroke of good fortune, Dr. Gerson, in January of 1946, was able to arrange with Dr. George Miley, Medical Director of the Gotham Hospital in New York City, for accommodations for his patients. Dr. Miley had carefully observed Gerson for some time, and was keenly interested in working with him at close hand, so he extended hospital facilities to him and his patients, including a special diet kitchen for a control study, and observation of his work by physicians.

The end result was like a run on the bank. But Gerson was not exactly making points with the medical hierarchy. He would commiserate with himself, repeating his frenetic story: "On one side, the knife of the AMA was at my throat, and on my back I had only terminal cases. If I had not saved them, my clinic would have been a death house. Some of the cases were brought in on stretchers. They could not walk, they could no longer eat. . . . I was forced into it!"

Of course, he, himself, contributed much to the patient explosion. Like Dr. Josef Issels in Bavaria, he suffered from that happy but highly communicable state—supreme optimism. And it proved an essential ingredient in the healing process, often serving in the crisis to turn around the course of the disease. He inspired and nurtured that most precious of all mental states: the will to live. This was not euphoria, nor was it self-hypnosis. It was that confidence, that surefootedness that marked the genius that was Gerson. His mere presence at the patient's bedside was often enough to spark the process of recovery. Its happy contagion spread to the discouraged patient's family, rekindling new hope and effort.

Dr. Alvan R. Feinstein, in *Clinical Judgment,* says: "Unless an investigator recognizes that these biologic and psychic causes can change the course of a human illness, he may fall into the frequent, widespread, and traditional clinical fallacy of *post hoc ergo propter hoc* reasoning: the clinician gives a therapeutic agent, the patient gets better, and the clinician concludes that the agent must have been responsible. In the specious self-deception of *post hoc* clinical reasoning, many a drug, diet, or device of ancient and modern medicine has been given false credit for improvements that *really were due to nature or to man himself.* . . . Living material has inherent biologic capacities to grow, heal, or otherwise change itself. *Living human material, moreover, has psychic properties,* not present or noteworthy in the study of lower animals, *that can affect many reactions and sensations in the state of human illness. Hence a patient's improvement after treatment may often be due not to the therapeutic agent, but to his natural powers of recuperation or to diverse psychic effects."*

Max Gerson, through sheer heart and intuition, knew and applied these laws. His calm assurance lifted up faltering spirits; his sparkling blue eyes, ready smile, and firm, confident bedside manner often accomplished what nothing else could. Just the "placebo effect" of his presence was often enough to turn the scales for a sick patient. Coupled with demonstrable improvements, it removed the hopeless looks from the faces of the patients and—just as important, if not more important—served to efface the heavy atmosphere of gloom and the funereal looks of family and friends.

This represented a physio-psychological attack of no mean proportions, triggered more by the presence of this "giant mind," as Schweitzer called him—a pillar of strength—who had somehow come down from his own Mount Sinai with a set of healing tenets set forth in imperishable stone.

In his methodical, step-by-step therapeutic regime, Gerson would not tolerate disobedience. The highly volatile condition of a cancer patient permitted no errors. It was no easy task to probe the subtle weaknesses of each organ and function. Challenging problems in diagnostic work were ever present, sometimes requiring hourly monitoring and emergent changes in administration of the assorted dietetic and therapeutic agents that composed the treatment modality.

He had never forgotten old Dr. Sauerbruch, and the now memorable incident that had almost destroyed their famous lupus experiment, i.e., when the overgrown nurse attending the patients in the lupus ward was discovered to be secretly feeding them on knockwurst and beer. This lesson Gerson had learned well. He would not, could not condone infraction of his strict instructions, because he knew the tragic consequences.

He found it best simply to send patients away if they would not comply, rather than prolong the agony of an intransigent patient or his family. Bitter experience had shown him that, if the patient disobeyed, he would die. Gerson felt compelled to direct his attention to those who had a chance at survival—and to these he gave his whole heart, mind, and devotion.

As things progressed, Gerson discovered the need for certain educational work. He realized as a teacher that disobedience is often the result of ignorance—a lack of understanding of the treatment, of the principles of health involved, of the goals to be achieved, or of the consequences of infraction. To obtain maximum understanding and cooperation of patients and their families, he decided—on a trial basis, at first—to institute a series of Saturday evening lectures. The results were so rewarding that Gerson made these meetings a permanent part of his overall program.

14

Enfant Terrible

Beware the jabberwocky that whiffles and burbles,
The jubjub bird, and the frumious bandersnatch,
But most of all, beware the vorpal blade that goes snicker-snack!

Gerson was a hot potato. Even more. Word of mouth alone was fanning out like a brush fire, helped by the favorable winds of alert and excited journalists and announcers. It was rare in medical annals to find such a hospitable alignment of the public media for a renegade with the mark of Cain upon him.

In the past, the maverick, the outsider in medicine, rarely survived his first winter. One malcontent among the sick—just one unhappy patient who was willing to bear witness—served exceedingly well to achieve that permanent quietus, devoutly to be wished. But, in Gerson's case, the hierarchy was hard put to find a formula that would work, and that would make this very unpleasant phenomenon go away: a physician whose life was exemplary, his credentials unassailable, and his competency unchallenged. And—to add insult to injury—he was doing what they could not: curing cancer patients! If not checked, Gerson-ism could become epidemic, threatening the very life structure of the medical establishment.

One physician, observing Gerson's clinical treatment, had remarked, "If this thing works, we can chuck millions of dollars worth of equipment into the river, and get rid of cancer by cooking carrots in a pot!" Though rather simplistic, this comment nevertheless stirred up contemplations of nightmarish quality: like beating scalpels and hypodermic needles into ploughshares and pruning hooks; exchanging batteries of drugs for fruit and vegetable seeds; and the arsenal of space-age mechanical monsters littering intensive-care units, for herbs and nuts. It could transform medicine—even in the configuration of its educational process—by changing its emphasis from pharmacology, for example, to the study of soil science, even—ugh!—including earthworms! Or to the giving up— no matter how traumatic—of much of the dehumanizing electronic gadgetry in diagnostics, compelling physicians once again to feel and intuit with their patients—as people—not as computer printouts, or ominous graphs full of frightening mountains and valleys; vibrating lines and dots dancing on TV screens; or dark-field X-ray plates with eerie white structures of spinal columns and rib cages, and vague-looking blobs of elusive protoplasm, morbid and worrisome.

All this was not just disturbing. It was positively alarming. The structural timbers that supported the medical edifice were being threatened. Even the very key of the arch was in danger, challenged by implications of revolutionary changes blowing in the wind.

Dr. Alvan R. Feinstein, in *Clinical Judgment,* confirms that "the methods of laboratory research provide neither the technology nor the judgment for the *clinical* study of people. . . . The clinician's experimental material in therapy is distinctly different from the cadavers, human parts and substances, animals, and inanimate systems of the laboratory; the clinician's material is an *alive,* whole, sick person. . . . The human symptoms, signs and personal properties that distinguish patients, occur only at the bedside and are discernible only by clinical methods of examination."

This served only to confirm the remorseless searchlight of Professor Kussmaul's pronouncement: *"Der Erfolg am Krankenbette ist entscheidend,"* the result at the bedside of the patient is decisive—with Gerson's results showing ever too clearly the cracks and fissures in this tightly knit hierarchical—almost feudalistic—closed-circuit system.

So, now, the medical establishment stood, unhappily, between a rock and a hard place. Its dilemma? How, exactly, to compound an appropriate bowl of hemlock? The hunting parties that staffed the five investigations were having atrociously bad luck. The examining doctors and commitees had mounted a virtual perpetual game of hares and hounds, commuting between the headquarters of the New York County Medical Society and Gerson's clinic—but to no avail; they kept returning empty-handed. When it appeared that this travesty, out of sheer, frustrating exhaustion, had reached an impasse, "the vorpal blade"—that most ominous of threats to beware—went "snicker-snack!"

Ironically, the shaft that was finally loosed and found its mark was not one from their own quiver. A twist of fate closed the trap shut when Dr. Max Gerson, innocent of its possible consequences, appeared on Long John Nebel's all-night talk show. Long John, himself just as guileless, and unequipped with a fail-safe device for such confrontations, became the innocent victim of a power play.

The blast that was triggered by Max Gerson's appearance, actually claimed two victims. The first and most obvious one was Gerson himself, who was standing at ground zero. But lethal fallout, ironically assisted by a flood of excited letters and telephone calls, which followed the broadcast, enveloped Long John Nebel full force, too.

So the mills of the demigods ground slowly, but small. On March 4, 1958, Dr. Max Gerson was suspended from membership in the Medical Society of the County of New York.

In the afterphase, inquiries concerning the reasons for his suspension met initially with puzzling ambiguity. For example, the New York County Medical Society said at first: "It is not within the province of the Medical Society of the County of New York to pass upon the efficacy or adequacy of any doctor's treatment of his own patients." It next said: "Dr. Max Gerson's Dietary Treatment for Cancer was investigated by the Medical Society of the County of New York by a committee of physicians who went to his office. His records were inadequate and his claims unsubstantiated. After due investigation, he was suspended from membership for a period of two years. . . ." Finally, they admitted that Dr. Gerson was "presently under suspension from the rights and privileges of membership, as a result of *personal publicity.*"

The smoke fully cleared in this area when the AMA confirmed: "We have been informed that he has been suspended from membership in his local society for a period of two years, beginning March 4, 1958. *The specific charge was his use of radio interview to discuss his work in the treatment of cancer.*"

There it was, out in the open. No mention of the effectiveness of the Gerson treatment, no reference to the five investigations, or to the inadequacy of Gerson's records and claims; only extreme displeasure and censure for personal publicity. When asked by a member of the Board of Censors where he got all his patients, Gerson replied by firing a full salvo: "First they go to you, then to an osteopath, then to a chiropractor, and then they come to me. Why don't *you* cure them?"

In passing—to close this grimy chapter—it seems not uncharitable, under the circumstances, to quote from "Principles of Medical Ethics" of the American Medical Association.

> *PREAMBLE:* These principles are intended to aid physicians individually and collectively in maintaining a high level of ethical conduct. They are not laws but standards by which a physician may determine the propriety of his conduct in his relationship with patients, with colleagues, with members of allied professions, and with the public.
>
> *Section 1.* The principal object of the medical profession is to render service to humanity with full respect for the dignity of man.
>
> *Section 10.* The honored ideals of the medical profession imply that the responsibilities of the physician extend not only to the individual but also to society where these responsibilities deserve his interest and participation in activities which have the purpose of improving both the health and the well-being of the individual and the community.

15

Le-Hyeem

It was Saturday night at the Oakland Manor Cancer Clinic at Nanuet, New York. This was Dr. Max Gerson's weekly evening lecture to patients and members of their families.

"Dear friends," he began, "I want you to listen to a tape of a radio broadcast by Raymond Gram Swing a few years ago, July 3, 1946, the day after he attended a hearing of a Senate subcommittee where I presented five of my patients. If some of you heard it before, it is still good to hear again. Unfortunately, the bill which was under consideration for the appropriation of funds for cancer research, was not approved. However, the need for this research continues, especially in nutrition, and I believe, also, you will gain some hope for your own case from the encouragement of this famous Mr. Swing. Now listen to his own very words:

"I hope I have my values right if, instead of talking tonight about the agreement reached on Trieste by the Foreign Minister in Paris, or the continuing crisis of the OPA in Washington, or President Truman's signing the Hobbs anti-racketeering bill, I talk about a remarkable hearing before a Senate subcommittee in Washington yesterday on cancer and the need for cancer research in new fields.

"Let me first say that I well appreciate that one of the basic virtues of the modern medical profession is its conservatism. For without the most scrupulous conservatism in the statement and application of medical knowledge, there can be no confidence in the integrity of medical science. But for the very reason that the practice of medicine must be conservative, medical science must be bold and unceasingly challenging. Otherwise, medical science will not progress as it can and must, and will lose its integrity.

"A bill is before Congress, the Pepper-Neely bill, to appropriate a hundred million dollars for cancer research under Federal control. It proposes that the government go in for cancer research with something like the zeal and bigness with which it went for the release of atomic energy, turning the job over to the scientists with resources generous enough to solve the problem.

112

"This alone would make a good theme for a broadcast, just as an example of the use a great democracy can make of its intelligence and wealth. But the subject has been made peculiarly gripping by unprecedented happenings yesterday before the subcommittee which is holding hearings on this bill, and of which Senator Pepper is chairman.

"He invited as a witness a refugee scientist, now a resident of New York, Dr. Max Gerson, and Dr. Gerson placed on the stand, in quick succession, five patients. They were chosen to represent the principal prevailing types of cancer, and in each instance they showed that the Gerson treatment had had what is conservatively called a 'favorable effect on the course of the disease.' That in itself is remarkable, but it is the more so because Dr. Gerson's treatment consists mainly of a diet which he has evolved after a lifetime of research and experimentation. Today, that Dr. Gerson has been curing cancer by a dietary treatment, is medically impermissible, for the reason that there must be five years without recurrence before such a statement is allowed. Dr. Gerson has cured tuberculosis and other illnesses, with his diet, but he has only been working on cancer for four and a half years.

"Let me say right away that I am not discussing this Gerson diet as a cancer cure-all. It has produced remarkable results. It also has the failures in its records, which anything, as yet unperfected, is bound to show. It is not something that offers release from the most rigorous and conservative medical observance in its acceptance and application. Whenever something new and promising comes up in medicine, the temptation of the outsider and even some physicians is to run to glowing superlatives and expect too much from it. But anything that offers even a possibility of treating successfully at least some of the four hundred thousand existing cancer cases in this country is stirring news, no matter how conservatively it is formulated.

"There would be no Pepper-Neely bill to appropriate a hundred million dollars for cancer research if the existing research were coping with the need.

". . . I have spoken about this carefully and abstractly which is to lose some of the shock and delight of the experience yesterday at the hearing of the Pepper Committee. It is one thing to talk abstractly about chemistry and diet and vitamins, and other factors in medical science. It is another to see, as the Committee yesterday saw, a fifteen-year-old girl, who had had a tumor at the base of the brain which was inoperable, and which had paralyzed her. Yesterday, she walked without assistance to the witness chair, and told clearly about her case and her treatment. There was a sturdy man, who had been a sergeant in the army, had had a malignant tumor, also at the base of the brain, which had been operated on but needed deep X-ray treatment, and this it could not receive because of the danger to the brain. Yesterday he was the picture of health as he testified, and quite naturally he was proud of his remarkable recovery. There was a woman who had had cancer of the breast which had spread. Yesterday, she was well, and testified with poise and confidence.

"A few cases showing such improvement cannot, of themselves, affect the outlook of the medical profession. But they are attested by facts and not flukes, and as such they have to be accounted for. And there are many, many more cases which could have been cited. It would seem to be the business of medical research to leap on such facts, and carry every hopeful indication to a final, conservative conclusion.

"So the advocates of the Pepper-Neely bill can argue that unless we learn now how to deal successfully with cancer, many millions of persons now living in this country are condemned to die from cancer. A hundred million dollars is little more than a token payment for America to make to avert such a sweep of death, and they can then point to the Gerson dietary approach as a most promising field for research. Already it has achieved results, which while relatively few, are astounding and challenging.

"Dr. Gerson was an eminent if controversial figure in pre-Hitler Germany. He was bound to be controversial because he was challenging established practice in treating illnesses such as tuberculosis by diet. He has been assistant to Foerster, the great neurologist of Breslau, and for years assistant to Sauerbruch, one of the great physicians on the Continent. The Sauerbruch-Gerson diet for skin tuberculosis is well-known to European medicine; and the account of it is part of accepted medical literature.

"Dr. Gerson told the Pepper Committee that he had first come upon his dietary theory in trying to cure himself of migraine headaches. Later he treated others, among them a man with skin tuberculosis as well. Dr. Gerson was an acknowledged dietary authority in Weimar Germany, and was responsible for the German Army of his time being placed on dehydrated, rather than canned foods."

Gerson switched off the tape recorder, and was just turning to the blackboard in front of the group, chalk upraised, when three urgent raps sounded on the door of the classroom. It opened to a sharp thrust, and Johanna, Dr. Gerson's oldest daughter, breathless, her face ashen-white, rushed into the room to his side. Gerson had stopped in the middle of a sentence, and was still holding on to his piece of chalk. As Johanna whispered something in his ear, his hand with the chalk started shaking. He dropped weakly into a chair beside the blackboard. Before he could locate the handkerchief in his back pocket, tears had already started down his cheeks. For a few anxious moments, Johanna hovered over her father; then Gerson, somewhat more composed, stood up, patted her affectionately on the shoulder, and turned to face the solemn group.

Without preliminaries, he announced, "We just received a phone call with very bad news. I'm sorry I have to tell you that Mrs. Solomon just died!"

There were gasps of horror and shock; a few burst into tears. Mrs. Gladys Solomon, a gentle woman, endeared to them all, had come to Gerson with inoperable cancer. She had improved steadily on his treatment in the six months after she returned home. But sometime during this painful struggle with the malignancy, her husband had apparently left her. Just when it seemed she was well on the way to a full recovery, their marriage broke up. Mrs. Solomon had completely lost her will to live, and gave up the therapy.

Gerson looked angry, distraught. As he addressed the bereaved group, his unusually harsh voice and manner conveyed an undercurrent of despair. "There is no cancer where there is love," he declared vehemently, as if to summon the gods as his witnesses. Gerson's mind was pained with the recollection of other insecure marriages that had not weathered the cancer crisis. "I tell you, it's not only her husband. We are all responsible. 'Incurable!' Always frightening us with 'Incurable!' Words! Nothing is incurable—except, maybe, doctors. Let us try to learn something from Mrs. Solomon."

He pondered a moment. "Did I ever mention before, the 'wounded physician'? All of us who think, act, and work for our patients like they are our own flesh and blood—we are *wounded*. We share the pain and the suffering. Otherwise what are we? Who are we? Shadows! Why should we make cancer such a big secret? Such a nightmare, that the husband runs from his wife! We should face it. It's true. Even the patients—here in this room—trying to save us, the healthy ones, from their misery. They pretend it's nothing, it's not so painful, not so bad. Do you want to live? To win—*over* the cancer? Then you, as the family, must also bear the wounds, the pain. How many times have I told you that the practice of the treatment is a difficult task? In the hospital as well as in the home, it requires somebody's help all day long, particularly in advanced cases where a life is at stake, and the patient is very weak. The family has to give up some of the social life, and to do this humanitarian work with deep devotion. The decline in our modern life is evident by this lack of devotion for the sick members of the family.

"Everyone is responsible. I, also. It's true. Our society, too, is responsible for Mrs. Solomon, not only her husband who deserted her. So she gave up her hope and stopped the healing treatment. This is not so hard to understand. This is the heart of a woman! I recommend to you all today to read St. Paul. He knew about love. Do you like to hear what this Saint said—from his heart? 'Love suffers long and is kind, love endures all things, and love never fails.' Please, please try to love and help each other.

"The incurable is curable. I told you, so many times. So we don't have to hide in the dark. It should all be out in the open. This creates a healthy frame of mind. Then we can see the facts, straight in the face, and lean on each other; share with each other—whether it is pain or joy. If you keep everything dark, how is the light to come in?"

Dr. Gerson's voice hardened. "If you cannot give up something for your sick one, let her die in peace. Please don't leave her to die on my doorstep. I admit to you, very frankly, I have no power with the patient, without your love."

Gerson grimly picked up a piece of chalk and became the teacher again. In a renewed clear voice he began where he had left off. "I think I was talking the last time about the importance of carefully following—to the letter—my 'Combined Dietary Regimen.' You all have this booklet with you? Good. Now let's see how much you have learned. I think I will ask you a few questions to test you out. Who can explain to me about our diet?"

An older man, sitting in a faded blue terrycloth bathrobe, raised his hand and started speaking—at just about the same time. "First, we have to take out the poisons from the body, so that's why we drink lots of juices—apple and carrot juice, also green juices."

"What kind of a juicing machine should we use?" Gerson quizzed.

The eager patient now read with enthusiasm from the instruction booklet, "We use a separate grinder and a separate press, I think, because if it's a 'cert-er—if' . . . what is it?" he stumbled.

Gerson helped, "Centrifugal."

"Yes, center-ifical, that's no good, because the exchange of positive and negative electricity kills the oxidizing enzymes which we need."

"So I suppose these enzymes are important?" Gerson prompted.

"Oh, most important, they kill the cancer cells; they build up the cells in our bodies. Look at me, I could hardly stand on my feet when I first came here. Really, Dr. Gerson, it was no use living anymore. I was too much trouble to everyone."

The lady beside him protested: "That's nonsense, Morris, you were never any trouble. He is really a very good patient, Dr. Gerson. He does everything like you told him. At first I didn't like to make so many juices—then came the raw liver—I don't know which was worse; and—*worst of all*—those coffee enemas. Ugh! Who ever heard of it! It was so new to us. Who ever heard of coffee—*that* way! *Now,* I don't mind; especially when—look at him, he's a new man. Yesterday—Morris doesn't know yet—I even tasted some pressed raw liver juice myself. Imagine—raw liver juice. Ugh! At least the liver is for the mouth, but the coffee—you know, from the *other*—side!"

"All right, that's good. Now I would like to know something about pots and pans."

A dreadfully thin woman got up slowly, holding on to the chair in front of her. She was Dorothy, a schoolteacher. She had arrived by ambulance two weeks previously—in a coma. "No aluminum," she declared. "Absolutely no aluminum utensils, because there is a reaction with the food, and it damages the nutrients. Stainless steel is best to cook with."

"Yes, that's right, Dorothy. Also, glass, enamel, earthenware, cast iron, and tin can be safely used."

Dorothy continued, though it appeared an effort: "We should not scrape or peel the carrots, just brush them clean; also, the calf's liver should be fresh, but not frozen; and don't eat avocados or nuts, because they contain too much fatty acids. Also, no cucumbers, because they have too much sodium. And of course, no smoking, no drinking, no salt in any form; and no canned or preserved foods." Dorothy sat down with a happy smile for her contribution.

Gerson occasionally enjoyed an oblique pass. "Are you all vegetarians?" he inquired mischievously.

A young man ventured, "I think, yes! At least in the beginning, but later on we can start using a little butter, perhaps a piece of cheese or fish."

"Well, yes—but don't jump so fast. You must follow strictly my orders for the dietary regime." His tone and gaze were stern. "No animal proteins, no eggs, no butter, no cheese, and no fish—until I, myself, change your diet from the strict instructions in my booklet. You must keep studying this carefully each day and make sure you are following it without any mistakes, and without any deviation whatsover."

"Dr. Gerson," the young man inquired, "I would like to ask you a question about fasting. My landlord suggested this as a good idea. He heard about it from a fasting institute in Texas where they fast almost everyone."

Gerson eyed him stonily and sighed. He was caustic. "Everybody is a doctor these days. If your normal weight is a hundred and thirty-four pounds but you weigh over two hundred pounds—and your problem is simply of overweight, nothing more—then—under the supervision of a doctor—you can fast. Fasting may be indicated in some conditions, but we are here not speaking about obesity; we are fighting the worst: chronic disease and terminal cancer! Remember, the body's reserves are severely depleted. You need all the nourishment you can possibly get, to build up again the cells and tissues. My diet and medication are directed to restoring the liver function, especially; and to clearing out all the toxic waste material. We have to get vital energy back into the whole system to build up the body. This means *food!* The best quality of organic food, without chemicals or pesticides. The food prescribed in my combined regime is easily and quickly digested. It has been carefully selected for this first purpose. From years of experience, and hundreds of chronically

ill patients, I learned that the body needs larger portions and more frequent servings. You must eat and drink as much as you can, even
during the night when you wake up. It is dangerous to starve a body
by fasting, when it is so weak.

"In the beginning you will—naturally—not be able to completely
digest and assimilate everything, but be patient. By-and-by, and faster
and faster, your body will take up more and more from the juices, the
soup, the salads, fruits and vegetables. You will begin to gain weight,
instead of losing. It will all be turned around the other way. Do you
remember how thin and frail Morris was when he first arrived? Look at
him now, he gained ten pounds just in the last month. Dorothy, too. Today she *stood up!* And she's walking! Isn't this a miracle? Do you remember, two weeks ago—yes, two weeks—she was carried into this clinic
on a stretcher! All of you, even now, are maybe twenty, thirty, forty
pounds underweight. How can you think of fasting in such condition?"

A quick knock on the door interrupted them. Johanna stepped
inside and announced that Frank Wanamaker, the reporter from the
Riverview Press, had arrived for his interview. Gerson looked at his
watch and exclaimed, "Ach! Already half-past seven." He turned to the
group. "Well, my dear friends, we are finished for today. You are slowly
learning, but by-and-by. . . . We can't cover everything in one day."
His eyes twinkled. "And don't forget—if your landlord gives you medical advice, ask where is his medical certificate? Otherwise, let him eat
with you some of your freshly squeezed calf's liver juice. That will cure
him of everything—even giving advice!"

Gerson turned to Johanna, patting her hair, "Dear Johanna, what
would I do without you? Please ask the reporter to come in—and—oh,
Heinrich." He turned to a reserved-looking middle-aged man, in a dark
gabardine suit, who had been sitting in the audience. "Heinrich, you will
of course stay with me and Johanna for this interview."

A moment later, Johanna returned, followed by an open-faced,
lantern-jawed young man, of about thirty or so, introducing him as Frank
Wanamaker—first to Dr. Gerson, then to Dr. Heinrich Wolf.

Gerson arranged a few chairs comfortably in a circle. He was the
first to speak. "You have already met my daughter? I also invited Dr.
Heinrich Wolf, because he has some information which you will probably
find worthwhile for your interview. And now, young man, I must apologize
for asking you to come at such a late hour, but I think it will be important
for you, since you said over the telephone that you are anxious to learn
about my treatment methods."

Frank Wanamaker had already produced a steno pad and pencil from
his briefcase. He was direct and to the point. "I'll be very candid with
you, Dr. Gerson, my editor sent me to interview you so I could unmask
you as a fraud!"

Gerson smiled wryly. "My dear young man, you pay me a great compliment—to be so frank. So now, I suppose, you want me to tell you how honest I am?" A sardonic laugh rumbled in his throat. "I would like, first, to quote you from Emerson, who once said, 'The more he spoke of his honor, the faster we counted our spoons.' " Gerson reflected a moment, then exclaimed, "Why don't you ask my recovered patients if I am a fraud? I think your editor might find that more dangerous than telling it to me! Who is the real fraud? The real hypocrite? These doctors see their own dying patients recover by my treatment but keep their eyes still shut. Mr. Wanamaker, *the big hazard is when you tell the truth.* That is a real test. Maybe your editor should not so much speculate upon frauds, as upon truth. Or is that, maybe, too dangerous, no?"

Observing Wanamaker a bit nonplussed, Gerson eased into a somewhat milder gambit. "Believe me, Mr. Wanamaker, if you are looking for a fraud here, you will have to look for a very poor one, which doesn't make me such a successful fraud, does it? A fraud has to be selfish, no? What can be my selfish motive? To deceive dying people by making them better? That is a new kind of selfishness. You will be poor to work like me. *That* is my warning I give to any physician, if he is so foolish to follow me. He will never be rich.

"There is no money in my practice. As I testified before Senator Pepper's committee in 1946, ninety percent of my patients I treated without charge. I never refuse to take any patient who comes, irrespective of his condition. Until the present moment, every penny for my practical work and research work—for cancer as well as other chronic diseases, including tuberculosis—I financed from my own pocket. I did not ask or get help from anybody. Look at my clinic. Can you see how simple it is compared to your modern hospitals?" Gerson shrugged his shoulders. "Yet you will be surprised to hear that, even in this modest place, doctors —yes, Mr. Wanamaker, medical doctors—come in the middle of the night and beg me, 'Please, Dr. Gerson, please help my wife,' or 'Please help my sister,' or "Please help my mother, but don't tell anybody I was here.' Cancer specialists, too! Now tell me, who is a hypocrite and who is a fraud!"

Wanamaker's eyes had grown noticeably larger and wider as his pencil raced across the pages of his notebook. He held it poised a moment to ask, "Dr. Gerson, can you tell me more about your meeting with Senator Claude Pepper?"

"Yes, gladly. He was Chairman of the Senate Subcommittee in Washington. On July 2, 1946, I testified in front of him. I brought five of my cured patients to the hearings, and they directly reported to him that their own doctors gave them up, then they came to me. Would you like to know how it happens? First they go to their medical doctors, and then when he cannot do anything more for them, they go to an osteopath, then to a chiropractor—and *then* they come to Gerson—to me. Why don't the medical doctors cure them?

"Do you know that one of those cases—it has to be called a miracle, what else? This woman, Mrs. Anna Hanna—she was one of the patients before Senator Pepper. She had an operation because of her cancer—what we call a colostomy. In this operation, an opening is made into the colon through the abdomen; it acts as an artificial anus so you can have an elimination through your abdomen instead of the rectum. This means that, as long as you live, you will have to carry around with you a little rubber bag tied to your side, to receive the excrement, the feces. It is not very pleasant, but sometimes necessary. Mrs. Hanna had such a colostomy by her own surgeon, then she came for my treatment. Now, you want to know the miracle? Our Creator—God—or, if you like to say 'Nature'—it's up to you; God healed up her whole body and brought everything back to the beginning—to absolute normal. Yes, Nature closed up the permanent colostomy, so now her stool goes through the anus, because the tumor was entirely absorbed. Can you believe it?"

Johanna excitedly reminded her father, "Papa, why don't you tell him about the esophagus cure?"

"Oh, yes," Gerson remembered. "Yes, it is the first in the annals of medicine. This cancer was localized on the fifth vertebra of the patient, near the heart, and was inoperable. It became impossible for the patient to eat, and then to drink. Eventually he could hardly breathe. After the cobalt treatments, he came to me. His own doctor had told him he would always have to keep a tube in his stomach to take food. Eight days after the treatment started, he could swallow, eat, and drink. Will you believe me, he returned to his work as an auto mechanic? *Now*—his only complaint: every two hours, the enema!"

Wanamaker was overwhelmed. "Dr. Gerson, all this is like being hit with a piledriver. Look, I'm going to need a lot more help from you than I anticipated. Can you provide me with an outline of your therapy so that I can get a better hold of the concept; and also the methods you use so I can put my teeth into it? It's got to be radically different from what traditional medicine offers in the treatment of cancer patients?"

"It is—one hundred and eighty degrees different. The best thing—let me give you—here, first, a copy of my booklet, which I call my 'Combined Dietary Regimen,' which I give to every patient to study and follow. It includes also the medications which I use in the beginning of the treatment. The patient has to be close to it, it's like his own skin. Everything is in it, the medications, all the foods, the juices, the enemas, the liver injections, the potassium and lugol solutions, and so forth. It's for doctors, too. How I pray every day they will read it, and use it."

"Now, as I reported to Senator Pepper, since the end of January, 1946, I treat my patients in a hospital in New York, the Gotham Hospital.

But, first, let me explain more about the theory. In a nutshell, my experience leads me to believe that the liver is the center of the restoration process—we sometimes call it the biological brain of the body, the balance wheel of life. If the liver is too far destroyed, then the treatment cannot be effective. There are tests for this.

"I am aware, Mr. Wanamaker, of the imperfection of my theory as well as any other theory, but I shall try, nevertheless—if you permit me to be a little technical with you—to explain the end results of the Gerson diet. It is condensed in three surpassing components:

"First, the elimination of toxins and poisons, and returning of the displaced 'extracellular' Na- (sodium) group, connected with toxins, poisons, edema, destructive inflammation—from the tissues, tumors, and organs where it does not belong, into the serum and tissues where it belongs—gallbladder with bile ducts, connective tissue, thyroid, stomach mucosa, kidney medulla, tumors, and so forth.

"Second, bringing back the lost 'intracellular' K- (potassium) group combined with vitamins, enzymes, ferments, sugar, and so forth—into the tissues and organs where it belongs; liver, muscles, heart, brain, kidney cortex, and so forth; on this basis, iodine, ineffective before, is made effective, continuously added in new amounts.

"Third, restoring the differentiation, tonus, tension, oxidation, and so forth, by activated iodine, where there were before, growing tumors and metastases with dedifferentiation, loss of tension, oxidation, loss of resistance and healing power.

"You realize this is oversimplification, but let it suffice for the present. In a moment you will hear from Dr. Miley a more detailed description of my treatment. Besides demonstrating five recovered patients who came as witnesses for the Pepper committee,—and I will give you all that information in a few minutes—I entered, for the file, a document entitled 'Case History of Ten Cancer Patients, Clinical Observations, Theoretical Considerations, and Summary.' I have, now, for some time been working on a book for medical doctors in which I will present the fully documented case histories of fifty cancer patients—50 cases with X rays, every detail. These fifty cases I have selected out of hundreds, because they provide a complete spectrum of every type of malignancy—all hopeless cases, given up by their doctors, and which I brought to remission or cure.

"But before we listen to the five cases, I think it will be useful for you to hear someone besides me—Dr. George Miley, Medical Director of the Gotham Hospital. He loaned me his facilities with diet kitchen, and speaks completely as a doctor. He is not going to make any money out of his testimony. He came to the Senate hearings only to speak what he saw with his own two eyes. Here on this tape, I have prepared his statement made before Senator Pepper at the hearings on July 2. Listen for yourself. He will tell you better about my regime than myself!"

Johanna brought over the tape recorder, which she placed beside Frank Wanamaker, on an end table just outside their small circle, and turned it on. They listened quietly to the words of Dr. Miley:

"I wish to congratulate you, Senator Pepper, on the bill. It is a wonderful thing, and I indorse it wholeheartedly.

"My name is Dr. George Miley. I was born in Chicago, 1907, graduated from Chicago Latin High School, 1923, graduated with B.A. from Yale University in 1927, from Northwestern Medical School, 1932, interned at Chicago Memorial Hospital in 1932 and 1933, University of Vienna Postgraduate Medical School, 1933, 1934, following which I visited the hospitals in India, China, and Japan.

"Next practiced medicine and surgery in Cedar Rapids, Iowa, until January 1934, when I moved to Philadelphia to enter the department of pharmacology at the Hahnemann Medical College and Hospital of Philadelphia. Received doctor of medical science from Hahnemann in 1941 for original research in ultraviolet blood irradiation therapy. Have been in medical research as clinical professor of pharmacology and director of the Blood Irradiation Clinic of the latter institution.

"I am a fellow of the American Medical Association, National Gastroenterological Association, and a member of the New York State and New York County Medical Societies, Pennsylvania State and Philadelphia County Medical Societies, Philadelphia Physiological Society, American Rheumatism Association, and American Association for the Advancement of Science. I hold a national board certificate and am licensed to practice in the states of Iowa, Illinois, Pennsylvania, and New York. Since August 1945, I have been Medical Director of the Gotham Hospital, New York, in charge of blood irradiation research, and am acting as the representative of Dr. Stanley Reimann, its head of oncology (science of tumors) and pathology (science of abnormal anatomy), to observe and control, as necessary, the experimental work of Dr. Max Gerson in the study of the clinical effects of diet on cancer patients at the Gotham Hospital.

"I first met Dr. Gerson in 1942, at which time I was interested in the effects of the Gerson diet on tuberculosis. I visited his office at 667 Madison Avenue, New York City, with Dr. Charles Bailey, outstanding Philadelphia and New York chest surgeon, and we observed several tuberculosis patients who had made remarkable recoveries following the use of the Gerson diet. During this visit Dr. Gerson mentioned to me, for the first time, the potential use of the Gerson diet in cancer, an idea which then seemed rather fantastic to me, but no longer does. In the last four years I have found Dr. Max Gerson to be an honest and ethical practitioner of medicine, interested in bettering modern methods of treatment, as the result of many years of clinical study of the effects of diet on various disease processes. Since January 1946, we have, at the Gotham

Hospital, extended hospital facilities, including a special diet kitchen, to Dr. Gerson, for a controlled study and observation of his work by physicians. The results are, in my opinion, most encouraging, but a tremendous amount of work needs to be done as yet before statistically significant conclusions can be reached.

". . . I feel that the Gerson dietary regime offers a new approach to the cancer problem. We do know experimentally that diet definitely does influence cancer. There is a lot of experimental work done to substantiate that. I will run through this statement rather briefly.

"I do not think Dr. Gerson has mentioned what the diet consists of particularly. The Gerson dietary regime is quite harmless and consists of a low salt, low fat, low animal protein and high carbohydrate diet, plus frequent injections of crude liver extracts and the oral administration of adequate amounts of minerals and vitamins to supplement those vitamins missing in the diet. The diet consists chiefly of large amounts of fresh fruit and fresh vegetables, and does not allow any meat, milk, alcohol, canned or bottled food. Tobacco in any form is prohibited. The diet burns down to an alkaline ash and in general is a combination of many well-known and approved dietary nutritional discoveries by many other workers. It is reasonable to assume that the closer one's diet is to nature and the soil, with fresh fruit from the trees and fresh vegetables directly from the garden, the nearer one is to normal health. Primary biochemical investigations by Dr. Rudolph Keller indicate that the use of the diet is soon followed by certain definite electrochemical changes, notably, shifts toward normal of markedly unbalanced sodium, potassium, and phosphorus ratios in the blood serum and the body tissues. Dr. Keller, as a result of his investigation of the diet, believes that this type of electrochemical reaction can very well change the entire metabolism of the body in cancer patients. A preliminary paper by Dr. Gerson describes the diet in detail and cites ten cases of cancer in which it appeared that the Gerson dietary regime favorably influenced the course and symptoms of the disease.

"There are certain definite problems to be overcome before any type of treatment of cancer can be considered partially or wholly successful, problems which are not solved by surgery, radium, or X ray. A survey made by Dr. Stanley Reimann of cancer cases in Pennsylvania over a long period of time showed that those who received no treatment lived longer than those who received surgery, radium, or X ray. The exceptions were those patients who had received electrosurgery and lived approximately as long as those who received no treatment whatsoever. The survey also showed that, following the use of radium and X ray, much more harm than good was done to the average cancer patient. This is a conclusion which is not generally accepted and is highly controversial among leading cancer workers. It would appear that none of the routine measures employed today to combat cancer are as effective as their proponents would have us believe.

"These problems and . . . new approaches to their solution are described as follows:

"*The abolition of pain* has been possible only by the use of narcotics, which are deleterious to any patient's general health when administered over a long period of time. This problem, in my opinion, *has been solved more by the Gerson diet than by any other method today. We have observed marked relief of pain in approximately ninety percent of the patients who entered the hospital with severe types of pain due to cancer.*

"*The further spread of cancer processes have been apparently retarded by the use of the Gerson dietary regime in several cases observed.*

"*A reduction in the size of the original malignant growth has been observed to occur in certain instances following the use of the Gerson diet.*

"*The reduction of metastases or secondarily disseminated cancers* from the original growth has not been observed in the Gotham Hospital series, but, in certain instances of private patients seen in Dr. Gerson's office, *there was an apparent disappearance of metastatic nodules.*

"*The control of acute pyogenic (pus forming) infections* in areas eroded by cancer, which is one of the chief causes of death in cancer. The only type of treatment in my experience that has been of any use in the control of this type of infection is ultraviolet blood irradiation therapy, . . . and this, though only offering a temporary relief of three to four weeks duration, is of extreme importance to the welfare of the individual patient, especially where the patient's general health must be raised to a level high enough to allow the institution of other treatment such as the *Gerson dietary regime.*

"*Hemorrhage due to erosion by cancer masses* is a frequent cause of death. Its control is only possible if there is no spread from an original cancer or there is a reduction in the original tumor or its metastases. To date, *the Gerson diet is of value in the control of hemorrhage* to the extent to which it limits directly the encroachment of cancer masses upon important blood vessels.

"*General debility, and especially loss of weight, have been frequently overcome by the Gerson Dietary Regime.* As a result, many formerly debilitated patients were able to do normal work again.

"*The maintenance of the morale of the cancer patient is of primary importance at all times. When any one, or any combination of the (aforementioned) problems are solved for the individual cancer patient, his or her morale is enormously improved* so that the practical solution of one or more of these problems must be accomplished wherever possible, regardless of whether the patient is considered a hopeless case of cancer or not.

". . . It is obvious that the many potentialities inherent in the Gerson dietary regime for cancer patients should be explored and exploited to the fullest extent for the common good. In order that this new and highly encouraging approach to the problem of cancer cure and prevention be utilized on a statistically significant scale by both laboratory and clinical workers alike, sufficient funds must be made available for this work. . . . These observations have become apparent to several distinguished physicians who have witnessed the effects of the Gerson diet on cancer patients and whose signed statements are also herewith enclosed.

"Therefore, it is my carefully considered opinion that in view of the success so far, and the excellent future promise of the Gerson dietary regime . . . it would be unthinkable not to give major consideration to these new avenues of approach to the cancer problem in the research program contemplated by Bill S. 1875."

Wanamaker, who had been listening intently, now leaned back and automatically reached into his jacket pocket for a pack of cigarettes, then shamefacedly replaced them, explaining, "If I listen to much more of this, that might be the last pack of cigarettes I ever buy! . . . Helps me relax!"

Johanna interposed, "Look, I have a better idea, let me bring out papa's favorite drink . . . for *all* of you!" She had a mischievous sparkle in her eye, and, as she left the room, she threw a broad grin in Gerson's direction.

Gerson had a guilty look about him. "Gentlemen, how can I stop my daughter? She knows my one weakness. I am sure you will keep my secret, especially from my patients; I love a cup of coffee now and then. So now you know my big sin!"

Johanna was soon back with a large percolator of coffee and some cups. One of the cups already carried hot water and a teabag, which was rapidly turning the contents a mild green. "This one is for me, peppermint tea," she said. "After all, it's my father's suggestion—*for me!* Good for quieting down the stomach. Would you rather have tea, also, Mr. Wanamaker? Dr. Wolf?" No, both opted for the coffee. Wanamaker savored the blend with relish before he reopened with his next question.

"Dr. Gerson, did you actually present case histories to Senator Pepper?"

Johanna picked up his question, allowing her father a little quiet time. "Oh, yes! Not only case histories—ten of them—but actually five of his cured patients came to testify for his treatment! My father has made up complete copies of the case histories and X-ray photographs. They are for you, here, in this large envelope. And now, let me—you can listen to the proceedings which I have here on tape. We also made a typewriter copy for you. We did some editing in order to report only the relevant parts of the testimony. These are five of the recovered patients who gladly came to testify for my father." Johanna started the recorder.

U.S. SENATE COMMITTEE HEARINGS
CASE NO. 1   ALICE HIRSCH

(This is one referred to by Raymond Gram Swing as the fifteen-year-old girl with an inoperable brain tumor.)

Dr. Gerson. This original statement shows that this was a cervical and upper thoracic intramedullary glioma, with an operation in the Neurological Institute, Columbia University. That is the only case arrested in two thousand years of medical science. The patient was operated on, she being a girl fifteen years old.

Senator Pepper. What is your name?

Miss Hirsch. Alice Hirsch.

Senator Pepper. Now what did the little lady have?

Dr. Gerson. She had intramedullary glioma. Glioma is a tumor of the whole cerebral nervous system, it could be in the brain or in the spinal cord; and this was in the spinal cord. The tumor was here (indicating). You can see they operated here, by the scar. They took the bones out, here, for inspection. They made a so-called laminectomy. It came out here, where you see the long scar.

Senator Pepper. You made the operation?

Dr. Gerson. No. It was made in the Newark Beth Israel Hospital, October 15, 1945.

Senator Pepper. That is where the operation occurred?

Dr. Gerson. Yes, here is the original operative record.

Senator Pepper. What did you do?

Dr. Gerson. The physicians told her father: "We cannot do anything; it is a tumor, and nobody can remove such a tumor from the spinal cord. She would die."

Senator Pepper. Was that before the operation?

Dr. Gerson. No. During the operation they saw that the tumor was in the spinal cord. It was inside—not outside. An extramedullary tumor can be removed; so they operated to look into it and to see whether it was extra or intra. When they found it was an intramedullary tumor they could not do anything—they closed her up, and sent her home, and told the father, "Please make her as comfortable as possible; that is all; we can do nothing else." That is all. So, when she came to me, and we applied the treatment, and here (indicating), she had a paresis in the lower right arm; the process involved especially the nervous ulnaris of the right hand and the right leg; she could not walk much; these portions became more and more paralyzed, little by little increasing if the tumor grows. It destroys the spinal cord, and stimuli from the brain cannot be carried to the muscles, which atrophy.

Senator Pepper. And by your dietary treatment you cured the tumor?

Dr. Gerson. We killed the tumor, yes; otherwise, you can understand, the muscles could not have been restored; she can move now the hands and arms . . . there is a little bit of weakness left here.

Senator Pepper (addressing the father). Is the statement that Dr. Gerson has made substantially correct?

Mr. Hirsch. Absolutely. She was to have been paralyzed by around December 1—she was supposed to be, according to the other doctors.

Senator Pepper. What was her condition when she went to Dr. Gerson?

Mr. Hirsch. Very, very weak.

Dr. Gerson. She could not walk.

Mr. Hirsch. We had to feed her by hand. We had to take her up out of bed when she wanted to go anywhere, and she could not walk to any extent.

Senator Pepper. Could you see the tumor?

Mr. Hirsch. No.

Senator Pepper. It was inside, was it?

Dr. Gerson. Only by the operation it is visible.

Senator Pepper. And that there was a tumor in the spine?

Mr. Hirsch. We knew before the operation that there was a tumor in the spine, and before the operation it was almost impossible to do anything for her.

Senator Pepper. Is this a true copy of the report of the Newark Beth Israel Hospital about the operation and all?

Mr. Hirsch. That is right. That is from the Beth Israel.

Senator Pepper. Would you like to leave a copy of this for the record?

Dr. Gerson. I have presented that for the record.

Senator Pepper. Now another witness, Dr. Gerson?

Dr. Gerson. Yes, sir; Mr. Gimson.

(Prior to questioning Mr. Gimson, Senator Pepper queried Dr. George Miley, Medical Director of the Gotham Hospital—who had been observing the progress of Gerson's patients at the hospital—about the Hirsch Case.)

Senator Pepper. Is it your opinion as a doctor that the cure, or the apparent cure, or improvement in the condition of Miss Hirsch which you witnessed, is due to the treatment that Dr. Gerson gave her?

Dr. Miley. Well, I cannot see anything else to account for it. It is the only change in routine which she has had at all. If it were an isolated case you would say, "Well, maybe she was going to get better anyway?" But if she had died, as apparently everybody who saw her thought she was going to die, everyone would have said, "Well, you see what happened!" But, taking it along with quite a few other cases—and it is getting to be too much—it is no longer a coincidence. *There are a good many people walking around that should be dead.*

CASE NO. 2   GEORGE GIMSON

(George Gimson was a former Army sergeant, also mentioned in Raymond Gram Swing's broadcast. A letter from the Veterans Administration Hospital, Lyons, New Jersey, is part of the record describing Mr. Gimson's malignancy, as "carcinoma, basal cell, skin back of right neck, of hair follicle origin and precursor of rodent ulcer.")

Dr. Gerson. Mr. Gimson came with a big tumor that was arrested. He was operated first when he was a soldier and was in camp.

Mr. Gimson. Fort Riley, Kansas.

Dr. Gerson. And then they operated, but they could not remove the basal cell carcinoma, because it was grown up into the skull, so they sent him for deep X-ray therapy to another hospital.

Mr. Gimson. Fitzsimmons, Denver, Colorado.

Dr. Gerson. He was sent to Fitzsimmons Hospital, at Denver, Colorado, for deep X-ray therapy, but there they decided that deep X-ray therapy is very dangerous for the brain, and the specialists there refused.

Mr. Gimson. They did not give me any treatment at all, so they discharged me.

Dr. Gerson. They discharged him, and sent him out and told him, "Sorry, we can't do anything!" Then it grew further, and the whole face was swollen, here (indicating). His left eye was entirely closed here; he could see very little with the right one . . . And I sent the case also to Professor Howe, the neurologist, and he saw it was growing into the brain. . . .

Senator Pepper. Go ahead, he came to you?

Dr. Gerson. Yes.

Senator Pepper. Now, Mr. Gimson, you tell us about your case. What was your condition, and what treatment did you get from the Army? When did you go to Dr. Gerson, and what did he do? And what relief have you had?

Mr. Gimson. I went to Fort Riley, Kansas, and I had something like an ingrown hair, you might say, on my neck.

Senator Pepper. Will you speak louder please?

Mr. Gimson. I went down to the hospital, and the doctor, the major, looked at me and he told me, "Have it off—it wouldn't take long," and

I could be back with the troop, and I wouldn't lose any time, I would be back in a day or two.

Senator Pepper. How long were you off?

Mr. Gimson. I was off four and a half or five months. Two days I had marching—to keep us busy, out of trouble. Then I went to the hospital. Down there they told me I would be back with the troop in two or three days. I went down and had the operation, the next morning, and I wound up in bed, and I could not move my head or anything— pulled away over on the side. They came in for inspection. This captain came in one morning and told me it was about time I had my head straightened out. I told him I could not move my head, because from the operation it pulled me all over on the side, so he just straightened it up—and he opened it all up again; and when he ripped it open like that, I told him, "I can't feel anything; I can't hear anything," so he looked at me, and he checked me, and he gave me an examination; then he told me, "We are going to send you," he says, "to Fitzsimmons, Denver, Hospital." I asked him, "Why should I go there? Why couldn't I go east?" He said, "Well, we haven't got the right equipment, here, for what your trouble is, so we are going to send you out there."

Senator Pepper. Where were you?

Mr. Gimson. I was in the regional hospital in Kansas; and from Kansas they shipped me out to Denver, Colorado, to Fitzsimmons, and when I went to Fitzsimmons they gave me an examination and took a hypodermic needle, and stuck me in the head with it to see if my feeling was there; so I did not have any feeling whatsoever, and they were going to give me this deep X-ray therapy, and they did not give me any. I put in for a Christmas furlough, and that was refused to me, so then they gave me a discharge the following week, and when I came home the tumor was coming up. Half my white shirt is all worn on one side from where this tumor swelled up behind my ear, here, where the scar was. It had started to come up again, so I went to the Red Cross about it, and I told them I could not sleep at nights, and I had pains; I could not even do a day's work. I would have to quit as soon as I put any pressure on myself; so she sent me down to Lyons, New Jersey; so I went down there, and they told me they had lost all my papers and records. I guess they did not want to tell me what was wrong; so they told me the only thing they could do for me was to send me to the Bronx, New York, and get a specimen; so I asked them, "You mean a specimen by opera- tion?" He says, "Yes." I says, "There is no more operating on me," and I refused all operation; so I came home, and my wife told me I was going over to see Dr. Gerson.

Dr. Gerson. Why did you refuse an operation?

Mr. Gimson. Well, they did not do me any good the first time, and my condition was worse; so I went over to Dr. Gerson, and he gave me this book, and that is what I am to do. There is no tumor. I can hear a lot in it. . . .

Senator Pepper. He gave you this book, to tell you what to eat and what not to eat?

Mr. Grimson. Yes; what to eat and what to drink, and everything.

Senator Pepper. And you went by this diet?

Mr. Gimson. Whatever is in that book, that is what I took.

Senator Pepper. And you followed strictly this diet?

Mr. Gimson. A hundred percent. I gave away my last pack of cigarettes just before I went up to his office, and from that day to this I never smoked a cigarette.

Senator Pepper. You quit smoking?

Mr. Gimson. I quit smoking and drinking, too. Last night I was best man at my brother's wedding, and I couldn't even drink.

Senator Pepper. How long, now, did you take this diet before you began to notice any improvement in your condition?

Mr. Gimson. Well, I would say about, oh, a month, two months, a month and a half to six weeks.

Senator Pepper. You took no medicine, or had no other treatment?

Mr. Gimson. No. Lilly's injection—that is, liver.

Dr. Gerson. Liver injections.

Mr. Gimson. Liver injections. Everything I am supposed to take and eat and everything is right there (referring to the little book).

Dr. Gerson. Here is the medication book.

Senator Pepper. So you are satisfied the treatment Dr. Gerson gave you has been responsible for the improvement in your condition?

Mr. Gimson. Every bit of it.

Senator Pepper. All right. Thank you! . . . Dr. Miley?

Dr. Miley. I saw this patient when he had already recovered to a great extent. I saw him after he had been under the treatment practically three or four months. I have been watching him, seeing him once a month, since. There is no sign of recurrence, certainly, and this particular patient had had a lapse, establishing it as a basal carcinoma, which is sometimes inimical to other treatments, but usually when it involves the bone, as it did in this case, it has gone pretty far. He had actual bone involvement, and apparently there are no signs of that at present.

Senator Pepper. Was the tumor that he had what we call a real tumor?

Dr. Miley. Yes; it was a tumor, starting with a hair follicle.

Senator Pepper. Was it malignant?

Dr. Miley. Yes.

Senator Pepper. Thank you, Mr. Gimson. We appreciate your coming.

CASE NO. 3   MRS. ANNA HANNA

Senator Pepper. All right, doctor. Tell us about Mrs. Hanna's case.

Dr. Gerson. In the Jefferson Hospital, an operation was performed on the patient. I read this original, here:

"We found an extensive carcinoma just above the rectosigmoid with infiltration of the mesentery of the rectosigmoid and descending colon. The growth was adherent to the vena cava and both iliac vessels, and there were suspicious nodules. Because of the metastatic involvement, resection of this growth was impossible. I took a specimen for biopsy which proved to be adenocarcinoma. Operative procedure consisted of a permanent colostomy."

Senator Pepper. Now, was that a malignant growth?

Dr. Gerson. Yes—carcinoma. When the lady came she was in a terrible condition. She could not eat, and her stool came here (indicating). Now, *the treatment closed the permanent colostomy.* The physicians thought it would be always there, but nature even closed the permanent colostomy, and now her stool goes through the anus, as the tumor is entirely absorbed. We have wonderful X rays. I have them here, but I have not shown them. The patient gained weight and is in good condition.

Senator Pepper. Is what Dr. Gerson has said substantially a statement of your case?

Mrs. Hanna. Yes, sir; absolutely.

Senator Pepper. Did you take any treatment except the treatment that Dr. Gerson gave you?

Mrs. Hanna. No, sir; not any; and they certainly came down and told my daughter there was absolutely nothing they could do, she was free to consult anybody she wanted.

Senator Pepper. (Here he addressed Mrs. Hanna's daughter to speak for her mother.) Will you tell us a little bit about your mother's case— what doctors she went to, and what they told her?

Miss Hanna. First she went to Dr. Vogel. . . . And he was suspicious of a tumor in the colon, and possibly cancerous, he said, from his examination; so he sent her to the Fitzgerald Mercy Hospital, in Darby, Pennsylvania, for X-ray pictures. These X rays confirmed his suspicions, and he sent her to Dr. Thomas A. Shallow, a surgeon, of Philadelphia. . . . Dr. Shallow placed her in Jefferson Hospital in Philadelphia for examination and treatment, and after eight days of examination and some treatment to build her up, he operated on her, with the hope that he could remove the tumor; but during the operation he realized that it had grown so extensively and attacked so many organs that it was impossible to remove it; so he performed a colostomy to afford her temporary relief, and the report that he gave to me was that she might live six months, she might live two years—he could not predict the time, and it was very definite that she would not live very long. That operation took place on April 19, 1945 . . . at Jefferson Hospital, Philadelphia. . . . While mother was still in the hospital a girl in my office who happens to be a friend of Mrs. Fleming, another patient who is here today, told me of Dr. Gerson, and I got in touch with Dr. Gerson, and he said that he thought that perhaps he could do something for her. But she had to remain in the hospital for two weeks or for five weeks, and she developed pleurisy and different difficulties, and it was possibly two months following the operation before I could bring her to New York to see Dr. Gerson, and he gave her the regular Gerson diet.

Senator Pepper. And she followed the diet at home?

Miss Hanna. That is right.

Senator Pepper. You live with your mother?

Miss Hanna. Yes.

Senator Pepper. And then you took her back every two weeks for a time?

Miss Hanna. For a time.

Dr. Gerson. The first time.

Senator Pepper. And later on?

Dr. Gerson. Once a month.

Senator Pepper. Did you notice, did your mother begin to improve in health?

Miss Hanna. Almost immediately; and at the end of five weeks I believe X-ray pictures show that the tumor was almost completely gone.

Senator Pepper. You went back to doctors and got X rays, and they reported?

Miss Hanna. Dr. Gerson takes X rays, and during all this time she has been under the constant surveillance of Dr. Vogel, and he is very much impressed and thrilled with her response. He says he has never witnessed anything like it.

Senator Pepper. And she has had no other treatment that you attribute her recovery to except Dr. Gerson's treatment?

Miss Hanna. Absolutely none.

Senator Pepper. All right. Thank you very much.

Dr. Gerson. I sent the patient back to Professor Reimann to see her, and sent her back to Jefferson Hospital, and the physicians were so impressed that they demonstrated her to the other students, and even called the case "cured." She was demonstrated by Dr. Engel.

Miss Hanna. That is right. Dr. Bucher, pathologist at the hospital, presented her to the Jefferson Hospital medical student body.

Senator Pepper. Dr. Bucher?

Miss Hanna. Dr. Bucher He is the pathologist.

Senator Pepper. At the Jefferson Hospital, he exhibited her to the students?

Miss Hanna. Yes, sir.

(At this point, Dr. Gerson introduced Dr. Miley into the case.)

Dr. Miley. I have not examined Mrs. Hanna recently, but Dr. Reimann and Dr. Kilingle, of Philadelphia, examined her and could find no evidence of a sigmoidostomy of any kind, nor of the original growth.

Senator Pepper. Was your mother able to walk around when she went to Dr. Gerson?

Miss Hanna. Just a little bit, Senator. She was practically laid down in a bed in the back of the car to make the first trip, entirely. She did manage to walk upstairs once or twice a day.

Senator Pepper. Thank you very much, and thank you, Mrs. Hanna, for coming and giving us your statement. All right, now who is next?

CASE NO. 4   MRS. KATHERINE FLEMING

Dr. Gerson. Mrs. Fleming had a lymphatic sarcoma. She had terribly big tumors here, in the abdomen, glands all over the back, neck, axilla, both groins, two big tumors from the rebro peritoneal glands, here, and mesenteric glands; and one tumor was removed, there. Biopsy was made . . . and slides were sent to two hospitals, to Dr. Stuart, in New York, and another professor, I think Yale, and all decided that it is a myeloma, more specifically a plasmacytoma, a kind of very bad malignant tumor.

Mrs. Fleming. Dr. Averett removed it.

Dr. Gerson. Yes; he removed a piece for biopsy, and the others examined it.

Senator Pepper. Now, let us get to Mrs. Fleming. . . . Will you just tell us what your condition was before you went to Dr. Gerson?

Mrs. Fleming. I started several years before, going around from doctor to doctor, and nobody seemed to know what was wrong.

Senator Pepper. And who told you you had a malignant tumor?

Mrs. Fleming. Dr. Leonard Averett, who operated the specimen.

Senator Pepper. And he told you that you had a malignant tumor?

Mrs. Fleming. He did not tell me. He told my people. . . . So after I came out of the hospital he ordered X-ray treatments. I took fifteen of those, and quit work; and so then he discharged me and told my people there was nothing more could be done, it was just a matter of time; and I went from a hundred and sixty-five pounds to a hundred and thirty pounds, and then they took me to Dr. Gerson.

Senator Pepper. When did you go to Dr. Gerson?

Mrs. Fleming. May, two years ago.

Senator Pepper. And Dr. Gerson gave you his Gerson diet?

Mrs. Fleming. Yes, sir.

Senator Pepper. And did he give you any liver injections?

Mrs. Fleming. Yes, sir.

Senator Pepper. Did he give you any other treatment?

Mrs. Fleming. Just the vitamins.

Senator Pepper. Have you had an examination lately? You consider yourself cured, now?

Mrs. Fleming. I was examined by Dr. Averett, January, a year ago, and he said I had no signs of ever having it.

Senator Pepper. You consider yourself cured?

Mrs. Fleming. I think so.

Senator Pepper. And you attribute your cure to the treatment that Dr. Gerson gave you?

Mrs. Fleming. Nothing else; positively.

Senator Pepper (to Dr. Miley). Do you know about this patient?

Dr. Miley. I sent this case to Dr. Gerson, as a test, because a couple of years ago he had made this statement to myself and to Dr. Charles Bailey of Philadelphia, an outstanding chest surgeon there, and he was in Seaview and New York. I went over to see his tuberculosis cases, and some of his results were very, very remarkable. He had several bronchial chest fistulas which had healed up, *which had no right to heal,* and he mentioned at that time the possibility of using this in malignant disease. Both Dr. Bailey and I smiled skeptically, thinking it was rather fantastic; *so I picked out the worst case I could find and sent him one, which happened to be Mrs. Fleming;* and much to my surprise she improved. She was supposed to live three to five months, approximately, and, instead, she is still here. The tumors have at least palpably disappeared; they may reappear, but at least there is no evidence now, so far as she is concerned. She has put on very many pounds.

Dr. Gerson. Twenty pounds.

Dr. Miley. Her sister is giving constant reports, and she says she continued to improve and she has remained improved, and it is two years now since that occurred. Certainly, something should have happened by now if it were going to. We do not know—we are still watching it. She has a two-year improvement, at least.

Senator Pepper. Thank you very much for coming, Mrs. Fleming. Now, doctor, have you another?

Case No. 5   Mrs. Beatrice Sharpe

Dr. Gerson. The patient was first operated three years ago.

Mrs. Sharpe. 1940.

Dr. Gerson. 1940—now six years ago. Later she had a recurrence on the breast, left breast operation, the breast was removed, but how much later?—Two years, about?

Mrs. Sharpe. Well, about 1941 I had a recurrence.

Dr. Gerson. You were at Memorial Hospital?

Mrs. Sharpe. Memorial Hospital, yes; taking treatments. In 1942 I had to go back and had more radium treatments. In 1943 I had X-ray treatments, and in 1944 they told me I couldn't take any more treatments, and that was all they could do for me.

Dr. Gerson. They sent her home.

Senator Pepper. Now, I have here . . . a letter from Memorial Hospital. . . . It reads, "Diagnosis: Recurrent inoperable carcinoma of left breast." . . . Mrs. Sharpe, just tell us about your case, will you? What happened to you after you went to Dr. Gerson?

Mrs. Sharpe. In 1940 I had a mastectomy, and in 1941 I went back and I had this recurrence in my neck, and I was sent over to Memorial Hospital for treatments. In 1942 I had to go back, and in 1943 and 1944 there was nothing more they could do for me, so I heard of Dr. Gerson, through a chiropractor. He gave me Dr. Gerson's name, and I thought I had nothing to lose, so I went to Dr. Gerson's, and in three weeks' time on the treatment the mass started to disappear. My head was stiff. I could not move my neck.

Senator Pepper. You had what—a tumor of the neck?

Mrs. Sharpe. Yes.

Senator Pepper. You had a big tumor that stuck out here on your neck?

Mrs. Sharpe. Yes.

Senator Pepper. And it finally has subsided entirely?

Mrs. Sharpe. Oh, yes.

Senator Pepper. And you have no more of the symptoms?

Mrs. Sharpe. And I am going to business all the time.

Dr. Gerson. She did not lose one working day. *Most of my patients, they do not lose even one working day;* they continue to work.

Senator Pepper. You attribute the recovery entirely to the treatment that you received from Dr. Gerson?

Mrs. Sharpe. Oh, absolutely.

Senator Pepper. Dr. Miley, have you anything to say about Mrs. Sharpe?

Dr. Miley. I saw her fairly early when she still had some tumor masses. Dr. Gerson was very enthusiastic in claiming they had gone down, and they had gone partially from the original, but, since then, they have really gone down much more, and I felt at the time he was a little overenthusiastic about it, but certainly his results today, six to eight months later, since I first saw her, justify the fact that there is certainly a steady subsidence of any signs of recurrence, and she certainly remained clinically better.

Johanna switched off the machine. "That completes the testimony from the five patients," she said.

They all looked at Frank Wanamaker, waiting for his reaction. For him, it had been a stunning experience, almost too overwhelming. He was churning inside with how he was going to handle his editor, who expected him to return with Gerson's scalp hanging from his saddle. He focused back to the group. "You know," he said, "it is difficult to understand, with all this evidence shouting at you, why you can't convince the medical community of the value of your treatment? Why they keep referring to your work as quackery?"

Dr. Wolf, who had been sitting quietly all this time, responded, "I think I can answer that. The history of medicine is filled with tragic errors which allow such a long time to elapse between the time of the discovery of a basic principle and the actual medical application of the discovery for the good of mankind. A recent paper by Hammett says:

" 'Nowhere today is this delay more unhappily evident than in the field of cancer research. The accumulated data of Rous, Shope, Coley, Bittner, Strong, Andervont, Green, Greene, Williams, Taylor, Furth, Twombly, Cowdry, Diller, Bawden, Pirie, Stanley, Wycoff, Kunitz, and others indicate beyond peradventure the path for getting at something of practical benefit to the cancer patient of the future other than surgery and radium.'

"Perhaps the answer lies somewhere in what that great man Winston Churchill once said: 'Men occasionally stumble over the Truth, but most pick themselves up and hurry off as if nothing had happened.' "

Wanamaker was troubled by a shadow of frustration. He knitted his brows, trying to put things together. "Dr. Gerson," he asked, "have you shown any of this work at all to the New York Medical Society—or the AMA?"

Gerson's hand, holding a cup of coffee, paused in midair. It remained in that fixed position, as his mild blue eyes hardened perceptibly. He very deliberately set the cup down upon the table, unfolded his long figure, and stood up slowly. With his head cocked a bit to one side, he examined Wanamaker, seemingly making up his mind; then started a slow pacing around the table, and began to talk—flailing his hands for emphasis. His voice carried a note of frustration, and poorly concealed fury.

"Five times! Five times they came here—the Censors and committees of the New York County Medical Society, to investigate my methods. In February 1947, they reviewed eighty-six case history records and examined ten patients; another time, at their request, I presented fourteen cases before two of their supervising doctors and about thirty other physicians who had been invited to attend! Again—on their invitation, I demonstrated twenty patients before them—out of forty cases which I prepared when I attended an International Cancer Congress in Berchtesgaden, Germany, in October 1954. Again in 1953 I complied with the request of their doctor—one of their Censors, to show films and records.

"If they wanted, they could see every single one of my patients—every X ray and test—and creep into all my records and files; it is alright, they are welcome—with pleasure." Gerson was almost shouting now. "But, instead, I have been deprived by them even of that common right of publication which every physician should have, and which the AMA should protect unbiased, especially in such an important medical problem as cancer. This right was suppressed since January 8, 1949, when the *Journal of the AMA* in a critique of several cancer treatments, ridiculed my treatment and placed it among others which they called 'frauds and fables.'

"What more do they need or want from me to prove anything? The same questions over and over. The same games every time. Is it honorable to play games with dying patients? God has more power than the AMA. He can do anything, but still, even God, as Einstein said, does not play dice with the universe, like they do!"

Wanamaker interjected, "What happened with these investigations?"

"What happened? Nothing happened! Nothing! Do you think they would be so quiet if they found out something wrong? Never! If there was anything wrong, they would find it—and very quickly. Mr. Wanamaker, nobody—and just try to find out, yourself, if you don't believe me—nobody can get one word out of them. It's like ghosts in a haunted house, with their games to frighten people."

Wanamaker just shook his head. Johanna, beaming with pride at her father, could not restrain herself. "Let me quote you something," she exclaimed. "Dr. Gerson" (she sometimes called her father "Dr. Gerson") "is very fond of 'The Rubáiyát of Omar Khayyám,' especially one particular verse. When he gets started with the medical society, he always recites it—and so loudly! . . . Please, papa . . . ?" Gerson demurred, so Johanna gave the rendition:

> *"Myself when young did eagerly frequent*
> *Doctor and Saint, and heard great argument*
> *About it and about: but evermore*
> *Came out by the same door where in I went."*

Gerson, for a moment, had stopped his mad pacing to listen—but he was hardly finished with his diatribe.

"I did not make up my treatment like a bootlegger with whiskey in my bathtub, who puts a stamp on, 'Bottled In Scotland.' Everything about my therapy is tested." He laughed shortly. "It's real, like genuine Scotch. The carrot juice, too, is real—although not so strong. I have a medical license, and I have a history of experience which is not exactly talk; it is in many medical journals, mostly in Europe. Some I have written here, and they are translated. I don't practice behind closed doors in some secret office. My work is all out in the open. It is only necessary that you wish to look, and not to hide your head in the sand, afraid that you might find out the truth. *The great truth is that my system works, and that you can save lives with it. You save people! Human beings! Why* does my method work? Because it follows God's and Nature's laws of healing. God is alive in our heavens, and his laws are alive, and they operate, they work. Some of the big brains are planning and hoping some day to catch God in a mistake!" Gerson snorted. "It will be a long time to wait!" He was finished. He sat down.

Frank Wanamaker, who had been racing along with his notes, changed to a new shorthand book at this point. He removed a book of paper matches from his pocket and withdrew a safety razor blade tucked behind the matches. As he sharpened his pencils, which had grown noticeably smaller, he asked Dr. Gerson if there was any other practicing medical doctor besides Dr. Miley who had been in a position to observe his work and results closely, on a day-to-day basis?

Gerson smiled and said, "If your pencil is not yet tired, I will let Heinrich answer that question. Heinrich—Dr. Wolf—worked in the same office with me for seven years. We collaborated in treating many patients, his patients and mine. Heinrich, tell Mr. Wanamaker what you told Senator Pepper—but . . . ," Gerson concluded with an impish grin, "only the good things!"

Dr. Wolf smiled as he raised his eyebrows at Gerson. "All right, Max, so this was your grand scheme after all—to bring me into the newspapers!" He turned to Wanamaker and said, "Yes, I can tell you exactly what I said in my letter to the Pepper Committee, which is part of their record. But first, to make one thing clear from the start, I am not entering into the theoretical foundation of my friend's methods, but simply reporting from my personal observation of the facts over a period of seven years that I shared the same office with Dr. Max Gerson."

As Wanamaker looked at the man in front of him, he could see a special quality of integrity in the square-jawed, open face, disarming in its simple look of conviction. He listened attentively, pencil raised over his pad.

Dr. Wolf's next remark carried a strong show of feeling. "This man, Dr. Max Gerson, is one in a million. Do you know what twenty-four-carat gold is? It's one hundred percent pure! That's Dr. Gerson, pure gold!"

Johanna was hanging on to every word. Here was a respected professional showering plaudits upon her "papa."

Dr. Wolf continued: "I had every opportunity to observe nearly all the important cases treated by Dr. Gerson with his diet, many of them my own patients. I was intrigued and astonished at what was happening. The results of some chronic skin diseases, in some types of heart diseases, and in some dangerous cases of high blood pressure, were astonishing. In some of my patients the blood pressure that had been up to a hundred and seventy and a hundred and eighty, went down to a hundred and thirty permanently, and the symptoms of headaches and dizziness disappeared entirely.

"During the last three or four years, since Dr. Gerson paid particular attention to the effect of his dietary regime on benign and malignant tumors, I observed practically all of the tumor cases which he treated. I observed and supervised their X rays and saw the patients at nearly every visit. Let me tell you about some of these patients that I also reported to the Senate Subcommittee.

"One of the first cases of malignant tumors was a Mr. Baldry (1942), who, after surgical removal of a mixed tumor of the left side of the neck, developed a metastatic tumor of the right lung, which was diagnosed by X ray and bronchoscopy. The tumor disappeared after Gerson started treating him, and there was no recurrence when we last heard from the patient about one year ago (1945).

"In 1942 I saw one of his patients who had been operated on for cancer of the tonsils and subsequently treated by radium and X ray, which resulted in an X-ray ulcer about two inches in diameter. There were several metastases in the glands of the neck. Under the dietary treatment the ulcer healed, the glands became very much smaller. After a year the patient left New York. Later I read in the papers that the patient died, two months ago. Yes, I can answer your question, which I see in your eyes: I saw, also, a number of failures; not everyone survived, but in my opinion they were due to the fact that Dr. Gerson accepted for treatment patients who were so far gone that they were absolutely hopeless, even for the most optimistic observer. When you can effect remissions of thirty to fifty percent of such hopeless cases where the other physicians have given up, there must be something happening which is of value, don't you think so?

"One of my own patients, whom I referred to Dr. Gerson because she had been suffering from cancer of the stomach for half a year, is doing well. I saw her four weeks ago. Since then, I have observed many cases of primary and metastic cancer. I saw one patient with a colostomy which had been performed by her surgeon because the cancer had completely obstructed the lumen of the sigmoid and rectum. I verified this case history personally—by barium enemas carried out through the colostomy opening and the rectum. In this unheard-of case, after Dr. Gerson's regime, the colostomy wound closed up by itself, and normal passage of the bowels was established. If you are looking for a miracle, this is the case.

"Another case of Dr. Gerson's which I observed closely was a patient who, upon a laminectomy, was found to suffer from an inoperable malignant intramedullary glioma tumor. She has now regained the use of her arm which was paralyzed when I first saw her seven months ago, and, when I last saw her in the office two weeks ago, she was making gradual good progress.

"Also among Gerson's patients I saw four cases of malignant brain tumor, one of them metastatic. Two seem to be now perfectly well; both of the others had their failing eyesight partly restored; the progress was arrested. I also saw three women who had been operated for breast tumors, malignant and verified by biopsy, and had had a recurrence while being treated by their own doctors. After Dr. Gerson took on the cases, in all three, the metastatic tumors in the lymph glands disappeared.

"It should be mentioned that Dr. Gerson's dietary treatment is not only effective with malignant tumors but even with benign tumors, which are often very difficult to improve.

"And now I'll tell you what the real crime is: that there is no one to follow in Dr. Gerson's footsteps. Why should they? Dr. Gerson tried using a few young doctors as assistants, but they were soon frightened off by the medical people calling his work quackery. Ask Joseph Ziegler, the radiologist, how they threatened *him*. He was handling Dr. Gerson's X-ray work but he was warned that if he continued to do work for Gerson he would lose all his other business, so he was made to stop. Also, the pathologist who tested Dr. Gerson's tissue samples! They even canceled Dr. Gerson's malpractice insurance! Do you know what that means? How can you work under such conditions, without X rays, without tests, especially when every patient has both feet in the grave. *That* is the quackery of our condition today—and there will be no one to follow in Dr. Gerson's shoes—only a fool!"

Johanna interjected, "In case you are wondering about the malpractice insurance, it's a mystery to us. Out of a clear blue sky, the insurance company just said, 'We canceled your insurance.' No explanations— period!" She faced Mr. Wanamaker, "Can you work without your telephone or your typewriter, without your hands and feet? They are your working tools, so? My father's working tools are the diagnostic procedures which require blood and tissue tests, and X rays. Another shocking story, something unbelievable: my father was treating the wife of a *physician,* a doctor who was connected with a major pharmaceutical company with its own research laboratory—I better not mention the name. So, naturally, this doctor took the specimens *to his own laboratory* for examination. Do you know, they refused him? It came from Dr. Gerson, that is why! I don't know how my father can suffer so much and still continue. I am telling you frankly, even a saint would decide to go back to Heaven rather than work under these conditions. You can imagine, too, how my mother feels his disappointments. She takes it so personally, and worries so. Why does he continue?"

Gerson shrugged. "I continue because I must, what else can I do?"

"Excuse me, please." Dr. Wolf, who had been silent, now joined the conversation. "Max," he said, "there is one laboratory experiment which you performed that, in my opinion, is quite extraordinary—revolutionary is perhaps a better word; and which has not been covered in your discussion, but to me it seems of the utmost importance. I am referring to the tests you conducted with two rats you connected together—one of which had a malignancy! I feel sure Mr. Wanamaker would be most interested, not only in the results, but in the broad implications which this experiment has."

Wanamaker's attention came to a sharp and immediate focus at this development. "I certainly *would* be interested. It has the earmarks of an exciting story!"

"Exciting? It's the proof of my theory!" Gerson declared vehemently. "I had the idea to make an animal experiment in which we connected two rats—one cancerous and one healthy one. We cut them open along the side and connected a blood vessel, then sewed them together. The blood from the healthy rat circulated in the sick one day and night, and cleared up the sick body. Thus we showed that with a healthy normal metabolism you can cure cancer. We cured the cancerous rat with the healthy body of the normal rat. But—I must explain—we are only in the early stages of this experiment.

"However, I must tell you something further. It is what happened later. There was one patient, a Mrs. Schumann, whose husband heard about the experiment with the rats. When his wife was first brought to me, she had a very bad liver—with probably hundreds of metastases also in the rest of her body. I told them I didn't believe I could do anything for her, so that is when her husband—Frederick—I remember now, offered his healthy body. She said no because she didn't want to have him immobilized so long, next to her, with extensive nursing care, day and night. Frederick was such a determined one—he begged her to let him do it; how he struggled to save her life! Ach, that was big love, big love! I, also, did not want to experiment with human beings, it was too early yet. But, anyway, I gave her my regular treatment, and, in spite of her bad condition, she is still living, and improving.

"Perhaps you can imagine if such an experiment could be tried with human beings and succeed, it would be proof of my theory that cancer cannot survive in a healthy metabolism; and it would destroy the mistaken idea of today's medical doctors to treat symptoms instead of the total body. It worked with the animal experiment, so why shouldn't they give it serious attention in research with humans? Don't you think so?"

Wanamaker nodded. "I couldn't agree with you more. Did you go any further with it yourself?"

Gerson chuckled, "Only in my dreams! Ach, so busy, I was. So busy. I had many regrets that I didn't try it. It was so much in my mind that I had dreams for weeks about it. One, which continued night after night, was about Mr. and Mrs. Schumann connected together in a private room in my clinic. One morning, in my dream, I remember I came into their room on my usual rounds. I could not believe what I was seeing. Mrs. Schumann was *standing,* all dressed up! A surprise for *me,* she said! She was wearing a new green dress with red flowers—carnations, I think. Her hair was fixed up so beautiful. Her face was twenty years younger, and she looked in perfect health. Her husband, too, was dressed up—in a new suit. Their eyes and faces were shining like two honeymooners! You know the explanation? It seems that, in this dream, I had a medical assistant—a young intern. You know, you can do anything in a dream! You can even get medical assistants! Well, this imaginary intern had made the small necessary operation to separate them, because the case was finished! She was fully recovered! They packed their suitcases, and went on a long vacation. Such a happy couple!"

Gerson was enjoying his own story immensely. "I am also happy to tell you that, since it was a dream, it continued long enough for me to receive *two* Nobel Prizes. *One* for my spectacular experiment; and the other for my establishment of a 'Donor's Ward'; yes, that was another part: I established a special ward where volunteer donors are connected with cancer patients. It was the biggest ward you can imagine. It stretched for miles! From that dream I did not like to wake up—not without my Nobel Prizes!" Gerson broke into a contagious hearty laugh, in which they all joined.

Wanamaker had become emotionally involved in this moving tale, and could not contain his enthusiasm. "If you'll pardon my language, Dr. Gerson," he exclaimed, "that is one hell of a story! I'll say it again: That is one hell of a story; and I'm going to move mountains to try to get it published. Something really should be done about pursuing the research further."

Gerson nodded, although he was not optimistic. "I hope so, Mr. Wanamaker. I will be ready to provide you or anybody else with all the details. Just please let me know."

"I will, you can depend on it." Wanamaker smiled as he went on to his next question: "And now, Dr. Gerson, with all your heavy dreaming, and your impossible work schedule, do you ever have time for yourself and your family, a little rest from your demanding schedule? A concert, or movie, hobbies?"

Gerson pursed his lips and sighed. "You are joking. I have so many outpatients at my office in the city. How can they travel here, it's so far? Anyway, this place is so small. After hours, I must study and read medical journals, and I have to review each case carefully, to be prepared for everyday emergencies. I have medical notes to record, and then, when it comes to Friday afternoon, I take the train from my office to come here—it's about an hour and a half to ride, then all the rest of Friday, Saturday, and Sunday I attend to my patients in this clinic. You know, a friend of mine once joked with me and asked me do I like to know *how to work twenty-five hours a day?* I said, 'All right, please tell me, maybe it will help,' so he answered, 'You have to get up one hour earlier!' It's almost the truth!

"My dream one day is to see the Russian Ballet, to visit, once, the Metropolitan Museum of Art, but my fate is priority, priority of the patients. Priority is my fate, my duty, and my life. Schweitzer, my dear old friend, says the whole center of our spirit should be the reverence for life, and this is what I see all around me in my work. Someone much smarter than me has brought me to my duty, and here is where I stay with these hands and this head. If I know nothing else in my life, I know at least my duty—and that I must do. How my wife and daughters can bear with me, I don't know. They are angels in disguise." He sighed heavily, "I promised them, one day we *must* go to a concert."

"You sound to me like a very religious man," remarked Wanamaker.

"How I wish I could study the religions of the world! No, I am not what you call practicing any formal religion, you know, like attending the synagogue or the church regularly, but I feel things inside, and try to give expression to them through the people around me. I know my limitations. Trying to heal people is enough."

Wanamaker smiled. "So you heal the sick, but you don't preach the gospel or raise the dead!"

This drew a spark from Gerson, who considered carefully before answering. "They say that each human being is a reflection of one divine aspect of God himself. So, with every sick patient, I find myself looking for—and I find this reflection. It's there, believe it! It is, truly, if you look for it; the light of God is shining out of the eyes and in the face. An atheist will ask you, 'Did you ever see anyone come back from the dead?' When a doctor gives up his patient with one week to live, and that patient recovers, is that proof for the atheist? No! *What is dead?* What kind of miracle will satisfy him? How many miracles will satisfy the medical doctors? I have no power to bring back a man from the dead, so I cannot convert an atheist with such proof. But many patients were given up for dead by their doctors, then they recovered with my therapy—but still no doctor came to be baptized with this treatment!"

Gerson sighed heavily. "Mr. Wanamaker, you reach a time in your life and your work when you wonder who is listening. *Doctors should listen more closely,* because they are very sick, too. Yes, you will be shocked, but it is true: medical doctors die fourteen years younger than the average of our general population. Maybe they need the Gerson treatment more than my patients!

"A very famous Indian Yogi, Sri Yukteswar, said, 'It is not a question of belief. The scientific attitude one should take on any subject is whether it is true. The law of gravitation worked as efficiently before Newton as after him. The cosmos would be fairly chaotic if its laws could not operate without the sanction of human belief.'"

Wanamaker changed the subject. "Let me ask you, do you also have a prevention treatment?" he asked.

Gerson responded with his own question: "If a treatment cures, why can't it also prevent disease? Isn't it common sense?"

"But isn't your therapy strictly for sick people?"

"Yes, but don't forget, there are underlying, unifying principles in everything. I think I can give you an example. Suppose you are on a long trip. You forgot your road map, so you lose your way. You turn left, you turn right, this way and that way. Wherever you go, it's wrong, taking you farther and farther into strange country. Finally you are hopelessly lost—like a cancer patient is hopelessly lost at the end. How can you find your way out?"

"I suppose you either have to get hold of a road map, or find someone who knows the way."

"Precisely. My combined nutritional regimen is the road map. And your guide should be a physician who is following my road map, to get you back on the right road. If you can retrace your steps to the beginning of the problem, where you first lost the way with wrong habits, poisoned food, smoking, drinking and so on—you can reverse the process with my regime. So now, exactly what is the situation? With cancer you are in the wrong place on the map. You will have to go back to the point of good health, to the crossroad where you made your first mistake—where you first became careless. That is the place where your journey to sickness started. Ach, but you are such a young man still, and healthy—so you don't know, Mr. Wanamaker. It is not so easy to follow as an engineer's map.

"Everything with a map is exact: so many miles on Highway 66, or 75; you go north, you go south, up and down. All is precise measurement, with mechanical slide rules and aerial photographs. But with the human situation it is not an exact science. With each individual—his body is so different, one from the other. I regret to say, but my therapy is not a 'do-it-yourself' treatment; it must be directed by a medical doctor who will give his mind and heart over *to learn his patient like a road map,* and slowly lead his body back to the point at the crossroads where he made the first mistake—but this time he must show him the road to good health—not to cancer."

"Well, you've made that clear enough, but aren't we still talking about the *sick* patient being brought back to good health? I'm not sure I get your message regarding prevention."

"Ach, it is right under your nose. I have already answered but you do not see it still. Look, now you are back at the crossroads, standing in good health—and you know the right road, so you continue by going straight on this road in front of you." Gerson smiled. "You have now the 'Gerson Road Map,' so follow it!"

"But if I read you correctly, your road map only shows us the way back from sickness—which includes medications. If I'm enjoying good health, why do I need medications?"

"Excellent! Excellent! You don't need any medicines at all. What you need is only the nutritional diet in my instruction book, the general principles to be followed, a modified program. It is simple, no?"

Wanamaker was coming up for some air, so, smilingly, he tried a tongue-in-cheek queston. "Don't you have any shortcuts?" he asked.

A cluster of chuckles broke through the heaviness. Johanna mused that everyone wanted only that magic bullet that would shoot disease right out of the saddle. Dr. Wolf's dry comment was that it was time to replenish the coffee.

Dr. Gerson, however, could not be so easily dissuaded from the serious import of his subject. He had, in fact, latched on to his second wind. "No! No! Positively no shortcuts! Why is it everyone wants to see a doctor perform magic tricks—with pills and shots, always complaining that the road map is too difficult to follow? With a carbuncle, a sprained ankle—or, maybe, even migraine—of which I have, unfortunately, some experience—yes, I can do some magic, but it's not so easy to be a magician with cancer. The healing process takes a long time, maybe two or three years. You must ask yourself how long it took you to *get* the cancer!"

Johanna lightened the mood as she freshened up the coffee. "My father, you must know, is a dictator with his patients. If I use a crude expression to say it, you will excuse me; I know my father doesn't like it, but anyway, you know the one I mean? 'Shape up, or ship out?' The patients must obey him. This is absolutely necessary to save their lives. This my father learned from bitter experience."

Wanamaker, it seemed, was still unclear. He wanted to make sure. "Do you mean, Dr. Gerson, that by following just the nutritional part of the diet which you prescribe in your booklet, I can stay well?"

"It would be so easy to say yes to your question, but it is necessary for me to explain something further. For the healthy person, it is permitted to have, occasionally, some cheese, a piece of fish or chicken, but sparingly. The danger is when you decide by yourself that you change *this* a little; then you change *that* a little, soon you will lose your way again.

"Even I will permit—sometimes—a cup of coffee, or a bit of seasoning. It depends—on the physician—*not* on the patient to make such decisions. Always we should remember, too, something which we must call psychological satisfaction. Everything is not only physical. But the fundamental trouble is a common mistake made by patients. They feel that 'a little bit' of one or another of the forbidden foods cannot do much harm. This is an entirely mistaken notion; besides, these little bits tend to become larger and more frequent; they do not fail to produce harmful results.

"One cocktail on Saturday night, then two cocktails Sunday afternoon. You eat first steak and potatoes once a week, which changes soon to twice a week—with a little chicken. Ach, it tastes so good, how can it be bad?" Gerson hammed it up a little. "Just a small piece of Boston cream pie, please, so . . ." showing his forefinger and thumb spread minutely apart! "Then a coffee for—what do you say, a 'pick-me-up'— *with Danish!* You must never even think of it.

"Fix everything into a habit until it is like your shadow, always sticking to you. There is a saying, 'Habit is like a cable, and you weave a strand a day, until it becomes almost unbreakable.' *That's it!*" Gerson took a sip of his coffee and allowed a twinkle in his eyes. "My diet is not so bad! After you try apples and carrot juice once or twice, or oatmeal with a little honey, your suffering will not be so much. Don't forget, for the prevention diet, at least you don't have to drink the raw liver juice!"

Wanamaker laughed aloud. "You've convinced me! I think I'm ready to take the pledge right now for the Gerson course! Dr. Gerson, please excuse me, but I have just one or two more questions, if that's agreeable? You have been most generous with your time—you and your daughter, and of course, Dr. Wolf—and I appreciate it very much."

"Please, let us finish," Gerson agreed.

"I have heard that some doctors seize on one point or another to criticize your program. For example, they say that it is absurd that anyone can eliminate pain with coffee enemas."

Gerson leaned forward, raising his forefinger. "Here is my answer: You should ask that doctor when is the last time he gave a dying cancer patient a coffee enema to relieve his pain? They won't even look—just like the scientists in the time of Galileo. Nobody would look through the telescope, because they thought it was nonsense to expect to see

anything up there in the sky! How does any doctor know ab
enemas if he never even tried it? You heard what Dr. Miley
Senator Pepper? Exactly I will repeat: 'We have observed marke
from pain in approximately ninety percent of the patients who enter the
hospital with severe types of pain due to cancer!' Which do you choose,
if you are the patient, Mr. Wanamaker: morphine every two hours,
which will eventually destroy your defense system, or a coffee enema,
which will help you eliminate the pain—and the toxins—at the same time?

"Ah, but you must understand something more than this about
pain. You should know something more about my therapy which relates
to this point. Now it is time to discuss with you something fundamental
about my theory. Please listen closely. During my years of research and
clinical experience with hundreds of patients, the idea occurred to me
that there are two components in cancer which are of particular importance. One is the whole body, the general component. The other is the
local one, the symptom. Really, the local one, the symptom, is just the
tip of the iceberg, to speak plainly. The treatment has to be applied to
the general component. When we are able to bring this into balance, the
local one disappears.

"The general component is the digestive tract and the liver. The
digestive tract is very much poisoned in cancer. How then can we handle
that? The most important first step is detoxification. It is easy to say,
but very difficult to do in cancer patients. These cases, when they are
far advanced, can hardly eat. They have no stomach juices, the liver
doesn't function, the pancreas doesn't function, nothing is active.

"Where do we begin? Let us go into that: First, we give some
different enemas. I found that the best enema is the coffee enema as it
was first used by Professor A. A. Meyer in Göttingen. This idea occurred to him when, together with Professor Heubner, he gave caffeine
solution into the rectum of animals. He observed that the bile ducts
were opened and more bile could flow. I felt that this was very important
and I worked out coffee enemas. We took three heaping tablespoons of
ground coffee for one quart of water, let it boil for three minutes, then
simmer ten to twenty minutes, and then gave it at body temperature.

"The patients reported that this was doing them good. The pain
disappeared even though we took away all the sedation. I realized that
it is impossible to detoxify the body on the one hand, and put in drugs
and poisons on the other, such sedation medications as demerol, codeine,
morphine, scopolamine, and so forth. So we had to put the medication
aside. One patient was worried. He said he was taking one grain of
codeine every two hours and he also got morphine injections. . . . How
can you take these away? I told him that the best sedation is a coffee
enema. After a very short time he had to agree with that. Some of these
patients who had been in severe pain didn't take coffee enemas every

our hours as I prescribed—*they took one every two hours.* But no more sedation! After just a few days there was very little pain, almost none.

"I can give you an example. A lady came to me not so long ago. She had cancer of the cervix and then two large tumor masses around the uterus. The cervix was a large crater, necrotic, producing blood and pus, and the poor lady couldn't sit anymore. The condition was inoperable. She had been given X rays and vomited any food she took in. She couldn't lie down anymore. She could not sit. She walked around day and night. When she came to my clinic the manager told me, 'Doctor, you can't keep her here. This moaning and walking day and night is keeping the other patients from sleeping. *But*—after four days—she was able to sleep with no sedative whatsoever—which had not helped her much anyway. The sedation had worked for perhaps half an hour or so only.

"These patients who absorb the big tumor masses are awakened with an alarm clock every night, because they are otherwise poisoned by the absorption of these masses. If I give them only one or two or three enemas, they die of poisoning. I did not have the right as a physician to cause the body to absorb all these cancer masses and then not to detoxify enough. With two or three enemas they were not detoxified enough. They went into a coma hepaticum (liver coma). Autopsies showed that the liver was poisoned. I learned from these disasters that it is impossible to give these patients too much detoxification. When I didn't give these patients the night enemas, they were drowsy, and almost semiconscious in the morning. The nurses confirmed this, and told me that it takes a couple of enemas till they are free of this toxic state again.

"Now, Mr. Wanamaker, I am going to astonish you!" As Gerson made this surprising remark, he turned to Johanna and asked her to bring in "the specimens." Johanna excused herself a moment and soon returned with a large glass jar in which reposed the most hideous-looking soft lumps. Gerson smiled, handing it over to Wanamaker, who looked puzzled, as he swallowed hard once or twice.

"It is perhaps unbelievable to you, Mr. Wanamaker, but it is a fact— what I am going to tell you. Sometimes during the detoxification treatment, tumor destruction occurs by what I consider 'parenteral digestion,' that is, by absorption of the cancer cells and tumor masses through the bloodstream. But these specimens—these dead pieces you see in the jar—were detached from their sites, and eliminated by the body's renewed energy and activities—from the rectum, cervix, bladder, vagina, esophagus, tonsils, intestines, or wherever they found their way out from the bodies of my patients.

"Once the body gathers strength, it is so wonderful to behold; so powerful is its action if you give it support to work against this terrible cancer." Gerson grinned with satisfaction at Wanamaker, who simply stared agape at the gruesome contents, which he kept turning round and round. There was no comment in him, only awe.

Eyebrows raised, Gerson nodded his head knowingly. "So—you saw enough?" Johanna took the jar from Wanamaker and put it aside, as Gerson continued.

"I cannot stress detoxification enough. Even so, with all these enemas, this was not enough! I had to give them also castor oil by mouth, and by enema every other day, at least for the first two weeks or so. After these two weeks you wouldn't recognize these patients anymore! They had arrived on a stretcher, and now they walked around. They had appetite. They gained weight and the tumors went down.

"You will ask, 'How can such a cancerous tumor go down?' That was a difficult question for me to understand. I had learned in my treatment of tuberculosis patients that I had to add potassium, iodine, and liver injections to help the liver and the whole body to restore the potassium.

"Now, as far as I can see, this is the situation: At first, we give the patient the most salt-free diet possible. So, as much salt (sodium) is removed from the body as can be. During the first days, three grams, five grams, up to eight grams a day of sodium are eliminated while the patients receive only about one half gram of sodium component within the food diet itself, and no sodium is added.

"You will excuse me, Mr. Wanamaker, but I hope this is not too much medical talk for you? It is necessary for me to make myself clear on these points. Anyway, the patients are given thyroid and lugol solution. I learned, first through the so-called Gudenath tadpole experiment, that iodine is necessary to increase and help the oxidation ability. Then we gave the patients large amounts of potassium. It took about three hundred experiments until I found the right potassium combination. It is a ten percent solution of potassium gluconate, potassium phosphate (monobasic), and potassium acetate. From that solution, the patient is given four teaspoonful ten times a day, in juices. That large amount of potassium is introduced into the body. At the same time five times, one grain of thyroid and six times, three drops of lugol solution, half strength. That's eighteen drops of lugol, which is a large dose.

"Nobody was observed to develop heart palpitations from this, even though some patients told me that they could previously not take thyroid because they would develop heart palpitations. And all allergies disappeared! Some patients claimed that they previously could not take even one teaspoonful of lemon juice or orange juice—they were allergic. But when they are well detoxified and have plenty of potassium, they are not allergic. Allergies and other hypersensitivities are eliminated.

"When introduced into the system, thyroid and lugol solution go immediately into the cancer mass. These ripe cells take it up fast, and they perhaps grow a little faster, but they soak in more with great greed—as much as they can—together with a little bit of sodium, probably. But then there isn't much sodium left. So then these cells pick up potassium and the oxidizing enzymes, and die by themselves. You have to realize that cancer cells live essentially on fermentation, but potassium and oxidizing enzymes introduce oxidation. And that is the point at which we can kill cancer cells, because we take away the conditions which they need to continue to live.

"A cancer metabolism starts where the body is no longer able to produce a healing inflammation. This regime begins to return the metabolism to normal so that, instead of na (sodium), potassium and the oxidizing enzymes are brought into active cooperation with the return of the healing inflammation.

"This reactivated power of the detoxified body had to be perfected to the highest degree because the cancer cells with their highly negative electrical potentials have the power to repulse forcefully whatever is counteracting their life process, maintained by fermentation.

"The fresh calf's liver juice contains the highest amount of oxidizing enzymes, most of the minerals of the potassium group, especially, a high content of iron, copper and cobalt, as well as hormones and vitamins in the best activated composition.

"In my opinion it must be assumed, as a rule, that sodium and iodine favor undifferentiated, quicker growth seen in embryos and cancer; while potassium and iodine assure a more differentiated slower growth with normal cell division. The derangement has occurred very slowly by chronic intoxication with the ensuing edema, but, in our regime, sodium and potassium are the exponents of two mineral groups with opposite electric potentials, keeping the body in a controlled equilibrium, of course, with the help of the visceral nervous system, hormones, vitamins, enzymes, and so forth.

"From my own clinical experiments I have learned that it is necessary to change the metabolism, not just with one substance or another, but also to change the intake of proteins, enzymes, vitamins, and so forth—simultaneously—to activate all natural healing forces which we need for our therapy. This is the whole basis of my dietary regime which includes some medications at the start. These changes seem to force the cancer cells to a higher metabolic rate. In my opinion, the mineral metabolism, united, of course, with a number of other revived processes, brings about the decisive role for the death of the cancer cells.

"Cancer cells can ferment only; therefore they are unable to adapt to the new intensive changes—they break down and die.

"Man in his character and disposition reacts to his food like the soil to fertilizer. As a garden can be improved with the right fertilizer, so can man be helped with the right food. 'Mother Earth' is such a true expression; we are really her children whom she loves, so why shouldn't we return her love by taking good care of her—and of ourselves? Diet must be the basis of all medical therapy, and, in the hands of the physician, nutrition can be the highest and best remedy. I don't say that it should be a treatment in itself, but it will enable Great Nature to unfold its own healing power."

"Your explanation of your theory is so clear, even to me," Wanamaker commented. "Why won't doctors give your methods a chance?"

"Such a long story you ask me to tell," Gerson shook his head. "Today's medical mind will not accept it after the brainwashing in medical school. I should know! You think the American schools are bad, you should see the German university professors—with heads like stone, so hard and stubborn. With drugs you kill pain, they say, but an enema? Never! It's impossible! Why? 'Because it is not here in the medical books, only in the mind of Gerson, the quack!' " Here Gerson made a circular motion with his right forefinger, alongside his temple, indicating insanity. "Besides, who wants to sell fruits and vegetables like a street peddler, when you can be a medical doctor with a shiny brass plate in front of your door? It would bring down the profession. They think that way!

"Suppose, Mr. Wanamaker, seventy-five years ago—before the radio— you told somebody that one day it will be possible to hear people talking and singing—in Paris or London—their voices coming through the air on some invisible waves? He would report you to the boobie hatch!

"Let them read my published books and papers. Let them witness the patients, see my case histories. I didn't write these to be sold like some cheap comic book. I wrote for serious physicians so they could see the worst cases you can imagine. Even the names can frighten you. Listen: prostate carcinoma with metastases in lumbar spine, adenocarcinoma of sigmoid colon, thyroid cancer, intramedullary glioma, spreading melano-sarcoma, adenocarcinoma of uterus and metastases in urinary bladder and vagina. . . . You want to hear some more? No? I thought so. But, with these terrible cases, I had so many long-term remissions and recoveries. So, if the doctors would only be serious, they could examine my case histories and the hospital records; then they could realize the proof of my theories, and how I succeeded where they have failed, and where they are failing this moment. How can a doctor refuse to read my treatment—when he is failing and I am succeeding? When *his* patients are dying, and mine are living?

"I will never stop to repeat, from Professor Kussmaul, a great truth: *'Der Erfolg am Krankenbett ist entscheidend'*—the result at the bedside of the patient is decisive."

Wanamaker raised his finger. "Another question, please. I have read there is a school of thinking which maintains that you suffer a severe loss of nerve energy when you administer an enema?"

Gerson snorted with disdain. "Loss of nerve energy? You can say also loss of nerve energy when you breathe, or blow your nose! What nonsense are we talking about? These patients are in the last moment— dying. Any remedial measures must be considered, even the most radical. It takes nerve energy to pull the string of a parachute before you are smashed to pieces! Or to climb down the ladder from a burning building; or to swim to the shore when your boat is sinking! Loss of nerve energy! Ach! Is our clinic a class for kindergarten children?" Gerson's eyes glared balefully through his spectacles. "You know, Mr. Wanamaker, these days I think it would be much better for me to grow flowers in the country." Gerson appeared to have decided. "Definitely! *That* I will absolutely do in my next life! Nerve energy! What next?"

THE JOHN GUNTHER STORY

Wanamaker changed the subject. "Now, if you don't mind, I would like to ask you about the Gunther case—the son of the famous author John Gunther. The boy's name was Johnny, I believe?"

"Ah, yes, Johnny, such a fine boy. I don't mind, but it is a very hard story to tell."

Johanna interposed, "Papa, let me tell him, *please?* Mr. Wanamaker, I was very close to that case, from the beginning. Do you have some special point in your mind about it?"

"Yes, the common gossip is that Johnny was treated by Dr. Gerson and that finally he died; that your father could not help him!"

Johanna harumphed. "That's what I thought—well, the other side of the coin is quite different from how you heard. But first I want to tell you about Mrs. Seeley and her nursing home. Mrs. Seeley was one of my father's successful patients. Out of gratitude, because she wanted to help him, she started this nursing home where my father's patients could have a continuation of the complete diet therapy. For a while, Johnny stayed with Mrs. Seeley after he left the clinic. He was so sensitive—so smart, with such a sense of humor. I used to help Mrs. Seeley with the patients, and usually I brought my little daughter with me. Oh, but let me tell you first this wonderful story—about Johnny, in Mr. Gunther's own words. This is from his book *Death Be Not Proud,* which I have here. Now I will read: 'Johanna's little girl, aged about six, was fascinated by Johnny, and often came in to see him. He was polite, but bored. Girls of six were really not his dish. Once the little girl tiptoed in and asked if it were all right to stay. Johnny replied, "Okay, if you don't compromise me. Keep the door ajar." '

"Such a boy! By the way, Mr. Wanamaker, do you know John Gunther's book *Death Be Not Proud?*," Johanna asked. Wanamaker had not heard of it. "All the details are in the book. Such a moving story which he wrote after Johnny died.

"And now I will make my explanation as short as possible, but I don't want to leave out any important point. You know the announcer Raymond Gram Swing? Well, he was a good friend of the Gunthers, and he recommended them to my father. When Mr. and Mrs. Gunther came to see him—I can quote you? they had *'thirty-three doctors,* maybe more, including some of the most famous specialists in the world.' You want to know Johnny's condition when they brought him to Dr. Gerson? Mr. Gunther says that one doctor told him 'that the reason he had seemed so casual when Johnny entered the Gerson home was his conviction that he could not possibly outlast the week anyway.'

"So you know his condition. He was dying. Thirty-three doctors, Mr. Wanamaker. Do you like to fight with those doctors? My father was a saint. Some of them never let go their fingers from this case, upsetting Mr. Gunther, and nagging my father continuously with their interferences —even when everything was going so well. Do you know something? before Johnny was placed under my father's care, he had received injections of mustard gas. This drug was in the early stages of development, not highly refined, so Johnny was one of the first guinea pigs for this drug, but his malignant tumor continued to grow. They operated, but it still got worse. It was deep in the brain, and they could not cut it all out.

"I don't want to be so technical, but let me cite you from the book: 'In particular, what is known as the polymorphnuclear count of Johnny's blood was staggeringly low—down to three percent, and the red cells showed a profound anemia. One specialist told us later that he has never known of a recovery with such a blood condition.'

"So now you know when they come to Dr. Max Gerson—like they always come—when it is already too late. When my father first saw Johnny, his condition was so bad. His arm was all swollen from the mustard gas injections, and, as you already heard, his blood picture was badly deteriorated. So you now can understand Johnny's desperate condition—all the thirty doctors failed. They gave up! *But,* after my father started, listen to what Mr. Gunther says in his book: 'Within a week, Johnny was feeling, not worse, but much better! The blood count rose steadily, the bruises were absorbed with extraordinary speed; the wound in the bulge of his head healed, and miracle of miracles, the bump on the skull was doing down!'

"You must read *Death Be Not Proud;* you will find out that my father eliminated the brain tumor without surgery, without X rays, and without chemicals. He brought Johnny back to recovery. But, before my father's treatment even had a chance, Gunther's experts again had that poor boy on his way to the operating table. My father loved Johnny, as much as anybody, and desperately wanted to save him, so he was fighting against all those specialists like a tiger—*against the operation!*

"By now, the bump looked like two tomatoes, exuding large amounts of pus every day. My father's theory, from the beginning, was that the tumor was now *dead,* killed by the diet, and that the suppuration consisted of nothing but dead matter. In other words, the tumor was sloughing itself slowly out of Johnny's head. But *who* agreed with Gerson?

"John Gunther himself says that the 'battle of the doctors' almost destroyed him and his wife. 'I have never known such stress,' he says in his book, so you can just imagine the courage of my father to fight the doctors like he did—because, if he was wrong, and if Johnny died, he would be in the worst kind of trouble. Finally, it was the Gunthers themselves who decided to go ahead with the operation. And, now, I'm going to read you Mr. Gunther's exact words: 'The operation was scheduled for the afternoon. Early that morning the bump spontaneously opened of itself, *as Gerson had stubbornly predicted it would,* and Mount" (that was their family doctor) "—*summoned by Johnny himself* —who realized exactly what was happening, did the evacuation right in Johnny's room, because there was no time to move him. Mount called me at about eleven in the morning, his voice fairly choked with joy, saying that he had successfully drained an abscess that went five centimeters into the brain beyond the table of the skull, and had got out a full cup of pus and fluid. . . . [Gradually] the pear-shaped sac in the brain slowly closed with healthy granulation tissue. . . . That horrible, ferocious bump was altogether gone. It had disappeared. Mount had sucked it out completely. Johnny's skull would be as smooth and normal as mine, except for the scars of the original incision which the hair would cover!'

"So my father was proven to be right. Just as he told those doctors he was always fighting, the tumor was sloughing off, and the cancer cells were dying—to give it a chance. But nobody listened to him. Then the tumor broke of its own accord, and spilled out all the dead cancer cells. The brain was clean—and every cell which they examined in the laboratory was dead and sterile!

"You can just imagine the surprise of those doctors! And you can just imagine how my father smiled—as big as the whole sunrise! He was wild with joy. And for us, the whole family, when we heard, we were so happy to see his joy!" Johanna wiped a tear from her eye. *"That* was the battle of the century!

"Then what happened?" Johanna posited. "No, they didn't give him any medals! I'm sorry to say, the doctors so suddenly became busy with bandages, and this and that, looking so important, and who got the

credit? Not my father. He was, how do you say it, lost in the shuffle. Would you like to know what the patient, the seventeen-year-old boy— Johnny—joked to one of his visitors, he was so gay and confident by this time: 'The doctors are fighting among themselves now as to who cured me!'

"But *still,* Mr. Gunther was a worried father. He continued overly anxious, even when so many good things were happening, and he never stopped looking for more doctors, more specialists. He didn't believe in his good luck. There was always interference, and problems for my father from the doctors in maintaining the strict Gerson therapy. They still refused to believe it. On top of that, Johnny was so anxious, so restless to return to school, that when he was a little better he started working on his studies to enter Harvard University.

"My father was considered by Mr. Gunther to be a dictator. Yes, he was a dictator—about his patients' good health. His demand was for Johnny to *rest, rest, rest,* but did he? No! He was so anxious and restless to return to school that, when he was improved a little, he started working heavily on his school studies. For such a sick boy— where you need two to three years of absolute rest, and the strictest adherence to the regime—that is not too much in this type of case— but it didn't happen that way. Listen to John Gunther himself if you want to see how much rest this sick boy was getting. I will read: 'Johnny worked on and on. He was utterly obsessed about getting into Harvard in the fall. But to achieve this he had to complete making up his work at Deerfield and graduate, as well as pass the college entrance exams, a double task that seemed impossible. Then on March 18, we learned that he had caught up with the history course at Deerfield— though he hadn't been there for eleven months—and on April 7 he had a letter from Mr. Boyden that gave him radiant happiness: he had passed his English examination satisfactorily and so was abreast of this course, too. I took him to the science room in the public library, where he did some advanced work, and he proceeded to write up no fewer than fifty-four chemistry experiments!'

"Mr. Wanamaker, even you can guess, by now, the outcome? Johnny's condition was aggravated by his utter exhaustion, and the tumor came back. He was taken completely out of Dr. Gerson's hands now, so even the dietary regime was destroyed. His father wrote that one 'evening he ate steak and more or less anything he liked. He kept gripping a huge piece of hard cheese . . .' and so on. Johnny wrote in his diary April 13, 'Yesterday, I took seven hours of college board exams!' In May (the day is not mentioned), he wrote, 'Back to Neurological Institute! A second operation. . . . But I can eat again! Steak, ice cream. Cream of mushroom soup!'

"Can you see the beginning of the end, Mr. Wanamaker, in this story?

Johnny himself had a divine kind of prescience, and continued to ask his father—when there were changes in his routine—whether this had all been cleared with Gerson! One of the last entries in his diary: 'I go back to Memorial Hospital for nitrogen mustard treatment.' That was June 12. He died June 30."

Gerson at this point was having his own problems controlling his emotions. He touched Johanna gently on the arm and said, "Mr. Wanamaker, all that my daughter said is correct and true, but I cannot entirely leave the blame where it is from her story. I, also, have a direct responsibility for his death. It has been on my conscience. I will tell you now why this poor boy died. He had a terrible brain tumor growing out of the skull, larger than my fist. I cured that. It's written in the book. But, after that, the boy had an eczema and this eczema was of a special type which can usually be cured by giving the interior lobe pituitary extract, a hormone.

"The family doctor, Dr. Traeger, said, 'Why don't you give it to him?' But I told him that this is a terrible risk and I don't like to take such a risk with the life of that boy. When we give the pituitary, like many other hormones, we may kill. But finally I gave in, and it was my fault. And for a long time after that, I couldn't sleep nights. I gave him the hormone and the tumor regrew. I'm sorry, but that is the true story."

It was quiet for a while. No one wanted to speak. Johanna finally broke the silence, addressing her father: "I'm sorry, but I don't think you should take all the blame. The pressure from the doctors was too much, it never stopped, otherwise you would never use hormones, never. My father has too much terrible experience with it, even if other doctors use it. What more is there to say? The tumor recurred. His family doctor and the other consultants took Johnny completely out of my father's hands. They even took him off the diet! Johnny himself was so surprised, he asked his father, 'Does Dr. Gerson know about this?' even when my father was no longer involved in the case. What other result could you expect with all that? He died. That's the story in a nutshell!

"One more thing I want to tell you. It's so sad. Johnny kept a diary, you know, and they found his last words written inside the back cover of this diary. His mother had told him the story of the ancient Hebrew toast 'L'Chayim.' Johnny's notation was 'Hebrew Toast: *Le-Hyeem—to Life!'* "

Wanamaker stirred in his chair. "Thank you, Johanna, it's a moving story. I'll get a copy of the book, as you suggested. Dr. Gerson, just to change the subject a bit. An idea just occurred to me. Are you familiar with AA?"

"Oh, yes, Alcoholics Anonymous."

"What do you think of a group, say, 'Gerson Anonymous,' or 'Nutrition Anonymous,' where each member could give the other close-in support to stick to your regime? Of course, for cancer patients—but also the general public as a preventive measure?"

Gerson chuckled. "Well, it's a good idea, but, in such an organization, I would like to see a medical doctor, also a nutritionist, someone who understands about medicine, and about nutrition."

"Let me think about that for my article. May I ask you, Dr. Gerson, as I observe your full schedule, I'm struck by your energy and strength. You are not exactly a young man, yet you put out like a big old Mack truck. I echo your daughter's concern and amazement. In the face of so many obstacles and problems, how do you manage to continue your work at such a high energy level?"

"It's from my patients; *they* give me strength," Gerson said simply.

"I would like to add something," Johanna volunteered. "I have watched my father work, and I have worked with him and his patients very closely. His life is his work. These cancers which are eating up the people, killing them before your eyes, begin to disappear and go away. So you see, my father is literally giving new life to others. The great inner peace is his source of energy. I would like to say that his own life's energy depends upon it—giving life to others. With this inner life force he can surmount all the difficulties, all the attacks. Look how he is now." All turned to Gerson, whose face was radiant, in the aura of a quiet smile.

"Yes, I can understand that," said Wanamaker. "It still puzzles me, though—surely a few medical doctors must know what is happening here at your clinic. Aren't they impressed with your results?"

Johanna carried on: "Oh, yes, if you could be here some night when a medical doctor comes to see my father when nobody knows who he is and why he is here. Yes, Mr. Wanamaker, you will be shocked, like my father already told you—how they come in the middle of the night— cancer specialists, no less—and they beg my father, 'Please Dr. Gerson, help my wife,' or 'Please help my sister,' or 'Help my mother, but don't tell anybody I was here!' It's a great shame; there is so much politics in this medical business. It's sad but it's true.

"I wonder, why doesn't God do more for the dying? Sometimes, when a patient dies—oh, yes, some of them die here, too—he will ask, 'Dr. Gerson, isn't there a better way for the others?' You see, at that last final moment, he can forget himself, and he is thinking about other people. Yes, I heard them worrying about the other patients many times.

One night a dying patient somehow crawled out of his bed to put a blanket over the patient beside him. It is something wonderful to see. Some of them turn into saints—trying to help each other.

"Are they somehow trying to make up for their lost lives, at this very last minute—their lost love, their lost affection? Are they saying that they should have loved each other more? Maybe they get a glimpse of God's kingdom, of what is over on the other side of the veil? I really don't understand it. Maybe they already can see through a glass darkly, and it is their last chance on this earth to open the door a little for someone else to behave like real human beings in our depraved society. It catches you here, deep inside. You have to burst into tears; otherwise your heart will break.

"There was one patient who took my father's hand—he knew he was dying. He saw the tears in my father's eyes, and it is so hard to believe: that dying man could not bear to see my father's suffering, so he whispered to him—he was so weak—'Dr. Max. . . .' He even never before called my father by his first name, but I suppose he could call him 'Max' now—as a special privilege for the one who dies? And he said, 'Dr. Max, please, I'm so sorry to disappoint you, but don't be sad. It was too late for me. Your way is better than those butchers. Do your best for the others. They need you. Everybody loves you. I love you, too.' Then he closed his eyes. Yes, Mr. Wanamaker, there must be a better way, and my father is trying his best to find it, to build a bridge for the others who will come later."

Wiping her eyes, Johanna remembered something. "Oh, I almost forgot, but here is the best time to give you Mr. Markel's report, which he made to Senator Pepper's committee. Mr. Markel, he is just a private citizen who wanted to speak up for my father. You will find some surprising information here." Johanna handed him three typewritten sheets. "You can keep it for your reference."

Wanamaker decided to read it.

PREPARED STATEMENT BY SAMUEL A. MARKEL

"My name is Samuel A. Markel. My residence is 3410 Monument Avenue, Richmond, Virginia. I am a citizen of the United States, having been born in Elizabeth, New Jersey, United States of America.

". . . Millions of dollars have been and are being spent in cancer 'research,' and while it is unknown how much of the actual dollar finds its way into research as compared with other expenses, the amazing fact is that the medical profession is apparently still 'researching' on the subject matter of cancer, while there resides in New York City an unassuming physician who has long since passed the period of research on animals and is actually treating and, in my humble opinion as a layman, curing cancer in human beings.

"I have seen patients who appeared to me to be so far gone as the results of the ravages of cancer as to be beyond the pale of anything but miracles. These miracles are in fact being performed by Dr. Max Gerson.

"I have seen some of these results.

"The wife of one of my friends underwent an operation for cancer at the Walter Reed Hospital in Washington where her breast was removed, and which appeared to aggravate her situation and it appears that cancer had thereafter spread over her lungs. After a visit in New York for several months under the treatment of this scientist, Dr. Gerson, she had returned to her home in Richmond, Virginia. She says she has never felt better in her life. Her name is Mrs. W. G. Wharton. Her address is 2806 East Franklin Street, Richmond, Virginia, and her husband is presently the building inspector for the city of Richmond.

"I myself was relieved of a very serious case of osteoarthritis by Dr. Gerson after my own doctor had pronounced my condition incurable.

"My only interest in this matter is a humanitarian one, having lost my wife with this dreaded disease, and I feel that the least I can do is to add my voice and such funds as I am able, to the eradication of cancer, and I have therefore given freely to the various campaigns for research. It appears, however, that some doctors are fighting Dr. Gerson. I can readily understand that, when results so fantastic are obtained, such claims can hardly be believable. My quarrel with these gentlemen is the fact that they will immediately say such things are impossible or the doctor is a fake, without even stopping to inquire what is being done. I have had the same experience with my own doctors, who merely throw up their hands and say that anyone claiming to cure cancer is a fake.

"I understand, also, that the medical profession considers it unethical for any doctor to say that he cures any ailment unless that cure has been in effect for five years or more. I understand further that the oldest patient in point of treatment of cancer which Dr. Gerson has in the United States, is about four or four and a half years, and I hope that the good doctors of the medical profession will excuse me, if I as a layman say that I would not deny the results that I have seen on account of six months or so, and I feel that it is worthy of investigation and certainly of further research.

"The very fact that the patients treated by Dr. Gerson are living today when they were destined to die three or four years ago, according to the statements of these good doctors who treated them, I say it is a sensational result and the least that can be said for it is that Dr. Gerson has accomplished something that no one else in the medical profession has accomplished with respect to the treatment of cancer, so far as I am able to ascertain. I would hate to think that the antipathy to Dr. Gerson would be in any manner associated with the fact that his treatments are dietary and not surgical. . . .

"We are still researching with animals, while, here, an unassuming scientist in New York—and I hope the medical profession will pardon me for using the word 'cure'—is curing cancer today.

"Now, I understand that a patient must have been free of a recurrence of disease for five years before an ethical doctor would be permitted to say the patient was 'cured.' Well, fortunately, nobody can take my license away, because I am an ordinary layman. I am not a scientist, I am not a doctor—and I will not cloud the results on account of six months. I say when a patient has lived four and a half years longer than the time allotted by reputable doctors, I am willing to say he was cured. At least, he has not been buried when he was designed to be by the hospitals that sent him home to die, Mr. Chairman. They were told that they could not live but a few months. That is four years ago. Something has been done for them. It has not been surgery. It has not been radium. It has not been X ray—and those are the only three things, if my information is correct, that the millions of dollars had been spent upon. I say, if there is another avenue, a nutritional avenue—which this is—or anything else which gives promise of the cure of cancer, these research artists at least should be willing to condescend to look at it, Mr. Chairman. In this case there have been outstanding scientists, I am told, who have been told of this, and they do not even want to look at it. I do not ask them to admit that it is true. At least take a look!"

Just as Wanamaker finished perusing the statement, a telephone jingled in the next room. "Oh, papa, who can it be so late?" asked Johanna. She walked over to the extension line on a small end table near the window. She picked it up, listened for a moment, then turned to Gerson. "It's George Mansfield, from the Cancer Foundation—you know, *that* one, he's incorrigible. He says that he just arranged for you to be on a radio program."

"A radio program?" Gerson was startled.

"The Long John Nebel night show. Millions of people listen to it every day, he says."

Gerson pleaded. "Darling, what kind of program?"

"They feature exciting new personalities, people with unusual hobbies, scientific discoveries, things like that. George says many medical doctors have appeared on this show. It's for tonight—eleven o'clock!"

"Tonight! Impossible! Tell him no. It's too much. Is not the day long enough?"

Johanna turned back in desperation to the phone, but with a feeling of hopelessness. George was a bulldog. A recovered patient of Gerson's, he was the spark plug of the Foundation for Cancer Treatment, which had been formed by grateful patients of Gerson's. George had appointed himself chief evangelist in preaching the Gerson gospel. Johanna was floundering desperately as she listened to George's verbal barrage. She turned again to her father. "He says he's been working for three months and finally, through a special introduction yesterday, he made the arrangements for you. There will not be another chance, he insists."

Gerson observed Johanna's distress. "I'll go. That settles it." Gerson decided. "Find out where we are to meet him." Gerson turned to the others, "Well, my good friends, it seems there is no rest for the weary."

Wanamaker packed his notebooks into his briefcase and picked up the envelope containing the X rays and case histories. "The Long John program," he commented, "draws a large audience." Dr. Wolf had listened to it once or twice and agreed, although he was not so sure about its desirability as a platform for a professional man of Gerson's caliber. "Anyhow," he concluded, "it's done. I think we are finished here. If you like, Max, I will be happy to drive you. I have my car outside."

"Yes, that I would appreciate." Gerson rose heavily from his chair, and turned to the reporter. "Mr. Wanamaker, I thank you for being such a good listener. I hope you have learned enough so that you can come to a good conclusion. As a journalist, that is your department. I leave it to you. Telephone me any time if you need any more information; it will be my pleasure."

Wanamaker thanked Gerson, then took his leave.

Gerson spoke to Dr. Wolf. "Heinrich, if you don't mind, I'll go upstairs to change. Maybe a quick hot shower. It's good of you to help me today." Showing his weariness, he patted Dr. Wolf's shoulder as he passed by him on the way to his bedroom.

"Such a long day," he said.

In the preceding chapter, a number of scenes have been dramatized. The incidents and episodes in this chapter are presented in the author's own style and improvisation. Frank Wanamaker, the reporter, is a fictitious character, but the basic facts presented in his interview with Dr. Gerson are true and represent an integration of several news stories by many reporters who interviewed Gerson over the years.

16

"The Moving Finger Writes..."

Gerson had not the remotest inkling that his status as a physician in good standing was hanging in precarious balance. His guileless, uncomplicated mind simply could not anticipate such a catastrophic result as suspension. Other doctors had appeared on the Long John Nebel program, without being penalized. He himself had openly presented his papers, his case histories and findings, without complaint, to the investigating committees. Nothing he had discussed on the broadcast was at all different from what was already known, published, and presented to every public sector that might be interested. Nevertheless, as it turned out, he had been living under a Sword of Damocles.

Johanna was the first to sort the mail that morning. Among the accumulation was a routine-looking letter from the New York County Medical Society. It appeared no different from many others Gerson had received in the past. "Oh, no!" Johanna groaned, "Not another investigation!" Then she trimmed the end of the envelope, and unfolded the letter.

Her breathing literally stopped as she read the notice of Gerson's suspension from the Society for a period of two years. "I can't believe it! I can't believe it! How could they do this to papa! Oh, my God! Why?" Her distraught mind raced in mad circles. Maybe she could telephone the Society? There must be some mistake. She spun nervously back and forth in her chair, back and forth, in a frenzy of hysteria. At one point she lifted up a heavy onyx elephant in a passion, and only by the strongest self-control did she prevent herself from hurling it on the floor. Finally, she stood up and walked slowly upstairs. She had better pass this bad news first to her mother.

Margaret—Mrs. Gerson—quietly read the letter, then commented stoically, "Thank God!"

Johanna was stunned at her reaction. Mrs. Gerson continued: "I see this as a sign from God. It's a blessing in disguise. How much more oppression and suffering can poor papa take at his age? How many more patients can he help, working his heart out from morning to night? Johanna, let's face it. He's not so strong or so young as you think. I notice such things. You know how close I am to him, after all. And, while there is yet time, let him finish his book, which is so much more important than treating one or two more patients. How many years has he already been writing? Late in the night; many days before the sun comes up, but still it is not finished. His whole life will be meaningless if he does not publish this work for the medical doctors. Maybe only a few will read it, but maybe it will be enough to start a change. Anyhow, he must try. There is no doubt what must be done." Mrs. Gerson took Johanna by the hand. "Come, wipe your tears. We are now going to tell Dr. Max Gerson to finish his book!"

Margaret and Johanna walked downstairs to Gerson's office, and knocked imperiously on his door. Gerson called out, and in they marched —like a roll of thunder! He took one look at the duo and sensed trouble. "I'm sure I do not get my coffee this morning?" was his first probing thrust.

"Your coffee, you will get!" Mrs. Gerson responded, "But I'm not so sure I will give you any honey!"

Gerson hadn't a clue as to the problem. He chuckled and remarked, "I have been, somehow, a bad boy?"

"No! A *good* boy! *Too good,* in fact. Now we are going to change all that."

For the first time, Gerson noticed the letter in his wife's hand, and felt a tremor of apprehension. "I have some trouble?" he asked.

"Max, *we* don't think it's trouble; *we* think it's a blessing in disguise." She came right out with it: "The Medical Society has suspended you from membership!" she announced precipitately, thrusting the letter toward him.

Gerson remained cool as ice, his blue eyes raised quizzically, as he took the letter and leaned back deliberately to read its contents. A moment later he spoke to Mrs. Gerson, with a pathetic undertone in his voice: "You know, Margaret, for this I *need* the extra honey in my coffee!" She burst into tears.

"Don't take it so calmly, those . . . those monsters!" she raged. "No different from the SS; no different, Max, I'm telling you, only another kind of uniform. *Please get mad!*" she implored.

"Margaret, I have been mad all my life—it is all a bundle of pain inside of me. The burning started from the day I saw that pale young man trampled to death on the train platform in front of my eyes in Germany—that was April Fool's Day, remember? It's an ulcer eating at my heart. I found only one way to control it: by changing it over to the love of my patients, and of my work. It's what I have to give, for all the hate I have, even inside my bones. So now I just have to give them more—*without* the Society membership!"

"*You will not!*" Mrs. Gerson fairly shouted at him. "You will do nothing of the kind!" She walked around the side of the desk, and placed her hand on his shoulder. "Max, darling, listen to me—carefully. It is now necessary to write your book. To tell your story; or what will be the use of it all? You must give all your strength and all your will to this task. You have played with it long enough—late at night, early in the morning, with no sleep or rest. All your life, you have carried your cross without complaint. Look at your clinic. Where are your doctors to help you? They worked for a few days, then ran away. Where is Dr. Miller—who used to do your X rays? They frightened him away, too. To what laboratory can you go for your blood and tissue tests? When is the next investigation going to be again? *Who? Who* is helping you, Max, please tell me? Who cares about you? You are now seventy-five years old. Spring and summer are only an echo now, like the song of the meadowlark. The smell of winter is already in the air, and the autumn leaves are piled high against our door. Which is now more important, a few more patients to treat—or to publish your life's work for the whole world to know?"

She paused briefly. "Look at us—me, Johanna, Lottie, and Gertrude. We are the living, who also need your love and care. Please, dear Max, take *us* now as your patients. Yes, we, too, are patients. We have suffered —with you, and for you. So many hard years you spent for others—and we do not complain about that—but now please spend a little time for us—for your own sake, too. Make your family your patient now, we beg you, before winter comes with its cold winds."

Max Gerson, always sensitive, had turned pale. He was stunned by the depth of Margaret's impassioned outburst. And now, slowly, he turned in his swivel chair, until his back was to them. With his knuckles he wiped away a tear as he sat for perhaps fifteen seconds in perfect silence; then—slowly—his chair turned back so that he faced them again.

He seemed almost detached as he started speaking. "Time flies like a bird. The moving finger writes its story without coming back to change even one line. . . . You are right," he declared. "I have been selfish with my career." He paused briefly. "How deeply I love you all, you surely know. My heart has been troubled too long about my lost time from you. Forgive me. While there remains a little bit of autumn, let us begin to live like a family again; to do a few things together; to enjoy each other. And, now, I will seriously write my story; otherwise they will ask one day, 'Who was Max Gerson?' and only the wind will be there to answer."

Gerson stood up, took Margaret round by the shoulders, walked over with her to Johanna, where he brought them together, and hugged them close. "I promise: From now on I accept you as my full-time patients—my *only* patients!"

"Oh, papa!" Johanna fairly screamed with delight, and kissed him. "We must have a celebration!"

"Yes," Gerson agreed. "It's unanimous, let's have a celebration! We'll get everybody together. This Saturday night—positively—we all go to the concert!"

Johanna was elated. "Papa!" she exclaimed. "Leonard Bernstein is conducting at Carnegie Hall, with Arthur Rubinstein at the piano. Dr. Wolf says the critics are raving about the program!"

"Ach, my beloved family—just like old times! So what is there to talk! Johanna, you get the tickets. It's settled!" He released them both from his grip, and returned to his desk. "I have work to do now. It will not be easy to finish up with my patients, but I will make the best arrangements for each one. Dr. Wolf—maybe one or two others will cooperate with me to help them. Somehow, we will manage." He picked up the letter from the Medical Society. "What shall we do with this?" he mused. Johanna and Margaret held their breath, waiting.

"Here, Johanna, you take care of it. I think it belongs in the 'miscellaneous' file."

17

A Cancer Therapy

Dr. Max Gerson was deep in thought, chewing the end of his pencil. It was late one evening in February 1958, and late in the evening of his life. He sat at his desk writing *A Cancer Therapy*, the book that was to crown his life's work, and destined one day to emerge as one of the greatest medical treatises of all time on the treatment of malignancies.

On the picture screen of his mind, the past flowed softly by: his childhood experiments in the garden with its green roses; his schooling among gimlet-eyed professors; his pioneer work with Dr. Ferdinand Sauerbruch and the lupus patients; the successes and the failures.

Then his sudden flight from Germany; the uncertainties and hazards that pursued him through Austria, France, England; and, finally, America, a refugee come-lately on a surging new wave of immigration, but beckoned still by the long shadow of the Statue of Liberty in New York Harbor, still extending her welcome to the lost and tempest-tossed, and still with her lamp lifted beside the golden door. That was over twenty years ago. And, since he had first sat with his classmates in Albert-Ludwigs Universität in Freiburg, Germany, over fifty years had passed.

As fancies fled, through heart and head, he saw himself, his first year in America, toiling through English language grammars, trying to grasp the abominable syntax; reviewing schoolboy material in medical textbooks; boning up on old test papers, then sitting like the youngest fledgling student for his medical examinations.

How awkward—to wriggle behind ink-stained school desks—a wise old walrus—with his still new Savile Row tweeds vying with the young Ivy Leaguers in dapper gray and blue flannels—some of the students with hardly the fuzz off their cheeks—all aglow with their Walt Disney World, where every day new wonder drugs exploded in the medical marketplace— running neck-and-neck with the James Bond-type of medical equipment and, equally exciting, innovative surgical technology.

It was disheartening irony that a medical doctor, seasoned in the highly disciplined environment of Germany's most respected universities, and rigorously tested in the crucible of life-and-death clinical

166

experience, should have to strain and cram, cram and strain, as he wrestled with the torturesome convolutions of biochemistry, microbiology, and pharmacology in that devilishly frustrating new tongue—English!

But he had finally received his license to practice medicine in New York, January 27, 1938. He smiled sourly as he recalled that, had he arrived in the United States just a few months earlier, he would have been allowed, under then prevailing law, to hang out his shingle without this laborious, grinding apprenticeship.

Gerson now opened his eyes, thought for a moment, then leaned forward and started to write Chapter 1, "The Secret of My Treatment." And what were the first words with which he began this chapter about his "secret"?

"Of course, there is none!"

But this question of his "secret" was the one most frequently asked by inquiring physicians. In this respect, they differed hardly at all from their anxious patients who were always searching for that magic shot in the arm—that wave of the wand that would melt away this vale of tears, and all the aches and pains that flesh is heir to.

He thought deeply on the approach. He wanted desperately to make his book readable, and his theories easily understood. So he began by explaining that it all started from an uncomplicated premise, a cohering principle, which recognized that each form of life is a biologic entity, with a prime purpose of growing and reproducing, by using the foods at its disposal. As long as the body remained in a state of healthy equilibrium, it would prosper; but the onset of metabolic disturbances constituted the beginning of disease.

What was desperately needed—and that was the whole reason for the book—he observed to himself, was an understanding of nature's law of totality as it affected the workings of the human body. This meant, in essence, a clear view of simple cause and effect, of those elements—good and bad—to which the human body is exposed in its *outside* environment—he called it the "external metabolism"; and/or which are introduced *into* the body, the "internal metabolism." Sickness, he reasoned, starts with the contamination of the body through the elemental poisoning of the air, food, and water supplies.

"The soil dominates. It is the meeting place of the living matter of the surface and of the mineral matter beneath the surface; of the atmosphere above and the solid rock underneath. Essentially all living matter depends upon it, directly or indirectly—and is, in fact, a part of those processes that produce the soil upon which life depends." Man, he reasoned, has somewhat the same relationship to the soil, and it is not by chance that this "living organism" is called "Mother Earth."

In *The Essene Gospel of Peace of Jesus Christ,* Edmond Bordeaux

Szekely translates from the Aramaic and Old Slavonic texts: "Keep, therefore, her laws, for none can live long, neither be happy, but he who honors his Earthly Mother and does her laws. For your breath is her breath; your blood is her blood; your bone is her bone; your flesh is her flesh; your bowels her bowels; your eyes and your ears are her eyes and ears. . . . She has given you her body, and none but she heals you . . . for your Mother loves you. . . . Honor your Earthly Mother and keep all her laws, that your days may be long on the earth. . . . For your Earthly Mother is love, and God is love."

Thus wasn't it logical to assume that, if we are able to reverse the order—to mitigate or eliminate these abuses of the external environment—and simply restore the blood to its original pure state, and consequently the cells, tissues and organs, the sick patient would recover? Not as simple as it sounds with terminal cancer, but . . .

"A normal body," he elaborated, "has the capacity to keep all cells functioning properly in an organized way. It prevents any abnormal transformation and growth. Therefore, the natural objective of a cancer therapy is to bring the body back to its normal physiology—or as near to it as is possible. The next task is to keep the physiology of the metabolism in that natural equilibrium. The normal body also has adequate immunological reserves to suppress and destroy malignancies. But not in cancer patients, where the cancer has embarked on a path of growth without encountering effective resistance. What forces can head off such a development?"

How to convince those who really counted—the physicians who formed the first line of defense on the long gray line of battle? Where could you find this new breed of doctor who would accept the soundness of Ganzheitstherapie so that the fatal disease process could be reversed? Otherwise the undertaker, and the grave, would continue to be the ultimate beneficiaries.

He laughed to himself as it occurred to him that perhaps an errant gene could be stirred into the dead air of a medical university, which would infect one of the students, and mutate into a whole genetic chain that would inoculate all the future progeny with an irreversible case of Ganzheitstherapie. Something Alexis Carrel had once said popped into his mind: "If the doctor of today does not become the dietician of tomorrow, the dietician of today will become the doctor of tomorrow."

But how could the medical schools survive on such dull fare as intensive studies of nutrition? Enzymes, proteins, fats, starches and carbohydrates, minerals and other nutritional factors? Could they give up their front-page headlines with dramatic heart and kidney transplants, coronary bypasses, colostomy resections, or intensive care units with all their awesome equipment and snakelike clusters of colored wiring?

Perhaps the most forbidding prospect of all: How could the committed physician resign himself to being as poor as a country doctor who traded his services for chickens and eggs? The average terminal case could never afford the physician's time, the wearing twenty-four-hour-day vigils the treatment necessitated. Where could you find this kind of doctor? Only in the medical schools. It demanded a whole new educational process. Isn't that where everything begins? In the schools?

He was startled to find that he had been doodling, and that his pencil had automatically written "Gerson Health Institute"! Odd, he thought, but he smiled with some satisfaction at the idea. Then he carefully underlined it. Yes, it would probably have to start with the medical universities. With a sigh, he disengaged his mind from the problem. "Leave it alone," he counseled. "Let someone else solve it." He had his work to do. . . .

And so . . . as his thoughts continued in ferment, gathering force and momentum, his pencil raced more swiftly across the pages, his attention hypnotically fixed on its moving point. Page after page of script materialized under its persuasive pressure, and fluttered to the floor, one after another, with only a number he placed on each page to keep the order. Gerson made occasional reference to books, notes, and papers that surrounded him in unkempt piles, but for the most part his photographic mind retained all the vital essentials. It was rare for him to pause, and that only when Margaret—who was by now his close day-long companion and ally—would knock gently to tell him it was time for lunch or dinner.

One day, as she came in to serve his coffee, she caught him impatiently opening and shutting his desk drawers. She gave him a pixy smile, as she concealed something behind her back with her right hand. "Max, did you lose something?" she asked with pretended innocence.

He straightened up abruptly. "What could I possibly lose when you are looking after me like a mother with a new baby?" he joked.

"I thought . . . maybe, a book," she coyly mentioned.

"Ach! So *you* are the guilty one. Where is it?" he demanded.

"Max, I always count the pages you write when I pick them up. The last few days I was suspicious because there was not such a blizzard of pages on the floor, and I was right! You have been naughty! You have been cheating! I found this in your bottom drawer!" She produced a book from behind her: *Dr. Zhivago!*

Gerson leaped on the prize. "You, Margaret! How can you do this to me, your own husband?"

"Max," she said seriously, "you are not only my husband, now. You must remember that you are also an author. I now have *two* loyalties."

Gerson smiled at her as he sipped his coffee. *"Dr. Zhivago!* Such a fine book. I am at the place where he has deserted the Red Army to look for his family, and he finds they have been deported to France. Such

problems he had. Yuri reminds me of another doctor with big troubles—
Max Gerson!" Gerson chuckled. "Margaret, don't worry, everything is
going well. I'm almost finished with *Dr. Zhivago,* and I'm happy to report
to the supervisor of husbands and authors that, in this month, *A Cancer
Therapy* is finished, no doubt! And the publisher is waiting this moment
for the manuscript."

He now began to flip the pages in the novel feverishly, apparently
looking for his place. Margaret just stood there in front of him with a
poignant look that spoke of years of quiet patience and fortitude. "You
stopped at page 235," she said. "You'll find a bookmark there." She
waited for him to find it.

"It's *not* a bookmark!" Gerson exclaimed, as he fingered an envelope
he found tucked between the pages. "It's a letter. Feels like a card!"
He raised his eyes, quizzically.

With a hint of sadness in her voice, Margaret said quietly, "Read it."

As Gerson picked up her vibes, his mood turned somber. He lifted
the flap of the envelope and drew out a card. As he slowly read the
message, tears welled in his eyes. He reached into his back pocket for a
handkerchief and blew his nose mightily as he swiped clumsily at his
eyes. Then coming from behind his desk, Gerson walked over to Margaret
and took her in his arms.

"I forgot," Gerson apologized. "I always forget, don't I? I'm sorry.
Please forgive your old dog, who never changes." He paused a moment,
lifted her chin, then kissed her. His voice choked a little as he said,
"Happy St. Valentine's Day."

⊱ ⊰

A Cancer Therapy was completed and published in 1958.

⊱ ⊰

Mr. S. J. Hought, a reporter who had interviewed Gerson the year
before, and who had grown to respect him, was remarking upon one of
Gerson's patients: "I remembered the case of the woman crippled by
arthritis for so many years, semiparalyzed, who had been brought to
Dr. Gerson after the long orthodox treatments had failed. Within three
weeks she was able to move her toes and fingers. Later, she returned to
the clinic in Baltimore and told her doctor what had happened. 'I suppose
you disapprove,' she said.

"His answer was startling. 'Not only do I *not* disapprove, *but I am
not surprised at the results. That man will probably not live to see it, but
they will be erecting monuments to him.* At the moment, however, he is a
thorn in their side.' "

On March 9, 1959, Mr. Hought sat at his breakfast, reading his morning paper, when he was stunned by the newspaper type, which fairly leaped out at him:

"DR. MAX GERSON, 77, CANCER SPECIALIST" was the heading. It was an obituary, which read: "Dr. Max Gerson, a specialist in the treatment of cancer and tuberculosis, died of pneumonia yesterday in his home. . . ."

A passage from John 14:2 occurred to him:

"In my Father's house, there are many mansions. If it were not so, I would have told you. I go to prepare a place for you."

There must be one mansion for Dr. Max Gerson, he thought.

THE LEGACY—THE WORK OF CHARLOTTE GERSON STRAUS

It would be difficult to find greater dedication or greater loyalty and devotion than that displayed by Charlotte Gerson Straus to the cause of her father, Dr. Max Gerson. Yet, despite her prodigious efforts to bring the Gerson message to the American people—through lecture programs and the publication and distribution of his books and literature—it often seems that for the magnitude and urgency of the problem, progress remains painfully slow.

Although there are some medical doctors in America who might be strongly moved to attempt Dr. Gerson's therapy under favorable conditions, there are none today who dare risk the consequential displeasure of the orthodox medical community. The situation is patently fraught with risk, not only the possibility of ostracism by one's peers, but also the hazard of malpractice suits in the event a patient or his family were dissatisfied with the results. Being, after all, a treatment procedure contrary to accepted medical mode, the errant physician would be easy prey for devastating damage claims.

In the face of this reality, Charlotte Gerson Straus (the last surviving member of the Gerson family), with dedicated abandon—and confronted more with alternatives than with options—finally decided on a path of least resistance. Or July 20, 1977 she opened the first Gerson Therapy Center, not in America, but in Mexico, six miles south of Tijuana. Last reports indicated that three medical doctors are in attendance.

She and Mr. Norman Fritz, her close associate, are providing guidance to the Medical Director and his staff at the clinic and assisting in their training in Gerson methods. Beyond doubt, Charlotte Gerson Straus is deeply knowledgeable on the subject of her father's therapy, as is Norman Fritz, a longtime pioneer in the field of nontoxic cancer treatment.

The center is a simple, austere, starkly appointed facility—no X-ray services, no laboratory facilities, no surgical or intensive care capability. And yet, withal, Charlotte claims remarkable results even in the short period they have been in operation. She maintains that even during a brief stay at the center, improvement is already evident, with a healing reaction noticeable between the fifth and eighth day after initiation of the therapy. For any permanent healing to be accomplished, however, the intensive nutritional and detoxification programs must be continued over a long term, often one to two years or more. A minimum stay of three to four weeks is recommended to allow time for patients to learn the methods and to observe improvement in themselves, in order to give them hope and inspiration to continue when they leave the center and return home.

Perhaps, the gravest weakness from which the clinic suffers—besides its lack of diagnostic and monitoring tools and capabilities—is its inability to follow up patients who leave the clinic after their indoctrination period. So, despite intrepid efforts and ofttimes impressive early results, regretfully, what is being accomplished cannot be validated under scientifically and medically acceptable standards and criteria.

The solution, quite clearly, is to establish a prototype clinic in the United States—with official sanction—so that adequately supportive medical facilities and a full, professional staff is available to carry out the therapy, document case histories, and follow up on a long-term basis; thus, convincing proof can be generated over a sufficient period of time to establish the validity and merit of this treatment modality.

Charlotte Gerson Straus deserves high praise for her valiant and devoted service. It is to be hoped that she may one day realize her dream of working in a fully equipped, fully staffed, modern clinic in America—where every necessary facility will be extended—as fitting tribute to her heroic efforts in the cause of healing and as exemplified by the life and works of her father, Dr. Max Gerson.

Part 3
Paths of Glory

18

Commonalities in Therapy

Thus far in our treatise, we have reviewed the challenging work of Dr. Josef Issels of the Ringberg-Klinik in the Tegernsee, Bavaria—with his whole-man concept, Ganzheitstherapie; of the Lukas-Klinik in Arlesheim, Switzerland, under the perceptive guidance and direction of Dr. Rita Leroi, following the precepts and methods of Rudolf Steiner's Anthroposophical or Spiritual Medicine; and, lastly, the bright flame of Dr. Max Gerson's illuminating genius, with his fundamentally nutritional approach to the clinical treatment of the malignant condition.

These three stalwarts were chosen from an imposing array of pioneers —all pleading for attention, as they toiled mightily in every corner and crevice of the world's healing establishment. Literally thousands of such native sons—men and women of pristine integrity were—and continue today—fighting sporadic front-line battles against heavy odds. They have challenged this paralyzing terror of all diseases, using a diversity of agents and modalities with varying degrees of success.

It was not easy to select just three from these awesome ranks—to omit many valiant contributions. Our viable rationale was that many had already won their laurels among their peers, and in the public domain. To avoid a work of unmanageable proportions, time and space clamored to leaven evaluation and selection. Also, reasonable judgment desperately searched for a sharp focus—on the forest, not the trees—no matter how noble and diverting these constituents might be. In the last analysis, we felt that nothing should compromise the clarity of our purpose: to present a challenging and meaningful document on the problem of cancer in our time, demonstrating the inviolable integrity of nature, man, and the universe. Total concentration on essentials was crucial, so as not to diffuse our theme, or the character or quality of our thrust.

A miscellany of more and more doctors—with assorted and diverse therapies—would not, we felt, add integral breadth or depth to our theme or purpose.

During the ongoing analytical process, we fell heir to a windfall. As we had suspected from the beginning, commonalities began to reveal themselves like precious jewels in a crown. Illuminating certain conceptual bases, we discovered common roots in the family tree—which nurtured the main trunk. This fallout of rich fringe benefits gave added meaning to our work in its broadest sense, and helped, further, to support the validity of our choices, assuring us that the stars were still in their heavens.

What became abundantly clear in the philosophical dimension was that Issels, Gerson, and Leroi had joined that great Builder of the bridge, helping to form and raise the healing structure on which countless others before them had labored in an endless procession of time and tide.

Today, our society has accrued a discordant amorphous entity, the specialist, who survives remarkably well behind an easily defensible Chinese Wall, proving that a certain kind of success attends exploitation of the microcosmic. Some resemble the ferretlike creatures who scampered unnoticed among the heavy-footed, myopic mammals of the Eocene Period. Like this mite-sized predator, which survived eons of harsh geological change, the specialist in today's medical world has, tragically, upstaged the lumbering generalist, who has so much more in common with that rare breed, the holistic physician, who not only subscribes intellectually to the theory—but also transmutes this postulate into a full-scale thera-peutic system, which excludes no agent or method from the possibility of application within the healing spectrum.

Yet our noble trinity, Issels, Gerson and Leroi, despite frustrating barricades erected by frenetic specialists in all the medical disciplines, have been able to overrun their positions, and to stand on the peak of the mountain, viewing the panorama of wholeness that stretches before them. All three followed a unified holistic theory, Issels calling it Ganz-heitstherapie; Gerson, the Systemic Approach; and Leroi, Spiritual En-largement of Medicine. Each placed varying degrees of emphasis upon certain components of the regime. Like climbers on the ascent, although each took slightly different paths, all reached the same top of the mountain.

Each one of these heroic figures imparts a dynamic presence to the physician-patient relationship: Dr. Josef Issels is remindful of the youthful David venturing into a no-man's-land between two mighty armies, and defying the Philistine Goliath—exposed, and apparently defenseless—except for a quite laughable, harmless-looking slingshot. Dr. Rita Leroi moves unobtrusively among her "children" at the Lukas-Klinik, like a living figure of "Our Lady," the Mother of all mankind, healing—as it were—by her mere presence, or the touch of her garment. As for Dr. Max Gerson, noble and serene, he towers above the medical landscape like an Easter Island monolith. Giants all, they have in their own way, challenged the mechanism, the dogma, and the rote of fossilized orthodoxy, and, with total devotion, applied their minds, hearts, and souls to fashion the supports of the science of true healing medicine.

It will become increasingly clear that they, separately, achieved a startling congruence of medical architectural form, reinforced by the structural timbers of comparable primal elements, which permitted them to come effectively to grips with the problem of malignancy in our time.

So, let us now have a close look at the "paths"—to uncover, if we can, the common denominators, and the differences, with respect to the therapeutic agents and measures used; and, also, the cast of their particular emphasis, so that we, too, may have a view from the top of the mountain.

}⊱ ⊰{

In our previous discussion of the traditional methods, surgery, radiotherapy, and chemotherapy, the weaknesses of a system centered in purely physio-chemical modalities have been clearly pointed out. In the same orthodox community, in contemplating the awesome vacuum in psychological implementation and spiritual support, the archaic structure positively groans in torment at its own derelictions. It becomes drearily repetitive to reiterate the sine qua non: that it is in the nature of the beast—symptomatic medicine—to ignore the whole person, and to address itself only to what is clinically evident and measurable.

We propose now to venture into a delineation, on a comparative basis, of the commonalities present in the three regimes we have chosen to illustrate, and the degree of emphasis given by each. Some differences will also be noted in the use of varying therapeutic agents and methods, but these differences are considered as wholly overshadowed and sublimated by the accent of the prime thrust—holistic therapy—which forms the precious inner core of each treatment method. For purposes of clarity, and organization of the material, we shall discuss each major factor in the three modalities separately, making our comparisons accordingly.

It is hoped that this evaluation will provide a clear and comprehensive overview of all relevant and vital elements inherent in each, result in a leavening of the differences, and achieve a harmony of the parts. Our bottom-line objective is to convey an accurate, unmistakable picture of the cancer problem today, and to permit the professional and lay reader alike to exorcise the pettifoggery and mumbo jumbo of today's dismally confusing mélange, thereby establishing a positive understanding and informed position based upon hard facts.

Alongside our three notable physicians and their good works, it would seem wholly redundant at this juncture to interpose analogous data of the orthodox establishment. We feel that the defects of commission and omission present in accepted medical practice will become glaringly apparent from our comparative discussion of the therapies of Issels, Gerson, and Leroi.

PRIMARY THERAPEUTIC METHODS

DR. JOSEF ISSELS

Dr. Josef Issels's central focus was a head-on course on the causal front, attacking the tumor, tumor sites and systems, with his aim and trajectory compensated or corrected, as necessary, by a close resonance with accompanying diagnostic and testing measures. His greatest reliance was placed on the intuitive powers of observation of the human frame, and on intimate daily contacts with his patients. He remained always on full alert, so that he could respond promptly to expected and unexpected reactions and developments, and chart a new course with applicable remedies in the healing process. Each subtle nuance of the patient's condition prodded his searching mind, supplicating constantly for any agent or method that could alter the pathology for the better.

This attitude resulted in accruing a number of unusual vaccines and techniques, such as haematogenic oxidation therapy (H.O.T.); ultraviolet irradiation of the blood; autohormone therapy (ultra-short wave); pyreto-therapy (fever treatment), and so forth. Issels incorporated in his regime a great variety of alternative therapeutics and methods, which he used with his fine physician's sense of discrimination. His medical arsenal encompassed a greater diversification of primary medicaments than either Gerson's or Leroi's, and it is precisely this expansive range of possibilities in the treatment process that brings into immediate focus the crucial problem, typical of such a versatile genius, and that is the extreme diffi-culty of compiling a precisely integrated and meaningful doctrine of medical practice. Hair-trigger decisions are constantly demanded on a dynamic battlefield where the enemy is so formidable and unrelenting as terminal cancer, and where death clings constantly to one's elbow. The clinical labyrinth, under these circumstances, and the dynamics of the variables become particularly challenging as more and more medicaments are added to the physician's pharmacopoeia. It becomes obvious, too, that, as one introduces more variables into the equation, the probability of error grows.

The medical sector of Issels's regime is an originally conceived and personally tailored one, which demands great force of character and will, absolute confidence, and the resoluteness to stay on course without wavering, in the face of disappointments and failures. And these are the very qualities of the personality that are markedly evident in Dr. Josef Issels. But, regrettably, it is also this very consonance of traits that makes it difficult to follow in his footsteps. Dr. Issels himself admits that it would take years of practical experience for another physician to absorb and apply his modality with the same perception and results. This refers, in specific, to the selection of the precise agent and methods, or combination of agents and methods, and the extremely important matter of timing.

The experienced medical doctor, especially the practicing oncologist, has usually already found a comfortable niche early in his career, and is quite content with an expectable flourishing practice. He is hardly likely to be drawn into new directions and paths. In the reality, too, Issels has found it difficult to draw many such associates into his vortex. There is little appeal in joining a front-line unit whose commander is a battle-scarred veteran, under perpetual fire, and who clearly shows the fresh wounds of the warrior forever in the field.

The young intern, likewise, even from premed days, has already made solid plans for his future. As a fledgling, he is understandably fearful of venturing onto unfamiliar and threatening terrain—to take up a position alongside a medical maverick whose ship of state seems perpetually oppressed and battered by mountainous seas of the entrenched opposition.

The answer appears to lie in organizing Dr. Issel's diagnostic procedures, therapeutic constituents, and methods and modalities into a viable system—and then into an effective working manual of clinical practice. Translating whole-body treatment into an integrated system should help establish its validity as a scientific approach, leading eventually to its ultimate refinement through extensive clinical application.

Moved by a burning desire to make this possibility a reality on the broadest possible level, Dr. Issels has already accomplished much in this direction—through his exhaustive writing of books, papers, and lectures on the subject. These easily furnish the requisite scientific and medical detail for the preparation of a practical and acceptable curriculum for teaching Ganzheitstherapie in medical universities throughout the world.

Dr. Max Gerson

Dr. Max Gerson's regime, as we have seen, was categorically nutritional. His deepest perceptions were anchored in the certain conviction that the best sustenance for the ailing body was the food that Mother Earth supplied her children. As written in Genesis: ". . . every earth bearing seed shall be for meat." Every fiber of his being responded to the summons. Both in the laboratory and in the crucible of clinical practice, his lifelong research of almost sixty years—and on two major continents—served only to confirm that there was no substitute for this ultimate of fiats.

In the case of Issels, nutritional support, though very important, played a secondary role to his medicaments and other therapeutic measures. In Gerson's case, whatever he added to the dietary program was designed to reinforce the pressing metabolic necessities that the food itself could not supply. In other words, where functional weakness or failure handicapped the organism's powers of digestion and assimilation of critically requisite nutritional elements, Gerson's first response was to introduce those foods and substances that could supply the missing elements and/or required energies and healing forces. Initially, these might act as a stimulant to charge up the failing batteries, but in due course the body's own strengthened systems would take over and carry on, discarding the incidental medical inputs—just as the astronaut jettisons his empty fuel tanks, or the construction engineer, his scaffolding.

For example, the administration of the potassium solution was to help replenish the potassium missing from the cellular component, nudging out the imbalancing excess of sodium. Potassium-rich vegetables, fruits, and grains helped this activity. In its turn, the liver juice gave a high degree of potency to the crying need for oxidizing enzymes, as did the fresh fruit and vegetable juices. Acting with gentle persuasion, these constituents presented the body with a variety of nutritious foods and substances, in a particular form and concentration, easily acceptable and immediately utilizable by the ailing body. All of these agents complied with Hippocrates' ancient dictum: "Do no harm." None caused pain or suffering; rather the opposite. As in the administration of coffee enemas (part of Gerson's detoxification program), agonizing pain was eliminated in the majority of the cases, where, previously, the strongest pain-killing drugs, like morphine, had been routinely used.

By any standard, none of the agents used by Gerson could be put in the same category as the cytotoxic drugs, such as cyclophosphamide, fluorouracil (5FU), methotrexate, and others, administered in a standard chemotherapeutic course. Out of all the "hard" therapeutics that Gerson administered, the few that might remotely approximate drugs, per se, were lugol, liver and thyroid extract, pancreatin, acidol pepsin, ox bile and potassium solution—although, even here, their classification as vitamins or supplements could sit more reasonably. All were administered as transitional agents, being simply higher potencies of normal food substances, designed to make up, as quickly as possible, life-threatening nutritional deficiencies. The liver injections, for example, were a concentrated extract providing that extra thrust to the liver, so vital to the cancer patient in the early crisis stage of his treatment.

Compare these mild measures with the harsh, cell-damaging drugs of orthodox medical practice; with the cruel assault of deforming radical surgery; or with irradiation damage to the cellular system and, not uncommonly, to the organism as a whole, including the suppression or erosion of its immunological defenses; and Gerson's tender loving care remains, by far, the treatment of choice.

Using the idea of parallel lines to illustrate the interface of Gerson's nutritional regime with his modest use of gentle pharmaceutical potions (almost all nutritional—or nutritionally related), the powerful thrust of nutrition is seen from the very start. This is ascendant throughout the treatment period, and, as the patient progresses, there is a falling off of the "medical" components, until finally only the nutritional regime remains—at that point where the patient has overcome the malignant condition and is rounding third base, headed for home plate. He has left far behind the foreboding environs of the dark forest, and emerged into the radiant sunshine on the plateau of good health.

In contrast, Dr. Issels's treatment shows a consistent heavy reliance upon specified drugs, vaccines, and physio-biological methods such as H.O.T., and pyretotherapy. From the very start, these would dominate the therapeutic process, even into the postclinical stage, when the patient was usually returned to the care of his own physician, with comprehensive instructions from Dr. Issels regarding postclinical medical care. Nutrition would play an accompanying important but subordinate role in his treatment, because Issels is diligently bent upon first eliminating the tumor and the malignant systems. This does not derogate the effectiveness of Issels's approach. It would be a grievous error to read such an assumption into Ganzheitstherapie, his whole-man treatment, because certain components of Issels's unified approach act as vital mechanisms to stimulate, strengthen, and restore the body's defenses, just as do certain nutritional components in Max Gerson's regime. Although not to be considered as exact equivalents, the blood oxidation treatment (H.O.T.), for example, as used by Issels, purifies and regenerates the blood on the cellular level, contributing to the rejuvenation of the body's biological systems. Issels might easily claim that his specified therapeutic measures are highly compatible with Gerson's use of fruit and vegetable juices, liver extracts, potassium and iodine, with either modality furnishing restorative, cell-nourishing nutrients and oxidizing enzymes—or their equivalent activities—and aiding in the elimination of the toxic materials, thus restoring the cellular balance. There being no substitute for victory, Issels's record stands honorably alongside Gerson's, an exciting challenge in the face of the dismal results of treatment of terminal cancer by orthodox means.

DR. RITA LEROI—THE LUKAS-KLINIK

As for the Lukas-Klinik's regime, this is somewhat closer to the Gerson imprint. Dr. Rita Leroi uses one primary medical agent—Iscador, a derivative of the mistletoe plant, with some occasional homeopathic remedies in mild form. Spanning several decades of administration by hundreds of medical doctors (especially throughout Europe), with extensive clinical experience in thousands of cases, Iscador has proven itself miraculously effective, completely nontoxic, and free of all side effects—a claim impossible to make for a single one of the harsh drugs from the chemotherapeutic arsenal of the orthodox cancer fighters. Working on biological rehabilitation, not only does Iscador act to eliminate the malignant cell structures throughout the body—harming no healthy cell—but at one and the same time its double-barreled activity also resurrects the body's natural healing powers, initiating a reversal of the malignant process. Yet this startling but proven premise today remains unacceptable to most leading oncologists and scientific researchers of the medical establishment.

In view of Iscador's highly satisfying results, orthodox therapeutics occupy a distinctly minor place in Dr. Leroi's naturally oriented modality. The Lukas-Klinik does not oppose surgery, nor does it, in a particular crisis situation, resist mediation by other orthodox methods and techniques. Such use, however, is so minimal, on the average, as to be considered rare.

Very special emphasis is given by the clinic to a well-balanced, optimally nutritious diet. Vegetables, grains, fruits, herbs, even flowers and the leaves of plants are incorporated in the regime, cultivated and grown in accordance with the science of Biodynamic Agriculture, which antedates—and surpasses—in any comparable thrust, even the early American pioneers in this area. This is a holistic system of soil science developed and perfected in 1924 by the versatile and gifted Rudolf Steiner, whose Anthroposophical teachings, as we have seen, laid the foundations for the impressive cancer work of the Lukas-Klinik.

Biodynamic farming addresses itself to the quality of wholeness in the plant kingdom, taking into consideration methods of manuring, cultivation of the soil, observance of cosmic rhythms, the interrelationships of farm and environment, and so on. "It is the aim of biodynamic production to bring to optimal development the potentialities of grain, vegetable or fruit in all their wholeness. A rational approach to nutrition based on spiritual science requires a concept of quality gained from the totality of the nutrient plants." It is not a stereotyped system, but a unified approach to agriculture that relates the ecology of the earth organism to that of the entire cosmos. The spiritual-scientific methods incorporated employ the selfsame principle of totality in ministering after Nature's precious soil as we have seen applied to humans through Ganzheitstherapie. Between the soil and the plant's roots, the methods and material employed in the biodynamic system build a living bridge of bacteria, fungi, worms and other organisms, which nourish Mother Earth. Here, too, the revealing discovery was that, in the control of plant disease, this form of cultivation supplies invigorating, health-gi. nutrients, remindful of the healing therapeutic agents that compose the medical regimes of Gerson, Issels, and Leroi. Biodynamic cultivation abhors the use of pesticides, herbicides, and chemical fertilizers, which do fundamental damage to the soil and its products, much as harmful drugs and medical practices abuse the human body.

Dr. Leroi, in describing some components of the Lukas-Klinik's dietary program, indicates that "we have a wide choice of cereals which, ripened by the sun, are rich in strengthening proteins and carbohydrates. We add salads and fresh vegetables which have been cultivated biodynamically. Roots activate the brain and thinking capacity, flowers stimulate the metabolism, and leaves are especially effective in stimulating the rhythmic system. Products of sour milk, such as yogurt and different types of light cheese, dark bread and fruit juices complete our meals. Honey or pear-syrup is used for sweetening. Fats such as olive and sunflower oils and some butter are used; we avoid artificially hardened fats like margarine. For seasoning we use herbs in great variety. Tomatoes do not appear in our vegetable list, as they are proliferating nightshade plants and unsuitable for cancer patients."

If we were to illustrate here again, with parallels, the course of treatment of the Lukas-Klinik, Iscador, the principal agent, would be the strong continuous line on our chart, with the nutritional regime closely paralleling its "medical" regime.

At its very heart, the science of Anthroposophical medicine practiced at the Lukas-Klinik breathes compassion. Its pulse can be felt in every room and corridor, and in the soft cheerful sound of friendly voices everywhere, literally beating: "Do-no-harm" . . . "Do-no-harm" . . . "Do-no-harm"!

SUMMARY

Without the reconstitution of the metabolism through the underlying biological dynamics of nutrition, the restoration of good health becomes formidable, with the hopeless prognosis difficult to refute. *With* nutrition as a full-time partner in the healing program, the dismal prospect can be altered. At the invisible atomic level, phenomenal activity is taking place in a mysterious universe of madly whirling galaxies, in a new frenzy of excitement and anticipation. When they are aroused from their toxic stupor, we can observe, at the cellular level, the individual cell structures losing their harmful fluids, constituents, and tendencies— and going through a process of reformation. The innate creature intelligence has been reawakened and asserts itself once again, with a fresh sense of hope and purpose, and a strengthening of its capability of differentiation. With renewed vigor it moves to commandeer the helm of the ship

ain steer a course to better health and recovery. Imbalancing
odium, which has been trespassing on the body's vital pre-
dispossessed, and in its place is a welcome flow of potassium
rich nutritional elements that help to create a stable, normal
cell, and to outlaw the neurotic and pathological cellular condition.

PSYCHOLOGICAL AND SPIRITUAL FACTORS
IN THE THERAPEUTIC SITUATION

Having discussed the commonalities of the primary therapeutic agents
and methods used by Drs. Josef Issels, Max Gerson, and Rita Leroi, we
now approach the direct heart of the therapeutic spectrum: the area of
the mind, where the psychological and spiritual factors lay claim to
seniority in the successful treatment of the cancer patient. These factors
lend coherence to the healing ferment, adding a critical quality of integrity
to the entire modality—a mucilage that binds together all of the parts.
One is reminded of Genesis, and the essential ingredient—the breath of
life—that transformed a piece of lifeless clay into a living soul.

Before venturing into the common denominators present in the psychological and spiritual content of each of the therapeutic programs
under purview, we ask here for an allowance of a moment or two to
touch base with the state of the science today in the scientific and
medical world. This seeming diversion has, in fact, a point: to examine
the impact of the mental and emotional content of the psyche upon the
physiology; the response of the human body to the skilled ministration
by the practitioner who understands their activities and influences, and
who can introduce such elements into the clinical situation as will
ameliorate the pathology and, in due course, stabilize the biological
systems, reestablishing a normal, healthy metabolism.

At the same time, as we examine the empirical basis for the belief
systems of the medical establishment, we can more readily perceive and
evaluate the whole-person treatment used by our three pioneer physicians who labor mightily in the Lord's vineyard of healing, as they
work with terminal cancer patients on the psycho-spiritual frontiers.

To all who are seriously involved in the healing arts—and who deign
to contemplate more than their navels—the mental, emotional, and
psychological factors in disease are no longer theoretical abstractions,
but have solidified into a body of medical belief systems and clinical
practice. The rigid skeptic, whether psychologist, psychiatrist or medical
doctor, may peremptorily dismiss miracles attributed to mystical forces
and entities, but he can no longer reject the accumulated empirical
evidence that confirms that worry, fear, and anxiety cause tension and
stress that adversely affect the human condition.

Dr. Roy W. Menninger, President of the Menninger Foundation, and a member of the Task Force on Prevention (part of the President's Commission on Mental Health), says that "between ten and fifteen percent of the people have serious mental illnesses today. If you add those who are adversely affected, from time to time, by what I term 'problems of living,' then as much as seventy percent of the population could be included—in other words, most of us." The "problems of living," Menninger says, can be "the tension resulting from marital or family discord, grief over the death of a loved one, troubles encountered on the job, difficulties in dealing with people, insecurity about one's state—these are the things that seem to bother most people. . . . Eighty percent of the complaints people take to their doctors are not physical ills, as much as they are psychosomatic reactions to problems of living. . . . Emotional tensions and anxiety contribute directly to the increasing incidence of serious illnesses. As people try to cope with new lifestyles, they often end up smoking, eating poorly, turning to alcohol or drugs. . . . Thus, although we have conquered such dreaded diseases as smallpox and polio, we are seeing more heart problems, cancer, accidents, strokes and lung disease—problems that can frequently be related to lifestyles."

In one hospital study reported by the American Medical Association—and this is not atypical—the one thousand patients examined had complained about a veritable supermarket basket full of physical symptoms, but only one out of six revealed actual presence of disease. More than eighty percent showed no detectable illness. Despite a full round of diagnostics with X rays, blood, urine, saliva, and other laboratory tests—even exploratory surgery—the results proved negative—*physically!*

Taking this a step further, into the metaphysical realm, we find thousands of serious investigators, and even some converts—many in the professional ranks—who genuinely believe that spiritual manifestations and influences can likewise affect the pathological condition. There is a growing respect for the Eastern mystiques of Yoga, Buddhism, Zen and—more recently in the West—the explosive Charismatic movement in the Christian community. Measurable effects of seemingly inexplicable phenomena are taking place on the physiological scale of observation.

According to *Newsweek* (May 1, 1978), "Seventy percent of Americans believe there is life after death, and sales of books describing near-death experiences, out-of-body flights and other psychic phenomena indicate that the public is hungry for almost any kind of proof. The scientific establishment remains stiffly skeptical, but some psychologists and psychiatrists are growing more willing to consider such phenomena."

Only a short decade ago, the West scoffed at acupuncture—a highly suspect Chinese import. Today, thousands of medical doctors, osteopaths and chiropractors employ it, with good effect. A few years ago, one hesitated to mention the subject of auras where one could be overheard.

Today, the auras of people, plants, animals, even minerals, can be confirmed by Kirlian photography; and their nature, characteristics and significance appraised—including medical implications.

Research is going forward at a frenetic pace on deeper and deeper levels—into far reaches of hypnotism, biofeedback, polarity therapy, extrasensory perception, and parapsychology. Science is only now beginning to give long-deserved attention and respect to the concepts embodied in the healing practices of the laughed-at mystics, gurus, and masters whose methods are firmly rooted in the great Eastern teachings of the Upanishads, the Vedas, and the Bhagavad-Gita, and reveal deep psychological wisdom. Schopenhauer praised the doctrinal basis of the Hindu religion for its "deep, original, and sublime thoughts," and said: "Access to the Vedas (through Western translations of the Upanishads) is in my eyes, the greatest privilege this century may claim over all previous centuries."

Striking an alliance with the mystics and healers of the East might still be termed questionable by the hard-case skeptic, who views all this through a glass darkly. But when the lives of hopeless cancer patients are being routinely extended, and they are being returned to a state of good health on a statistically significant basis, we are compelled to take proper note of these thought-provoking "miracles."

From the pen of Paramahansa Yogananda, in his great Yoga classic *The Autobiography of a Yogi,* comes a discussion of miracles: "A miracle is commonly considered to be an effect or event without law, or beyond law. But all events in our precisely adjusted universe are lawfully wrought and lawfully explicable. The so-called miraculous powers of a great master are a natural accompaniment to his exact understanding of subtle laws that operate in the inner cosmos of consciousness. Nothing may truly be said to be a 'miracle' except in the profound sense that everything is a miracle. That each of us is encased in an intricately organized body, and is set upon an earth whirling through space among the stars—is anything more commonplace? or more miraculous?

"Great prophets like Christ usually perform many miracles. Such masters have a large and difficult spiritual mission to execute for mankind; miraculously helping those in distress appears to be a part of that mission. Divine fiats are required against incurable diseases and insoluble human problems. When Christ was asked by the nobleman to heal his dying son at Capernaum, Jesus replied with wry humor: 'Except ye see signs and wonders, ye will not believe.' But he added: 'Go thy way; thy son liveth.' "

EDGAR CAYCE

While we are on the subject of seers, honorable mention is due here to America's own great mystic, Edgar Cayce. He was known as "The

Sleeping Prophet," because he always entered into a trance or auto-hypnotic state when clairvoyantly diagnosing and prescribing for patients —or when projecting a "life reading" (i.e., recalling the past and fore-casting the future), sometimes for patients thousands of miles away. In most cases he knew absolutely nothing about them, being given only their names and addresses—yet his diagnoses, prescriptions, and readings were remarkably effective and correct. During his lifetime, more than thirteen thousand stenographic transcriptions were made of every spoken word while in his trance state, making Edgar Cayce one of the most carefully documented psychics in the history of parapsychological research. All of these cases are now a matter of public record at the library of the Association for Research and Enlightenment at Virginia Beach, Virginia. These transcripts, encompassing scientific, theological, historical, pharmacological and other medical disciplines entirely foreign to his life on this planet Earth, transcended his meager education, knowledge—and even his comprehension in the *waking* state. From the hundreds of books and articles that have been written about this seer, we cull one modest extract that discusses healing:

> For all healing comes from the One Source. And whether there is application of food, exercise, medicine, or even the knife—it is to bring the consciousness of the forces within the body that aid in reproducing themselves (through) the awareness of Creative or God Forces. . . . All strength, all healing of every nature is the changing of the vibrations from within—the attuning of the divine within the living tissue of a body, to Creative Energies. This alone is healing; it is the attuning of the atomic structure of the living cellular force to its spiritual heritage.

Although he was almost completely without an education—he never got beyond the ninth grade—Cayce's esoteric but pungent prose is imbued with a strange quality. It arouses a haunting nostalgia, like the tantalizing sound of a remote temple gong, whose vibrations reach one from the inner recesses, stirring the mind with things once known, but long for-gotten, like the fragments of a dream hopelessly beyond recall. Cayce, many believe, could probe the depths of the great central intelligence file—known to mystics as the Akashic Record—and retrieve precious morsels of the eternal verities—seething with ideas and verifiable facts to shatter the equilibrium of even the most resolute closed mind.

KATHRYN KUHLMAN

In our own backyard in America are numerous luminaries deeply involved in the more controversial area of spiritual or divine healing, and this area, too, asks for consideration. Perhaps the most notable among these was the late Kathryn Kuhlman, an ordained minister, who for about two decades conducted healing services before audiences often numbering in the thousands. Other hundreds of thousands used to watch her weekly TV programs, listen to her twice-a-day broadcasts, and attend her Crusades and Rallies around the world. Uncounted healings took place, usually instantaneously, among the afflicted in her audience. Joyously tossing crutches, braces and spinal jackets into the air, the transported beneficiaries of these graces would come running on stage, literally flying up the platform steps to give their testimony.

In her books *I Believe in Miracles* and *God Can Do It Again*, Miss Kuhlman presents first-person accounts of perhaps fifty men and women, suffering from such appalling afflictions as multiple sclerosis, spinal disintegration, leukemia, hydrocephalus, and numerous cases of advanced cancer—where the patients were inoperable, and the malignancies had invaded lungs, liver, stomach, gallbladder, and pancreas—all cases considered hopeless by medical science, but who returned from healing meetings completely cured—most instantaneously—to amaze their own doctors and live new, joyful lives. A few examples: Mary Schmidt, who for thirty-six years suffered from a monstrous inoperable goiter. During a "Miracle Service," the sixteen-inch growth on her neck vanished instantly, never to return. Carey Reams, paralytic, and crippled World War I veteran, whose body had been shattered by a land mine in Luzon, the Philippines, walked away from services without his crutches, restored to full health. George Orr, who recovered perfectly the sight in an eye that had been splashed by molten steel, and literally cooked into a blinding mass of scar tissue; and Ronnie Crider, a little two-year-old, with a clubfoot (one of many such), who was healed perfectly by this "Power." All these cases are documented, and the medical records are available from the physicians and hospitals named in the reports.

Kathryn Kuhlman never claimed any personal powers. She believed that at the heart of her faith, prayers, and healings was the Holy Spirit, or the Power of the Trinity, and that "it is the same power that flows through our physical bodies today, healing and sanctifying."

Miss Kuhlman kept in close touch with Ronnie, the child with the clubfoot, as he grew to be a healthy young man. Her comments about Ronnie somewhat illumine the undercurrents of the phenomena that were taking place: "In all my experience I do not ever remember a child who was more conscious of the mercy of God in his healing; a youngster with a greater understanding of the spiritual truths; none more deeply grateful for two good legs and two good feet. It is as though God had anointed this child with a very definite insight into spiritual things when, in His tender mercy, He straightened the little clubfoot."

To Kathryn Kuhlman, the more profound result—more profound than the healings themselves—was the strengthening of faith, ties, and commitment to family, friends, and humanity by those who experienced or witnessed these healings.

THE CHRISTIAN MEDICAL FOUNDATION

As for the professionals themselves—the medical community—there is a strong groundswell among them too—radiating in all directions, and typifying the seething ferment that is taking place at the present time. Perhaps one of the best examples of an organization oriented in this direction is the Christian Medical Foundation, founded by Dr. William Standish Reed of Tampa, Florida. Dr. Reed is a cancer specialist who believes implicitly in the healing power of prayer. He says that "if a physician is to be a doctor of the whole man, and practice enlightened medicine, he cannot ignore the soul of the patient." Dr. Elmer Hess, while President of the American Medical Association, used stronger words to describe this imperative: "Show me a doctor who lacks faith, who denies the existence of the Supreme Being, and I'll say that he has no right to practice the healing art."

The Christian Medical Foundation has a large physician membership, and serves as a consulting center for patients with medical, psychological and spiritual problems, bringing medicine and Christianity into a wholesome partnership. Its membership comprises not only physicians and nurses, but professionals from diverse disciplines, as well as ministers and lay members of all faiths. Through the CMF, the healing message of the Gospel has reached thousands through counseling, evangelism, and the written word, and also through meetings and seminars at which medical doctors as well as the general membership share their clinical experiences, explaining how the theory has been put into successful practice in the treatment and healing of patients, even in difficult, and sometimes critical cases, underlying the desirability of reaching more and more practitioners in the future. The case of Karen Emmott will serve as a useful illustration of the therapeutic thrust of the CMF philosophy.

Some years ago, while speaking at a church in Oklahoma City, Dr. Reed stated that in God's eyes there were no hopeless cases. He was immediately challenged by a member of the congregation who explained the case of Karen Emmott, a fifteen-year-old girl, whose heart had stopped during a minor operation, but, by quick action on the part of the surgeon, was started again. However, brain damage resulted, and she remained in a comatose state, her functions being mechanically maintained: one tube emerged from her nose, another from her throat, a catheter in her bladder, and restraints on her arms and legs to prevent self-injury.

Dr. Reed was taken to Karen's bedside, and the first thing he suggested was prayer, asserting that, although the girl might not be mentally awake, she was spiritually awake. "We must not neglect the spiritual consciousness," he told her parents. "Bring Karen something pretty on your morning visits, comb her hair, talk to her about the day she will be coming home. No more despairing words in this room." And, of course, they all continued to pray, including the nursing staff.

Following Dr. Reed's counsel, her mother, Isabel, came each morning to the convalescent home (where Karen had been placed), bringing news from home, reports from school, stories of the funny things her baby brother did, and messages from her friends. She reported them as if Karen could understand every word. She prayed, too, both in Karen's presence and at home.

Day by day a gradual transformation could be observed, physically and mentally. Eventually intravenous feeding was discontinued as Karen began to eat. She also started to respond in other ways—and finally became completely conscious. She learned to speak, and began doing a few things for herself. The happy day came when she was taken home, where the entire family could now enthusiastically participate in helping her—teaching Karen new, simple tasks like putting on her socks and tying her shoes. Although not yet completely recovered, Karen was able to attend a special institution for the handicapped, doing her reading and arithmetic without difficulty, and acquiring better muscular coordination. She regained her lost weight, also, and at last report was the picture of health. "In time," Dr. Reed says, "patience, work, and faith will restore Karen to a useful life."

The case of Karen Emmott, and many others in comparable situations, warrants serious attention in applying these ideas to the treatment of difficult and even so-called "hopeless" cases, in such a way as to reach the deeper core of our being—those dimensions that lie, as yet, outside the parameters normally insisted on by precise scientific definition, and that are ignored by today's routine clinical modalities.

DR. O. CARL SIMONTON

On an independent basis, also, much work is being pioneered in the area of psychological therapy by many distinguished physicians, where the results being achieved can be appraised more readily by empirical standards. Dr. O. Carl Simonton, an internationally known oncologist, and Medical Director of the Cancer Counseling and Research Center in Fort Worth, Texas, is a leader in this area. He and his wife, Stephanie S. Simonton, are coauthors of an important paper entitled "Belief Systems and Management of the Emotional Aspects of Malignancy." In the *Journal of Transpersonal Psychology* (Vol. VII, No. 1, 1975), he is hailed as a pioneer "in the domain of mind-body communication, and getting remarkable results in cancer control by coupling visualization for physiological self-regulation with traditional radiology" (Simonton's speciality).

Dr. Simonton says that "there are over two hundred articles in medical literature which conclude that there is a relationship between malignancies and emotions and stress." He also asserts that the weight of medical evidence supports the conclusion that *there are predisposing psychological factors* in the development of *all* disease. With respect to the *cancer patient,* there is unanimity that these predisposing factors are (negative) personality characteristics such as:

(1) a great tendency to hold resentment and a marked inability to forgive;
(2) a tendency towards self-pity;
(3) a poor ability to develop and maintain meaningful, long-term relationships;
(4) a very poor self-image.

But behind these traits—which underline the cancer syndrome—is the psychological disorder due to rejection—feeling alone and deserted. Dr. Simonton says further that there are three belief systems characteristic of the personal, social, and medical milieu that need to be squarely addressed. The first is that of the patient's own self-image, which is usually very poor. The second is a relationship with his family, and the people who surround him, i.e., how meaningful this personal environment and communication system are; and, last, the belief system of the physician. "Most physicians," he states baldly, "are not aware of the fact that their thoughts about the treatment, and the patient's own ability, influence the outcome, but they most definitely do."

He had found that the correlation with improvement in the patient's condition is *"not with the severity of the disease,* but with the *patient's attitude*—which can influence the body's immune mechanisms."

In identifying those psychological factors that predispose the organism to disease and death, Dr. Simonton, as we have noted, declares that the most traumatic is the feeling of rejection. Under any circumstances, therefore, a vital aim of any successful program of cancer treatment must be to neutralize and overcome this morbid state of mind.

And what is the superlative antidote for rejection? Paul's message from I Corinthians, Chapter 13, tells us: "And though I speak with the tongues of men and of angels, and have not love, I am become as sounding brass, or a tinkling cymbal. . . . Love suffereth long and is kind. . . . Beareth all things, hopeth all things, endureth all things. . . . Love never faileth; but whether there be prophecies, they shall fail; whether there be tongues, they shall cease, whether there be knowledge, it shall vanish away. . . . And now abideth faith, hope and love, these three; *but the greatest of these is love."*

It is this heart-moving empathy for one's fellow creatures that brings forth those miracles that can and do occur in the enlightened doctor-patient relationship. Love is not a figurative abstraction that the ego lets drop casually from its ready stock of sage comments during an interlude at the monthly medical consortium. It is indeed the very beating heart of the therapy—which pumps lifesaving adrenalin into the patient's faltering system. Without this catalytic agent—the psychological transport system—the treatment will fail, no matter how brilliant its technological conceptualization and execution. A treatment without this quality of humanism cannot rescue the despondent patient from his conviction of death.

Indeed, like a living Christ, the wounded physician demonstrates his concern and involvement by suffering through the agonies of the patient. Every moment of every day his uplifting presence at the patient's bedside is actually manifest or strongly felt. The doctor's empathy literally envelops the patient in a protecting, heart-warming embrace. Such deep personal concern acts as a transforming influence. It may decisively influence the course of the disease, often rousing the first faint glimmer of hope in the patient, and surprisingly change for the better the attitudes of friends and family, who, along with the patient, have long since given up all hope.

Such dedication is of a highly idealistic and spiritual order. It exemplifies that quality of nobility of which saints are made, and is always characteristic of the divinely guided soul who realizes intuitively the eternal bond of body, mind, and spirit.

The three medical pioneers, Josef Issels, Max Gerson, and Rita Leroi, whose work we have discussed at length, shared these common qualities. For them, it was always there: a driving force in their lives, cultured by intuitive understanding and appreciation of its potential. As an instrument responds to the touch of its musician, they responded to humanity—the inner beauty of a sick, needy mortal—as naturally as we all do to the beauty of the flowers and the stars. Each arrived at the same destination—though from different starting points. There are others who can and do grow gradually into such an awareness—which may then turn into commitment through an intensity of desire; some by experiencing the trauma of the privation and death of a brave soul, which deeply stirs their inner being and transcends the imprisoning fetters of professional obloquy and protective callousness, demanding retribution from an awakened consciousness and conscience.

Over the years, the daily dramas and tragedies have played out their scenarios on the motion picture screen of their minds as if, throughout, they have been part of a dispassionate audience—far removed from the battlefield of fear, anguish, and mortality. But, suddenly, the drama becomes real as one actor steps from the screen and touches his heart with a soul-stirring message of their common fragility and divinity. It is an act of grace that has finally brought, to the doorstep of the stranger, a friend whom he finally recognizes and invites into his house. The Good Samaritan has now joined the ranks of the wounded physicians.

So, from now on, like our three bright spirits, Drs. Issels, Gerson and Leroi, there is an upward sweep of their eyes to new horizons, a buoyant step in their journey, a grandeur in their visions. All have arrived at the top of the mountain, where, in a sweeping view of 360°, the sum of the parts is revealed to them in the harmony of the whole: body, mind, and spirit. These three bright souls were brought early to that awareness and faith that moves mountains—that showed them how to combine all components into a total therapeutic regime. They realized the linkage of the human and cosmic scales, and knew how to understand and comply with the requirements of the whole law that governs the human condition. As Edgar Cayce put it, they found the means by which they could attune "the atomic structure of the living cellular forces to its spiritual heritage."

And so, finally, we come to the master key. Let us see how these wounded physicians, attuned to the psychological and spiritual factors in the pathological condition, applied the doctrinaire material to the realities of the doctor-patient relationship to overcome psychological problems, especially the one of rejection, through the dynamics of a living partnership with their patients in the clinical environment.

We have termed these factors "Psychological Support" and "Spiritual Reinforcement," and now turn to observe how skillful clinical management results in the improvement of the physical condition and in the acceleration of the healing process; how the body responds to the play of these mentally bound elements upon the patient's physiology. We may then note how these sensitive human beings have engineered subtle psychological and metaphysical premises down to the ground, and created an ambience in the everyday clinical environment through this intimate partnership, which can initiate a reversal of the pathological process.

PSYCHOLOGICAL SUPPORT AND SPIRITUAL REINFORCEMENT

DR. MAX GERSON

How much more can be said about rejection? About the loss of a loved one? About other serious trauma and influences affecting health that are nurtured in the obscure chambers of the mind? Let us see, now, how Dr. Max Gerson came to grips with this problem.

As we know, Gerson worked virtually alone in his office and at his clinic, practically without professional help, except for a nurse or two. His clinic was austere, with no spacious grounds or other special accommodations. Under these straitened conditions, when it is considered that ninety percent of his patients were in the last extremity, sometimes moribund when brought in, his success becomes the more remarkable. The importunities of these circumstances compelled him to be all things to all people: doctor, friend, comforter, and father confessor. Yet his heart was always big enough to respond to the necessities of his sick "children" with a ready smile, a story—or some little witticism sparked by the inspiration of the moment.

With respect to the psychological milieu, Gerson sums it up in his simple comment: "The mental condition of the patient and the psychological cooperation of the family and the environment play important roles in the restoration of the body. Every patient needs faith, love, hope and encouragement. To accomplish this difficult task, the patient has to see progress in himself, and favorable results on others."

As for faith—Gerson, along with Dr. Josef Issels, could well say, "My work is my prayer." His courage never faltered, though he stood with his patients always at the threshold of that grim, dark door. He exuded a quiet resoluteness and confidence that provided the sick and the hapless with strong shoulders upon which they could lean, until their storm-tossed craft could once again anchor in safe harbor and take on new "stores," to gather strength in this friendly haven for the voyage home.

As for hope—it shone from his eyes, and blossomed under his tender hands and gently probing fingers. There was no greater tonic for the spirit than the encouragement he radiated in unlimited abundance. It was ever present in his ready smile and in those sparkling blue eyes, which belied his so-serious brow. And what greater hope and renewal could there be for man or woman than the reality? Tumors seemed almost to melt away under his very fingers, and the patients' state of well-being improved accordingly.

And then, when the pain vanished, they began to notice things forgotten. Common things—all of which, likewise, bolstered their faltering spirits. For example, they began to savor the little joys that had been blocked out by misery and travail. The air had a special fragrance— it smelled fresher and sweeter; they could recognize and appreciate the songs of birds again. There was a new awareness of the gladdening voices of people around them, especially the occasional happy sounds of the high-pitched chatter and joyous laughter of little children. Life, they rediscovered, was really worth living, after all.

But there were also tears that Gerson shed: for every patient who was not responding—for every patient who died; for he had, in the process, become part of them. Tears were shed many times for Johnny Gunther. The first time, they were tears of joy—when Johnny began to recover; then tears of remorse—when, against his better judgment, the doctors had prevailed upon him to administer hormone therapy for Johnny's eczema. And tears of self-recrimination when Johnny died. He felt guilty. Somehow, he should have saved him, despite the medical doctors.

Perhaps, above all, a deep despair, which haunted his nights, echoed down the corridors of time. It was filled with frightening sights and sounds. A train lurching suddenly to a stop in the small hours of morning; military uniforms and shouted commands. The picture branded on his heart was that of a young man, a Jew—kicked and trampled to death by the SS on a railroad siding in Germany on April Fool's Day, so many years ago.

It came as a recurring nightmare, disturbing his sleep, churning at his conscience, and strangely stirring his troubled mind. Often he was startled into wakefulness, to find himself breathing heavily, as if from strenuous exertion. He had discovered that he could still this gnawing restlessness and return to sleep only when he committed himself, again and again, to save more lives for the sake of that dead youth.

Lotte, Gerson's younger daughter, recognized this drive of her father's. She said: "In a way, he was giving people new life. I would say that his own life's energy depended on it. He got new life energy to be able to give life to others. It made him surmount all the obstacles, the personal attacks, and everything. You know, that was his great joy and satisfaction."

Gerson, himself, instinctively realized this. He was convinced of an energy exchange between himself and the patient, because he observed that his mere presence was often enough to elevate the patient's well-being, and to bring a glow to his own heart. In a man who did not practice any formal religion, somehow he knew that it was all related. He remembered ageless wisdom from the Bible to keep the body sound in health because it was the temple of the Holy Spirit.

As for love—Gerson exuded it from every pore. His hearty, bluff manner literally sang with good humor. He was something of an actor, and his occasional mock displeasure, accompanied by some jesting gambit with the patient, was enough to lighten any heart, no matter how heavy. Typical of the light he brought with him into the lives of people teetering on the edge of eternity were incidents such as the following, as he made his way through his daily rounds in the clinic:

With a pleasant smile, he stopped at one bed. "So . . . I hear you have a complaint about coffee enemas, Samuel! Is this true?"

"Complaint? What complaint? I *love* them. The nurse says every four hours. Why can't I get one every *two* hours? *That's* my complaint!"

Gerson took Samuel's pitifully wasted hands warmly in his own. "You're a rascal, Samuel," he chided, as he smiled hearteningly, "but you really feel better, don't you?"

Tears erupted like a torrent and ran down this sad man's drawn face. "Dr. Gerson," he choked, "I have no more pain." The words could scarcely come out. He buried his head unashamedly in Dr. Gerson's open arms. "No more pain!" He sobbed without restraint.

Gerson stopped at another bed. He spoke to Katherine—a patient with abdominal cancer. She was a sweet young housewife, who was sitting up in bed, quiet and slight, like a hummingbird. "Katherine," he spoofed, "don't make yourself so comfortable. One of these days, we'll chase you out of here. Only sick people are permitted to stay here, don't you know?"

Katherine reacted with an unbelieving look, and a tremulous kind of hope. "Do you really mean that, Dr. Gerson? But I don't really feel good. My head hurts terribly, and I feel so weak and depressed, with nausea all day!"

Patting her head, Gerson beamed his delight—and spoke encouragingly, "My dear, it's your good luck!" He placed her fingers at a spot on her abdomen. "Here, press down. What do you feel?"

Katherine gave a little scream of delight. "Oh, Dr. Gerson, I don't believe it! There's nothing there. The tumor—I can't feel it anymore! What happened?"

"Your 'flare-ups' are a sign of good reaction to the treatment. It's a little crisis you will go through occasionally as your whole condition improves. This we can expect during the treatment. Yes, the tumor is definitely going down. And that means, also, that other good things are happening in your body. Look, Katherine, I have a good idea for you: When your husband, Peter, comes today, you can give him a big surprise. If everything goes so well in the next two or three weeks, tell him he can buy you a new dress for your homecoming! Now wouldn't you like to have such a new dress to show your children how pretty their mother is when she goes home?"

As with Samuel, Gerson's saintly tenderness had an electrifying effect upon Katherine. It was as though a dark vault of lost hope—a steel cocoon of discouragement that had entombed her mind—was suddenly shattered, to let in cleansing, healing light. With Gerson's touching words, an uncontrollable torrent of hope surged through Katherine like an electric current, and she, too, broke down and cried with joy. It was Gerson's remarkable gift that he could—with a word, a thought—touch these humans so deeply they had to cry—since they could not get up and dance!

Gerson well knew, however, that the crisis was hardly over when a patient's condition improved sufficiently so that he could be sent home. "The practice of the treatment is a difficult task," he said. "The treatment in the hospital as well as in the home requires somebody's help all day long, particularly in advanced cases where a life is at stake and the patient is very weak.

"At the time of their leaving home, patients often had been given up by relatives, physicians and friends, none of whom had been able to offer any further advice. Upon their return, they suddenly find that everyone has contrary opinions to offer, criticizing components and preparation of the diet and suggestions 'to make it easier.' One patient, when friends and relatives began offering contradictory advice and suggestions, asked them whether these opinions ever helped a patient who had already been given up. This question put interfering persons in their place.

"It is not easy to stick to the treatment if the convalescing patient does not have enough help. The family has to give up some of the social life, and do this utilitarian work with deep devotion. The decline in our modern life is evident by lack of this devotion for the sick members of the family, but where affection and devotion in the family exist, all difficulties are disregarded for the sake of saving a life."

There were indeed other deeper implications in the terminal condition. In the midst of the trauma of dying, which enveloped the victim, his family, and others around them, profound changes were taking place. In many cases the imminent prospect of death had led the sufferer and his family to a soul-searching examination of their consciences. Guilt, and repressed emotions, sometimes festering for years in the subconscious, now surfaced. With the casting off of these corrosive inhibitions, hearts were reborn, pouring out their sealed contents of rancor and aggression; of old hurts and grievances; of negative attitudes, habits, and actions—a freeing of their true nature, and their very souls—before it was too late. Characteristic of this salutary process were contrition, confession, and penance, affecting all who were intimately involved.

Many were often led to a renewal of faith because of the living example of Max Gerson—who came as a stranger, but who, nevertheless, demonstrated that divine compassion and unconditional love of which Paul spoke. The patient himself, who started with resignation, and without hope, had accrued, in the crucible of this experience, a wisdom through that illumination that comes in the moment of truth, when one approaches the last door. The patients, too, could now see the real meaning of their lives, and its necessities; and how it should be lived in harmony with their loved ones, and with all humanity.

To husband or wife, sister or brother, the miracle of recovery was taken as a sign of intercession by divine providence. Through this transforming experience, prayer for many became a way of life. One startling realization ignited their inner core with the fire and force of a thunderbolt: that the life that was saved was their very own. It carried the enduring quality of revelation, and the change it made in them was forever.

Albert Schweitzer—a giant in his own right, whose cosmic mind embraced the universe—in one of those rare compliments that never come lightly from the tongues of the wise, said, "I see in Dr. Max Gerson one of the most eminent geniuses in medical history."

What more is there to say about Max Gerson?

DR. JOSEF ISSELS: "FIGHT FOR YOUR LIFE!"

"Remember, you were not born to be a patient. That is not your destiny in life. Most important is to fight against your illness and its causes. We provide you with experience, assistance, and the means necessary for this fight. Use them for yourself. Fight—as we do—for your life!"

In his "Dear Patient" letter, which welcomed patients to his clinic, Dr. Issels ended with this rallying cry to the colors: "Fight—as we do—for your life!" Above all else, Dr. Issels knew how imperative it was to enlist the patient as a full-time partner in the struggle for recovery. Forming a solid front with his charges, he boldly planted the standard of his fighting legion in the heart of enemy territory, determined neither to seek nor to grant any quarter. What greater stalwart would one want, to stand at his side against the Angel of Death, than this one? He was like the brave Horatius, who, at the narrow bridge that spanned the yellow Tiber at flood tide, with Spurius Lartius at his right and Herminius at his left—these three—held off the Tuscan legions—an army of a hundred thousand—casting his defiance into their very teeth!

The healing dynamics of this union, which Issels nurtured between himself and his patients, was attested in January 1971 by a visiting team of cancer specialists authorized to investigate the Ringberg-Klinik by the British Government's Department of Health and Social Security:

"The doctor-patient relationship here is very remarkable, Dr. Issels and his patient become partners in a venture to try and save the patient's life. He tells them everything, including the sites of primary and secondary tumors, promises nothing, but offers with confidence to do his best. The patients respond and appear to be inspired and impressed with it all. They take their own temperatures and pulses, chart their own fluid intake and output, and assess vomit and are responsible for fluid replacement. There is no doubt about their feeling for Dr. Issels, *amounting to devotion at times*. . . . Analgesic drugs are carefully charted and are used whenever they become necessary. . . . Undoubtedly, however, *the force of Dr. Issels's personality is such that analgesic drugs are required less often than they might be elsewhere. With a few exceptions patients seemed relaxed and none that we saw were asking for drugs*."

Also, on November 3, 1970, in a remarkable documentary film, the British Broadcasting Corporation described Issels's formidable salient into the defense systems of the cancer enemy. The BBC's production and writing staff grasped the essential nature of the conflict, and dramatically sounded its keynote with the title it chose for its broadcast: "Go Climb a Mountain." Instead of the lonely isolation of a social outcast—the common fate of cancer victims—Issels routed his patients out of their beds.

Hitherto stagnating in depressing cancer wards, waiting to die, they were now marshaled out in the winter, into the snow-clad countryside of the beautiful Tegernsee, and up and down the grassy slopes and mountains in the spring and summer. This was Issels's very special inspiration, coupled with the force of an electrifying personality. What he instinctively sensed and felt about needful measures did not always satisfy the pedant's fundamentalism and rote. It seemed altogether mad, but it worked!

If anything could be called a master key, this was it: a binding partnership, which transformed ingrown pessimism, gloom, and foreboding into an outgoing, reenergized human being. Instead of withdrawal from the world, the resurrected patients were precipitated, full force, into it. Rather than experiencing abandonment, they once again plunged into the mainstream by becoming members of a meaningful, purposeful social organism—the "Team." Togetherness, not rejection. The unheard-of staff-to-patient ratio of 1:2, which obtained at the Ringberg-Klinik, further underlined Dr. Issels's dedication, and exemplified the reinforcement of the psychological milieu within the total healing modality. Only a totally committed practitioner, altruistically motivated, with optimism and hope, could provide such intensive professional attention. A stranger, visiting the clinic and observing, especially, the outdoor activities, could not tell the staff apart from the patients—so closely welded had the relationship become. They were all in it together.

It was difficult to think of dying when you were throwing snowballs, or shouting with a new kind of happiness, above the sound of the wind! Or jumping madly up and down in sheer joy, with newfound hope—of living, not dying. "Go climb a mountain," Issels ordered—and they did!

That Man from Bavaria

Dr. Robert J. C. Harris, Head of the Department of Environmental Carcinogenesis at the Imperial Cancer Research Fund, on February 6, 1970, made some revealing comments to the senior members of the BBC production team that was collecting expert opinions on Issels and the Ringberg-Klinik, when asked to evaluate a bulky BBC dossier on Issels's methods and abstracted case histories:

"I have read the research documents prepared by you. His definition of terminal patients is accurate, the figures he gets are remarkable by any standards. . . . *I would suspect there's also just as much psychotherapy in his approach as anything else.* I mean, look at it this way: here you have cancer patients in the accepted terminal stage, who go along to this chap, having been told by their own doctors there's nothing more to be done for them, and he suddenly says to them that he's going to have a go—and he does have a go. There's no doubt about that. *I mean he seems to keep them on the trot from early morning till late in the evening.* Well, that induces a feeling that something is going to happen. And so probably he triggers off a will to live in them. And that's a jolly good thing. Being quite frank, probably not enough is being done for cases that are terminal. But in the end it's all a question of priorities: there just isn't the money, and of course the time, *to do what Issels does with cases of this sort.* More power to his elbow. Much more should be done for terminal cancer patients."

So spirit transcended matter, and, incredibly, now, instead of conceding to the enemy's ultimatum of total surrender, the patients began to set their own terms. Suddenly, in that invigorating view from the top of the mountain, they discovered *options*—instead of being confronted with stark alternatives. Issels had turned despair into hope, doubt into optimism—and, as it developed—defeat into victory.

The miraculous nature of such a transformation was rooted, beyond contention, in the psychic realm. This is nakedly apparent in the fact that these patients whom Issels inherited were the walking dead— iatrogenic disasters, wholly abandoned by the medical profession! The report of the visiting team of British experts (a group hardly enthralled with Issels's unorthodox methods) confirmed this, observing in their report the horror of criminal abuse and abandonment of these patients by their physicians. Here, in their own words, is their "holocaust" comment on just a few of these inhuman outrages:

"Dr. Issels receives some patients who have been shockingly mishandled medically as well as psychologically. Some of his patients seem to us to have been grossly overtreated by drugs or radiation, the treatment having been continued or repeated only to make matters worse when reactions had been mistaken for signs of tumour activity. His supportive regime, without cytotoxic drugs for the first weeks in most cases, allows time for partial recovery from some of these *therapeutic disasters.* We were astonished at some of the things with which he had been presented, and with which he was trying to cope: A previous amputation of a limb for osteogenic sarcoma of the femur through the midthigh, a patient moribund with mouth ulcers and gross debilitation from long continued excessive and unhelpful chemotherapy, bilateral mastectomy advised for duct papillomas which were not very numerous and were *only suspect—on doubtful grounds—of malignancy,* oedema and extensive fibrosis from excessive irradiation, and repeated stories of *abandonment* by doctors who had no hope or help of any kind to offer to their dying patients."

In contrast to such naked barbarism, Dr. Ralph Crawshaw, in his paper on "Humanism in Medicine—the Rudimentary Process" (*The New England Journal of Medicine,* December 18, 1975), sensitively discusses the essence of humanity: " . . . This important yet ephemeral concept, that the weak also matter, is hardly a conscious idea, let alone a belief. . . . These quivers of social awareness, that the other person, though weaker, has feelings and needs, may not last, but they are the green shoots of maturing human understanding, the raw material of humanism, the budding ability to see a choice between what is best for me, and what is best for thee and me. . . . Being human is a process, not a static condition. . . . Medical humanism is an immediate experience of shared dignity not a theoretical debate in grievance committees."

Issels marched boldly where angels feared to tread, by accepting these "therapeutic disasters," and achieved an acknowledged 16.6% cure rate, while, with many, many more, he extended their life spans immeasurably, with a better overall state of well-being and peace of mind. As a uniquely humanistic and psychologically sound enterprise, the physician-patient partnership proved a profitable healing venture. Instead of brute torture, Issels brought them new and hopeful treatment; instead of abandonment, he gave them shelter; and, instead of neglect, friendship and compassion. And, in this process, he instilled the will to live. "This can only be done," he said, "if the patient knows the clinical picture and is prepared to fight with me. It is a two-handed partnership, building this bridge between doctor and patient, over which the treatment regimen crosses."

His fighting Samurai spirit was not an entirely accidental or spontaneous phenomenon. It was the natural evolution from childhood of a sensitive personality, through a faith instilled by his devout mother and tempered in the crucible of his experience. Gordon Thomas, in his notable biography *Dr. Issels and His Revolutionary Cancer Treatment,* explains that "from early childhood—when Adelheid Issels, his mother, taught him to pray for the animals of the earth, as well as its people—his Christianity developed into a deeply private faith. He was baptized and raised in the tradition of the Roman Catholic Church. . . . The basic elements of his beliefs were childlike in their simplicity: God and heaven were real images; at death there was a pause and then a moving on to eternal life; hell was a torment inside a person here on earth. He built on that foundation a structure rejecting the parochial limitations of religion: God intended no doctrinal boundaries; a Jew or Moslem has just as much right in his beliefs as a Christian."

Josef Issels was decades ahead of his time in this area of the mind and matter—molded to a degree by his intensive studies of the Eastern religions and teachings. Just as he upstaged symptomatic medicine on the physiological plane, Issels now upstaged modern medical science on this Western front, playing the starring role in a more subtle but perhaps even more significant metaphysical dimension. Desiring nothing more than to be a standard-bearer for better health for all, he had no secrets, and, deliberately—like an elephant in the snow—left his tracks for anyone to follow; yet, even to this day, with some minor exceptions, few are

paying much attention to his importunities. Despite an outward stern-
ness, his feeling heart was often unbearably oppressed by the grief and
travail all around him, especially when he knew in every fiber of his
being that so much could be ameliorated by a little show of charity. His
fervent prayer, uttered with tears in his eyes: "If God would grant me
His grace, it would be the fulfillment of my life's dream to teach my
methods to the physicians of America, and of the world."

During World War II, Issels was assigned as a medical doctor with
the 278th German Regiment, dodging bullets as he tended the wounded
on the battlefields and in the field hospitals. He was taken prisoner by
the Red Army while his unit was retreating into Czechoslovakia in the
icy winter of 1944. Later, in a prisoner-of-war camp, the Russians began
sorting out the medical doctors and aides preparatory to shipping them
to Russia. By posing as a physical fitness instructor, Issels barely escaped
being sent into the interior.

The circumstances that confronted him in this prison camp were to
be startlingly reminiscent of those that later confronted him among the
terminal cancer patients in his clinic. The men were physical wrecks,
totally exhausted, suffering from hunger and malnutrition. Dysentery was
epidemic, and mortality twenty-five to thirty percent. It was therefore
not surprising that, under these appallingly harsh conditions, many fell
victim to apathy and depression; they gave up the struggle for survival
altogether. Men died all around him because of lack of hope, an understandable consequence of the tragic vacuum in the human dimension.
Without friends or family, death was a constant companion of these
unfortunates—bereft as they were of lifesaving spiritual food: compassion
and love.

To Issels's bold spirit, this was a challenge—and an opportunity.
He reacted with the same audacity that he later displayed in the good
fight against cancer. Employing psychotherapy—about his only remedy
at the time—he relieved mass depression with telling effect. It was
brought home to him in this death camp that emotional balance directly
affected chances of survival. Gordon Thomas says that "Issels stimulated
a determination to live in others by encouraging them to make light of
their hardships, and to retain their sense of individuality. He led them
in walks around the prison compound, forcing them to reject not only
the idea of defeat, but also of illness and death. So steadfast was his
belief in his own survival that he made a sketch of what his future office
would look like: a blueprint showed a complex of eight consulting, treatment and administration rooms. He also had other assets in his makeup
that enabled him to look to a future beyond the barbed wire. . . ." Above
all, Issels "had a *sense of humor* that was spirited enough to offer another
form of salvation. He laughed at situations that others found oppressive.
Finally, he had his faith, which sustained him more than anything else

in the incessant struggle against the apathy and disease of camp life. Many years later that period as a prisoner was crystallized by a passage he read which Einstein wrote:

" 'Strange is our situation upon earth. Each of us comes for a short visit, not knowing why, yet sometimes seeming to divine a purpose. From the standpoint of daily life, however, there is one thing we do know: that man is here for the sake of other men, for the countless unknown souls with whose fate we are connected by a bond of sympathy. Many times a day I realize how much my own outer and inner life is built upon the labors of my fellow men, both living and dead, and how earnestly I must exert myself in order to give in return as much as I have received and am still receiving.' "

Nor was Josef Issels a stranger to personal tragedy. He lost his brother Helmut in May 1944 in a Soviet attack. His mother, Adelheid, to whom he was most deeply attached all of his life, died shortly thereafter of a heart attack, but Issels was unable to return in time for her funeral. Her loss devastated him.

As if these trials were not enough, another was soon in coming, and under the most dismal circumstances. On August 5, 1945, Dr. Josef Issels and fifty other fellow prisoners were freed by the Russians because of their pitiful physical condition. Suffering with a history of painful kidney stones, Issels was down to a hundred and twenty pounds—a walking skeleton. He returned home to learn of the birth of a son, Peter Hans, a month earlier. Within weeks the baby developed encephalitis, inflammation of the brain. Issels, however, was ordered by the Allied Occupation Forces to a work assignment far removed from his home in Stuttgart. His job: to clear the streets of bomb damage; later to clean out lavatories! Finally came what must have been, if not some extreme form of penance, surely, at least, an ultimate test in humility. The exalted position, this time? A tea-boy in NAAFI, the British Army's equivalent of the Post Exchange!

Shortly afterward, his wife wrote to tell him that his baby was dying. Issels obtained permission to visit Peter in a Stuttgart hospital, and found him desperately ill. He argued fruitlessly with the German doctors who had given him up, going finally to an American medical unit that occupied the other half-wing of the hospital. He talked his way past the MPs, and found himself in front of an American major. Issels indicated his son's critical condition, explaining that he was a medical doctor. He asked for penicillin, which he thought might be of help. The major looked at him coldly, and said, "Get out of here. We don't give drugs to Germans." A few days later, Peter died. He was three months old.

Such abrasive experiences might tend to coarsen and brutalize; to weaken faith in one's fellowman, and in humanity. But Issels's mother had done her work well. She had nurtured and strengthened the inner man. Not only did he meet and cope with these tragedies effectively, but his resolution hardened. He became even more certain of his path. The hardships only refined the temper of the steel that was the core of Dr. Issels's being—and made him more determined than ever to pursue what his knowledge, his intuition, experience, and judgment implored: that the treatment of cancer called for a new dynamics, a break from the moldering concepts and methods; and very particularly in the area of the mind, where he had observed the greatest need and results—in the prisoner-of-war camp, where psychic hungers tore at the physical body, and often destroyed it. When Issels's Ganzheitstherapie—the treatment of the whole man—finally crystallized into a body of doctrine and practice, its iron core—perhaps its most profound application—was in the psycho-spiritual dimension.

Professor Denis Burkitt, a member of the Medical Research Council of Great Britain, discoverer of lymphomatous cancer, was highly complimentary of Issels's faith:

"He believes, as I do, that love and trust, and never giving up hope, frequently counts more than peering down a microscope. As you know, I am a religious man, and I am not at all surprised to learn that Dr. Issels believes at times that he, too, can be guided by God when it comes to making what conventional cancer researchers would dismiss as no more than an intuitive guess at how to handle a patient. . . . After many years of working in the field of cancer research, I have come to the conclusion that there is a dimension outside conventional research. It would seem that Dr. Issels could well be working in that dimension."

Let us now examine, carefully, Issels's therapeutic blueprint in this "dimension."

1. Tell the Truth, the Whole Truth

Many physicians prefer that their patients remain ignorant of their condition. Issels violently objects: "I reject this on the grounds that a patient has the right to know the truth about his condition, and, more important, to know he could be successfully treated when other methods have failed. Knowledge alone does not, of course, conquer real, exaggerated, or imagined fears about cancer. Nor, indeed, does it play a direct part in the active treatment of the disease. But suspicion is a breeding ground for psychological stress—and that can affect the course of the illness. It is a fundamental principle of my whole-body therapy that adult patients should be told the truth; because the treatment offers them a real chance, a new way, after other methods have failed. This encourages patients to come to terms with their illness."

Patients were told the nature of their cancer because Issels believed that it was fundamental for their survival that they knew the truth. Patients who had been treated conventionally showed severe stress when they arrived at Ringberg-Klinik. They were imbued with a dangerous fatalism, which Issels was convinced could be alleviated only by total honesty on the part of the medical staff. "I have clinically observed," he said, "in the vast majority of my patients that being told the nature of their cancer has helped to instill a will to live. The patient knows the clinical picture, knows what must and can be done to improve it, and, having received the truth, is generally prepared to fight all the harder against his malignancy." To Issels, telling the truth was an open demonstration of the two-way partnership between medical doctor and patient. He saw his role as instilling ". . . a will to live. This can only be done if the patient knows the clinical picture and is prepared to fight with me. . . . This two-handed partnership, building a bridge between doctor and patient over which the treatment regime crosses, is of vital importance. In such an atmosphere patients feel their fear of cancer diminishing, and their will to survive returning—important factors in combating a disease which lowers bodily resistance and depresses the nervous system appreciably.

"It is axiomatic in my clinic, that, as far as possible, there are no secrets. Patients talk openly about their cancers. Peace of mind, engendered by knowing the truth, can help a diseased body. A lifetime of close clinical observation has completely confirmed for me the need for such an approach.

"It is never easy to achieve this parity with patients who believe there is nothing left open to them. It can only be done by the doctor building up a meaningful contact with those he treats. . . . Sympathetic and honest management of patients, and providing them and their relatives with a proper flow of information, must be always regarded as being almost as important as skilled help and the proper relief of pain. The psychological state of many of these so-called incurables is almost immediately improved. . . . The question is not *when* to tell, but *how* to tell. It needs a careful psychological assessment of the adult patient. Fear makes a person a patient in the first place." According to Dr. Issels, it is the responsibility of the attending physician "to understand that fear, and to gauge it in each patient before revealing the truth to him. Having done that, the best step is to present the clinical symptoms as succinctly as possible.

"Test runs indicate that seventy-five percent of the patients, at least, are relieved to have the diagnosis which they suspected, confirmed. The 'white lies' are over. Now they can resume a real 'two-way partnership' which is the essence of all good doctor-patient relationships, and one which helps toward recuperation. Knowing allows them to take a sensible attitude toward the illness, also to put their affairs—material, paternal, and spiritual—in order."

In funereal contrast to Issels's enlightened psychological management is the dismal common mode of conduct by the Establishment—no doubt viewed by them as above reproach. This is discussed by Dr. Bernard Dixon in an article in the *New Scientist* of May 15, 1975. Dr. Dixon quotes first a senior consultant surgeon from Liverpool Royal Infirmary, who puts forward what he considers to be the preferred condition to Issels's method of treatment: "The patient with advanced malignant disease is more or less guaranteed a dignified form of death with continued help under the state service." Dr. Dixon demurs: "In stark contrast to such bleak complacency, both friend and foe have been profoundly impressed by Josef Issels's warm, invigorating relationship with his patients and the tremendous psychological help he gives them in their battle with cancer. As anyone who has seen a close relative die from cancer knows, this element or the lack of it, can seem every bit as significant as the latest panaceas of science-based medicine."

2. *Staff-to-Patient Ratio*

The astonishing staff-to-patient ratio of 1:2 at the Ringberg-Klinik allowed superior care and management of the sick. It was added proof, if any were needed, that they were enlisted in the good fight for the duration, and that the thought of failure never entered their minds. They were in the struggle to win. It was a practical and salutary demonstration of medical humanism in action.

3. *Staff Instruction and the Positive Mental Attitude*

Dr. Issels very early learned the importance of proper training and indoctrination of his professional staff in their relationship with the patients. He knew that pessimism was deadly, that "gloom rubs off on the patient and relatives, and adversely affects the treatment regime."

The staff followed an inviolate rule: Never—whether by word or action—reveal any signs of emotional withdrawal from the patient. Their spirited, involved response in the clinical situation was in inspiring contrast to the somber hospital treatment of the terminally ill, where the pall of gloom lies heavily around the dead quiet of the sickbed.

"Thank God it's over, he won't suffer any more." This, too often, is just the last nail in the coffin. Leading up to the tragic end is a vanquishing of hope, a surrender to the demon death by the subconscious— the release of negative forces that abhor hope, which totally compromises the possibility of recovery. It communicates itself to the ill, for the worst.

Dr. Josef Issels invoked living dynamics, never discounting the miracle. The living force generated by the energy of optimism, and the two-way partnership, was often enough to create a physical and mental environment so distasteful to the shadow of death that it literally bolted off for easier prey!

"Pessimism," Dr. Josef Issels emphasizes, "is never allowed. Gloom rubs off on patient and relatives, and adversely affects the treatment regime. Medical and nursing staff are encouraged to shape in the patient's mind a positive attitude towards cancer; the attitude must be towards total realism that cancer is not a bogey only treatable with surgery or radiotherapy." The need for such an attitude is strikingly illustrated by a survey carried out among eight hundred nurses. Questioned about the effectiveness of standard methods in the treatment of a number of cancers, their answers revealed a depressing but understandable view that little could be done. It is horrifying to contemplate how easily this morbid fatalism is transmitted to the sick.

Dr. Issels helped solve this problem in 1954 by formulating a set of nine rules for his doctors and nurses that would serve to strengthen the patient's confidence, and reinforce his hope and will to live:

1. Never promise a cure to anybody.
2. In dealing with prognosis, tell a patient or his responsible relatives that the first step is to arrest the tumor.
3. *That* will prolong life.
4. The next step is to try and make the tumor regress.
5. That will bring a further prolonging of life.
6. The patient should be told that the eventual medical aim is to try and reach a stage where the tumor disappears completely.
7. Time itself is another factor. Patients should be told that cure is a matter of time—in their case, five years free of disease—the statistical yardstick used to measure cure rates.
8. Our aim is to try and achieve the situation. But we can make no promises. And we never talk of "cure" but "remission."
9. We always talk with the knowledge that positive treatment can be offered. That is much more precise and beneficial.

4. *Visiting Hours Abolished*

Literally creating a revolution in medical practice, Dr. Josef Issels abolished visiting hours! He made himself freely available at all times to discuss any matter with relatives and friends.

"Relatives can help," he said. "In my experience, the sharing of facts with relatives is positive. . . . I have always encouraged a policy of bringing relatives to the bedside of their loved ones, and, if need be, to remain present even during a ward round. In this way, a patient does not feel divorced from the outside world."

This open-door policy proved a valuable two-way street. In offering a sympathetic ear as he listened patiently, never condemning, Dr. Issels "gave the impression the problem was a mutual one, to be solved by the joint efforts of doctor and patient. Over the weeks, he came to understand the family life of the (patient's) community as he tasted the homemade wines or joked over a bowl of thick country soup. The knowledge he gained gave him a new approach to diagnosing: the patient was not isolated in a hospital bed, but could be reviewed against his normal family background and environment. Issels found that the interrelationships inside a family often added another dimension to be taken into account when diagnosing. Searching for the causal effects of an illness—as distinct from treating the immediate symptoms—often meant knowing the family history for several previous generations. He looked at a patient as a whole; cause became as important as effect. In that way he laid down another foundation stone for the system that eventually started him upon a heterodox career."

5. "Seeding" Meetings: Togetherness

Remindful of Dr. Max Gerson's Saturday night meetings, Dr. Josef Issels every week assembled his patients for a two-hour lecture in the dining room. Usually, long-term surviving patients were invited to give their exciting and inspiring testimonies. These lectures were ". . . a mixture of science, homespun philosophy, and shrewd psychology. After attending several such lectures, many patients felt their fear of cancer diminished, and their will to survive returned. At the lectures there were no secrets. Patients' case histories were openly discussed; for those too ill to leave their beds, the lectures were relayed on loudspeakers to their rooms. Much of what they heard had not been medically approved. But implicit in everything was Issels's belief that his concept was the correct one. Twenty years passed before the great cancer hospitals of the world began to recognize the potential value of intensive psychotherapy for cancer victims; there was a growing awareness that stress played a critical part in whether such patients improved."

6. Involvement of the Patient in His Own Survival

Dr. Josef Issels's soul-stirring "Dear Patient" letter extends a heartwarming welcome to the new arrival. It is especially helpful to those from other countries, unfamiliar with Germany, its customs, language, or people. In immediate contrast to the isolation and rejection these unfortunates have suffered for long, lonely months—sometimes years— it is the first unbelievable outstretching of friendly arms vibrant with hope and encouragement.

There are no more games, no more mysteries. All is shared with them, relieving the dread anxiety of not knowing. The "Dear Patient" letter explains the entire therapeutic regime at the Ringberg-Klinik. It lists all medications the patient will receive (with indications of possible reactions and side effects). It counsels regarding regular ablutions (i.e., with cold water), vigorous skin-brushing to improve blood circulation, and hot baths with rosmarine oil. The patient is told of the possible necessity for removing infected teeth or tonsils, and is encouraged to participate, to the maximum extent possible, in outdoor exercise and other activities.

Imagine—yourself—if you will, having been, during your lifetime, a robust, highly motivated, and independent individual—overcome in your prime by such a calamity—and, now, totally incapacitated. You are wholly dependent upon those around you, often total strangers, for your most elemental needs. In a state of utter helplessness, the most private personal functions are open to public view: being bathed in bed, attending to your toilet, or being cleaned and dressed after soiling the sheets, through mortifying incontinence. Purgatory, with all its fearsome threats of physical agonies, can hold no greater terror than this for the sensitive soul of tender disposition. Death is often preferred to such hellish mental anguish. Under these humiliating conditions and dire emotional straits, it is easy to imagine giving up, because this nether world of the hopeless is a world no longer beautiful, but an Inquisition—oppressive with drug injections, pain-killers, intravenous feedings, catheters, and enameled urinals—and blank countenances hovering about, with the faceless look of death about them. Truly it is in the nature of a resurrection that, out of this well of loneliness, you are met by a cheerful face and eagerly offered supporting hands and warmly welcomed into a bright, sunlit room overlooking grassy slopes and flowering shrubs, where bustling, cheerful staff are no longer observing one as a soon-eligible corpse.

"Come, dear friend," says the cheerful lady in white, "take my hand, and let us—together—walk just one step forward. Have no fear, you can do it. That's it! That's it! Now just try a *little* harder. See, you *did* it! I told you! Wasn't that easy? You have a smile on your face now! Happy? All right! Now I give you another surprise: *This time, you will do it all by yourself!*"

The summons to activity stirs old nostalgia and new hope. The patient rushes fervently into the vacuum, taking his own temperature and pulse—entering these on his chart; measuring fluid intake and urine outgo—cooperating in every way that serves to cement and invigorate the healing partnership. Gone is the old conspiratorial atmosphere, replaced by complete candor and sincerity. The ailing terminal patient finds himself involved in a family process where he is for the first time a participant in his own salvation. He has emerged from a shadow world where a dark web of silence and conspiratorial intrigue has been woven about his mind and body like an entombing cocoon. This nightmarish veil has now been torn away. Into the dungeon has come the light of compassion, showing him a golden door through which he can gain his freedom.

Summarizing now, the psychological therapeutic input: Dr. Josef Issels dispelled, first, the gnawing anxiety and fear engendered by the conspiracy of silence by telling his patients the truth. He and his staff opened their arms wide to receive these unfortunates who had been rejected and abandoned. The proximity of caring hands and hearts brought them out of a depressing loneliness. In a warmhearted and cheerful environment they were provided with the comforting presence of an exceptionally large and friendly staff of doctors and nurses who looked after every vital need through a well-organized and integrated program of clinical management. Interest in life and in living revived, and with it the motivation to play a meaningful role as family members in their society once again. Indeed, the care and concern that pervaded the Ringberg-Klinik made it more a home than a hospital.

All of these positive psychological factors created a true healing environment, which underlined the dedication of the Ringberg-Klinik. In effect, Josef Issels made each of his patients partners, according them a respected place and role. The patient was no longer treated as expendable but, instead, found himself a unique and esteemed human being, *who was expected to recover!* It stirred the patient to a renewed consciousness, which carried the inspiring message that he would soon be joining hands with the outside world as a normal, healthy, and participating member of the dynamic human family.

THE LUKAS-KLINIK—DR. RITA LEROI

The game is charades!

Your first view is of a gentle countryside, with eye-pleasing undulating hills. Nestling cozily amid this pastoral setting is a large, homelike, two-story structure surrounded by an arbor of trees, flowers, and shrubs. You enter, and are brought to the first of many rooms where cheering sunlight radiates through transparent chartreuse curtains. It is here that you are to observe and remark upon the activities.

Sitting at ordinary wooden tables scattered about the room is a group of older men and women perhaps from thirty to sixty years of age—with here and there a somewhat younger person. All appear relaxed, but completely absorbed in modeling forms and figures—with clay and other plastic materials.

Now, please make your guess. What, exactly, is this place where these people are happily involved in a modeling art form?

No, it is not an arts and crafts center! "A community hobby shop?" Wrong again! Let's pass this by for now, and proceed to the next room.

Here, a teacher is giving lessons in speech formation. You observe stammerers being helped, and compulsive rapid talkers coached in slowing down their pace. The importance of clear articulation is being emphasized.

"A school for correcting speech defects?" Sorry, try again! "For retarded adults?" Hmm . . . let's go on to the next classroom, and see if you can do any better.

This time it is a group diligently applying itself to watercolor painting. They are learning to shape forms corresponding to these colors.

No, not an art school, sorry! You're not even warm! Next!

We see a class engaged in a free-flowing kind of dance, remindful of ballet, but without the strict form and posture. This appears more elemental. The participants seem completely enraptured, with an uninhibited ethereal quality in their free-style movements.

No, this is not a new-mode dance studio! "School for Ballet?" No! Give up?

What we have been observing is artistic therapy being practiced at the Lukas-Klinik in Arlesheim, Switzerland. The students in the classes you have observed are all patients—most with advanced or terminal cancer. The modeling, the watercolor painting, the class in speech formation, and in eurythmy—spiritual dance—all this is a most important part of the holistic program that in diverse ways helps bring the patient to a more sensitive state of inner awareness—about himself, his illness, his role in society, and his place in the cosmos. The clinic is not just a hospital, but a school for life, revealing and unfolding the mysteries of self and the spirit, a vital part of the total therapeutic process that is designed to improve the patient's well-being and effect a remission of his malignant condition. It is all encompassed by Rudolf Steiner's Anthroposophical Medicine, and, as we previously noted, is part of the totality that includes good nutrition and medical therapy—with Iscador as the central focus.

Every patient participates in this art therapy program, but each art form has a particular application in the realm of the spirit for certain types of individuals. For example, the spiritual science of Anthroposophy postulates that formative powers are weak in corpulent, overweight patients, and, for this reason, as they fashion the clay material, modeling awakens their "forming" powers through the feel of vaulted and hollow surfaces. As Dr. Leroi joyfully observes regarding this therapeutic activity: "When we see a patient leaving his teacher with glowing cheeks and eyes, we know that the therapy has been successful.

"For thin, intellectual patients we prescribe painting therapy. By becoming absorbed in the luminous world of watercolors, they learn to shape forms corresponding to these colors. We start by letting them experience the blue shades, and then contrast these with sunny yellow in order finally to reach the rainbow colors. If the patient wishes to paint concrete objects, he can turn to landscapes or other things after taking part in the color exercises.

"It is striking to note how many patients have trouble in speaking with clear articulation. Many mumble, stammer, or speak hastily. Often the speech is not under control but pours out without thought and order. These patients benefit from lessons in speech formation, which teaches them to become conscious of consonants, and to master and mold the stream of respiration.

"The whole artistic therapy is aimed at the unfolding of the soul's creative faculties which often lie fallow nowadays. The development of such qualities *counteracts the misdirected creativeness of malignant growth*. The ego's initiative should again radiate through the entire personality. Of course, the physicians observe carefully the response of each patient to therapy, and sometimes changes are necessary. During his stay at the clinic the patient gains confidence in his doctor therapists. The often introverted individuals begin to speak about their inner difficulties, to ask about the real purpose of life."

In his book *Psychosomatic Medicine, Its Principles and Application,* Dr. Franz Alexander underlines the specificity of mind-body relationship: "The body, that complicated machine, carries out the most complex and refined motor activities under the influences of such psychological phenomena as ideas and wishes. . . . All our emotions, we express through physiological processes: sorrow, by weeping; amusement, by laughter. . . . All emotions are accompanied by physiological changes: fear, by palpitation of the heart; anger, by increased heart activity, elevation of blood pressure, and changes in carbohydrate metabolism; despair, by a deep inspiration and expiration called sighing. All these physiological phenomena are the results of complex muscular interactions under the influence of nervous impulses, carried to the expressive muscles of the face, and to the diaphragm in laughter, to the lachrymal glands in weeping, to the heart in fear, and to the adrenal glands and to the vascular system in rage. . . . The nervous impulses arise in certain emotional situations which in turn originate from our interactions with other people. . . . The originating psychological situations can be understood only in terms of psychology—as total responses of the organism to its environment."

Socrates, who did not have the advantage of computers, space-orbiting satellites, or access to CIA intelligence files, nevertheless came upon the truth of it, asserting that "there is no illness of the body apart from the mind."

Psychosomatic medicine has today belatedly confirmed Rudolf Steiner's underlying philosophical premise of the unity of *mind* and *body*. But Steiner has gone one step further—and will again—one day—prove his point: that the essential ingredient to recovery finds its real source and roots in the realm of the *soul* and *spirit*. This is not an abstraction disassociated from mind or body, but represents a more profound—but related—dimension with intuitive content, which ultimately manifests itself in positive healing responses from the patients.

The highly toxemic condition of the body, typical of the diseased organism, has thrown the cellular organs and systems out of balance. The biological transformation that occurs through this state of intoxication causes the cancerous cellular systems to regress to a primitive fermentative state. No longer capable of differentiation, they have become truant, and simply do not respond to the body's normal, controlled system of organization. This toxicity weakens the overall defenses, and eventually results in the malignant condition, with metastases—an invasion into more and more of the tissues and organ systems. Clearly, because each cell is but a part of the whole, including the brain and nervous system, this poisoning of the body can and does cause torpor, lassitude, depression; and has other disastrous pathological impacts, numbing the mind, and seriously affecting clarity of judgment. It is easy to see how the loss of will to live finds this poisoned environment a fertile climate for its virulent expression.

Having now been introduced, crablike, to the psychological and spiritual content of the Lukas-Klinik's therapy, let us take our Cinerama camera to a broader plain, and observe what is happening in the all-embracing picture.

A previous section of this book discusses the Lukas-Klinik's treatment program, and includes all the crucial psychological elements in a general way, but we shall here take a somewhat closer look at their therapeutic impact, as we have done in the case of the corresponding modalities of Drs. Max Gerson and Josef Issels. The similarities among them will be easily seen.

The patient starts by entering a completely cheering and cheerful natural environment—a veritable Garden of Eden, scenically idyllic, eye-appealing, and soul-gratifying. Mother Nature enfolds him comfortingly in her bosom, dispelling the darkness of his depressed state and condition. It is entirely understandable that there should be a quickening of the pulse in a first flush of welcome surprise. These grievously afflicted have just been disentangled from a suffocating world of noisome and terrifying wards, peopled by shadowy, white-clad, dumb ghosts—and tragically pregnant with recollections of goodbyes from loved ones who revealed, through their long, lingering looks and downcast faces, inexpressible grief.

Unbelievingly, the patient now glances out over a large flower garden —from a delightfully furnished room, painted in enlivening shades of bright color. It is not surprising that, in sharp contrast, he should now contemplate his exit from his former state of confinement as a reprieve from the threat of instant extinction—and breathe a deep sigh of relief.

The staff meets the patients with arms outstretched. They all have become emotionally involved through their studies of Anthroposophical teachings. This binding philosophy has brought them here to minister to the sick. Its imprint is manifest as they labor in this healing vineyard, expressing their faith, hope, and love. They clearly understand the emotional dynamics of disease, and are prepared to grapple with the malignant condition and its often painful and gruesome physical manifestations —to lift the ailing person from the depths of his melancholia and despair. From morning till night they bind themselves to the patients, helping with their food, their medications, their toilets, dressings, and other necessary clinical management. It would be difficult even for the most practiced eye to tell—from word or action—that staff and patients were not members of one large, harmonious human "family."

In the dining room—colorful and bright—meals are taken in common. Dr. Rita Leroi believes that this constitutes another therapeutic element, and adds: "Patients and members of the staff are intermixed; the topic of disease is forbidden, and it is the duty of all co-workers to keep cheerful conversation going. In view of our international patients, with differing languages and interests, this is not a simple task. When it is well solved, each meal turns into a refreshing and pleasant event."

It is a transcendent experience to observe the hush that attends Dr. Leroi's entry into the dining room, where—at her table, too—she sits with patients and staff. All wait expectantly, as it were, until Dr. Leroi is seated. The hush turns into an even more prescient silence—until Dr. Leroi tinkles a tiny bell, then recites a loving prayer of grace, which breaks the suspense, and the meal begins. The meals taken in this atmosphere satisfy more than simple physiological hunger. To the patients and staff alike it is nourishing spiritual food—bread and wine from the Lord's table.

Now let us more closely examine the particular components of the total treatment program here, which are relevant to the psychological and spiritual therapeutic activities.

1. *Natural Environment*

As an immediately salutary introduction, Nature starts the healing process by offering her precious bounty: rolling hills, trees, flowers and blue sky, a setting of breathtaking loveliness, its intrinsic harmony highly conducive to healing. Even the most heavy in heart are drawn to note her lavish display, and to drink from her generous fountain of nectar with a new vitality, and awakening recollection of forgotten charm and beauty.

2. *The Truth*

The patient is told, completely, the truth of his condition—just as Dr. Issels does with his afflicted. Dr. Leroi expresses their view in this way: "It is a principle with us that each patient is entitled to know what he suffers from, and what his chances are. It is a sin against human dignity to keep him in darkness about his diagnosis and to feed him on false hopes up to the last minute. Naturally, the physician will frame his words so as not to discourage the patient. The patient must join as a partner in the battle. He should feel that his doctor will always stand by him and never slacken his efforts to heal. In this way a healing spirit can be present even if the patient comes to us in the final stages of cancer. Conversation accompanied by such utter trust between doctor and patient will have to touch on fatefully grave questions."

Thus the communication channel is opened up completely between doctor and patient, and there are no longer any secrets that hang forebodingly in a dark cloud of anxiety over the patient's mind.

3. *Togetherness*

The commitment of the staff to the patient's welfare is absolute, and is reinforced through their embracing and applying the living principles and practices of spiritual medicine in the struggle for the patients' lives. The commitment to humaneness and love of fellowman is indelibly imprinted on attitudes, word, and action. In this battle, they are all wounded, having bound themselves to the patient as members of his "family" in a common struggle. Altogether, it is an uplifting experience, and a mighty ploy against the corrosive effect of rejection—which now finds itself blocked by a gargantuan "No Trespassing" sign, guarded by the formidable flames of passion and commitment protecting these sacred premises.

In the beginning, the evil forces, physical and mental, hang on to the diseased person like his very shadow of death. They peer hungrily in from the outer environs, but eventually these rapacious specters must abdicate this pure land for more accessible prey.

4. *Spiritual Cleansing—Metamorphosis*

The patients come to learn about themselves through the process of intimate personal involvement and activity. Dr. Leroi destroys the false notion of fatalism, and abjures guilt: "The patient must learn that his condition is not a punishment imposed upon him by God. He must learn to see the possibilities for inner development. Often hopeless, lifelong entanglements are solved by his disease. In order to reach such an attitude, the patient must recognize himself as a spiritual entity—whose native element is in the spiritual world, and who has to go through many incarnations in order to develop and be an instrument for the world's progress. Such fundamental exchanges are the crowning features of our therapeutic efforts. If they have real impact, a person's entire life may take a new turn.

" . . . Many patients regain, through this therapy, a renewed initiative, and rise out of their depression. Very frequently tumor growth can be retarded, and sometimes a complete standstill may be observed over the years. We have seen many cases in which histologically verified tumors have regressed and disappeared completely. Carcinomas of the bladder, genital and digestive tract and melanomas show the best response to Iscador. Breast cancer in women is a somewhat difficult field; our best results are in the post-operative phase."

5. *Art Therapy—Realizing the True Self*

As we have noted, the psychological factors, in conjunction with the physiological influences, exert their effect through clinically observable deterioration, progressing to that extremity where the pathology results in terminal cancer. Any therapeutic activity that can counteract or reverse this activity—without harm to the basic organism—is desirable in the healing situation.

Art therapy, often through subtle and intangible expression, makes a positive contribution in this direction—to the well-being and ultimate recovery—by reaching into the deeper layers of the patient's subconscious. It eliminates structured, stressful self-deception, imperceptibly unfolding the path to a healthy awareness of self and the inner nature. Establishing personal identity thus becomes part of the regenerative process.

Participating in the spiritual dance, and working with the plastic and visual arts, brings to the awareness the subconscious wrappings that bind and strangle the true self, and provides channels for achieving freedom of expression. The art form thus plays an important role in releasing the psyche from damaging physiological trauma, and contributes measurably to the overall recuperative process.

Comparison

Compared with Gerson and Issels, Dr. Leroi's spiritual parameters are more deliberately elaborated in the communication process between doctor and patient, and more consciously directed to the deeper psychological layers, based upon an organized body of doctrine: Anthroposophy, the spiritual science of Rudolf Steiner. It carries a bolder thrust in metaphysical terms in opening up the patient's receptivity to the influences of the etheric and other spiritual layers and forces. All of which suggests that the "consummation devoutly to be wished" is that utopian resolution that would introduce all healing truths into the science of medicine, even those infinitely subtle configurations such as the charismatic and faith-healing schools of the West, and the comparable esoteric teachings of the East. Obviously the precise input and manner of application must be dependent upon the intellectual and intuitive range and depth of the supervising medical doctors and clinical therapists, and upon the comparable attunement of the patient, each situation allowing for an inflow of substances, ideas, and influences that will marshal to a maximum degree the patient's individual physiological and spiritual resources for a victorious conclusion.

In summary, we have clearly observed two healing strategies collectively at work at the Lukas-Klinik: first, the dietary and medical phalanx, which operates essentially on the physiological level, gradually detoxifying the system and building up its immunological defenses and its intrinsic strength; and, second, the psychological and spiritual therapies in their various forms and dimensions. Both are orchestrated toward the achievement of a perfect harmony in which doctor and patient are part of the symphonics of healing. Together, this binding partnership of Ganzheitstherapie constitutes a total purification process that cleanses the bloodstream; ultimately weans the poisoned, refractory cells from their anarchistic state; and in the natural recovery process transforms them into normal, healthy cells and systems. In a very real sense what has occurred is a resurrection of the body's innate intelligence capabilities, which, in the poisoned pathological state, cannot be alerted to elicit the necessary directional and defense responses.

Simple, the struggle and the victory is *not,* but its essence, as Dr. Leroi declares, is a quality of courage and action that ennobles. Exemplifying this canon, this common transcending quality of courage, the Lukas-Klinik has found great joy in rallying to Dr. Issels's standard, and in responding to his rallying cry: "Fight—as we do—for your life!"

HUMOR

It is quite impossible to leave this subject of psychological therapy without discussing the heroic role of humor which was brought into the clinics—like the music of children, or the gods. Issels, Gerson, and Leroi could not live without the joy of laughter around them, which each imparted in abundance to their charges. There was always a ready joke, a witticism, to remove the dark mood of pessimism, the worried expression in anxious eyes. From Josef Issels one could expect an earthy jest—like the coarse farmer's bread and homemade wine that families shared with him; from Gerson, the lifting prod of whimsy and satire. As for Leroi, her warm smile and wit might carry the gay, motivating thrust of challenge, say, for the patient who appeared a bit awkward in his eurythmy dance exercises.

In 1960, that compelling writer Pearl S. Buck wrote *A Bridge for Passing,* in which she explained how her own despondency was oppressing her like a sickness. It was after the death of her husband, and she was still quite in the depths of despair. Hoping for some relief from sorrow through activity, she had undertaken participation with a Japanese film company in a coproduction of *The Big Wave,* one of her earlier books, with a setting on the island of Shikoku in Japan. Every night, in Tokyo, she found herself painfully alone when she returned to her hotel from the day's work of casting. She suffered so from pangs of depression that she took to an aimless walking of the streets, with sad notes playing always in her head. Common scenes like the romping of children, a young couple walking arm in arm, or soft music wafting from Japanese tearooms —all conjured up an overwhelming nostalgia of other, happier times.

Then one day—suddenly—a happy change occurred in this dirgelike routine. A comic figure, a grotesque gnome of a man, emerged on the scene in the person of the Japanese costume director of *The Big Wave.* Whether fat man or brooding villain, aged and bent grandmother, or ravishing young diving girl, his genius in modeling the role, created a lively, hilarious atmosphere. He could insinuate that extra comic bit— like a turn of the head, a raised eyebrow, a feminine twist of the body; or a shy cough, and lifting of a hand in front of the mouth with eyes downcast—which sent the staff into uncontrollable laughter. It was not just humor; it was great art.

Mrs. Buck happened to stumble across this "old man" one day, drawn by happy sounds exploding from the costume room. She describes her experience as she watched him:

"The model was a microscopic human being, male, of vague age, but certainly not young. He stood something under five feet and if he weighed ninety pounds, it would surprise me. He was skin and bone, and if the skeleton was a child's, the face was fascinating. Wrinkled, lively, full of fun and mischief, it was the face of an old faun. The top of the head was bald, but hair surrounded the large bald spot and stood straight out from the skull, as though the old faun were undergoing electric shock. He was certainly full of some sort of electricity for he was issuing orders without let, as he modeled a fisherman's outfit made for a man four times his size. He was a good model, nevertheless. He clutched the trousers in at his waist, gave a twist to the belt, arranged the Japanese coat, and became a fisherman. Everybody laughed, and I sat down to watch.

"He knew all the characters in *The Big Wave,* it appeared, and he modeled them all. When he modeled a man he faced us. When he modeled a woman, he turned his back. I recognized each character, even the young girl, Setsu. How an old man could pose so that he suggested a gay young girl, even from the back, is something I cannot explain. I wished for the millionth time that I understood Japanese, for whatever the old faun was saying, the audience was convulsed. Every now and again he was dissastisfied and threw off a costume, or rejected what was offered, and pawed among the confusion of the piled garments with all the fierce intensity of a monkey looking for fleas."

From that moment, the gag that had choked her soul with grief melted away. The old "faun" had worked his magic upon her with his own divine human comedy. "I laughed with all my heart," relates Pearl Buck, "and for an hour was healed. It was the beginning of something happening. I can report that I carried through my program for the evening; and went to bed at a reasonable hour, also, for the first time in all the weeks. The fact marked a beginning."

Gone was the morbid grief barrier that had wracked her mind, dispelled by a funny old man's lightness of soul. Gone the heartbreaking, lonesome wandering into the streets at night.

Paraphrasing an old piece of wisdom: "Whom the gods would heal, they first make laugh!"

IN SUMMARY

There remains little more to be added to our discussion of the primary common denominators that make up the whole of the treatment regimes of Drs. Josef Issels, Max Gerson, and Rita Leroi. With respect to the structured application of psychological and spiritual philosophies, Dr. Gerson, working virtually alone, was limited by the dimensions of time and space, so he spoke with his heart. Dr. Issels, always patiently available to those who needed his counsel or strong shoulders, fought against a merciless clock, too, battling in the trenches from morning until night. He, like Gerson, suffered from the difficulties of filling staff needs, and was oppressed with impossible caseload—one more desperate than the other. Yet, as with Brother Lawrence—a saintly French monastic of the seventeenth century—Issels, though without conscious formulation of the psychological elements, walked always in the "Presence of God," and for him, too, divine grace helped him fulfill, through word, action, and result, the ultimate of Christian fiats—to preach the Gospel and heal the sick. He, like the others, could be known by his fruits. As for Dr. Leroi, she operated in a somewhat less turbulent flux, and with the precious perquisite of a dedicated staff. She moved in a tranquil and quieter atmosphere where her motherly presence and treatment leavened the torments of the sick in a more compliant environment, reinforced by the viable spiritual tenets that were practiced at the Lukas-Klinik.

All three reached the same top of the mountain. In the final analysis, the differences, essentially, were few, and more a matter of variations in style and medical executive technique—of logistics of time, space, and staff—rather than any irreconcilable differences in the intrinsic thrust or content of their therapeutic regimes.

The common dominating theme that all shared was the dynamic of the holistic concept. This imposed its own immediate necessities for strict, ordered discipline in clinical management. The procedural details involved were painstakingly laborious, but they were an inviolate bond to successful treatment. It demanded unwavering purpose and resolution, and a sense of responsibility that was, so to speak, bred in their bones, and that each fulfilled with a rare degree of professional competence. And they shared another invaluable asset: open and reflective minds, and a creative imagination. Finally, and hardly the least, they were masters in the art of handling people. This combination of talents was more than enough to provoke envy, especially on peer level. Illustrative of this understandable show of human weakness by their confreres was the remark of one physician who testily complained about Josef Issels that "his patients think he's Jesus Christ himself!"

Psychologists interested in such matters might be hard pressed to affirm which came first—the talent or the creativity. The Hindu sages, on the other hand, would have no such problem. To them it was elementary that the receptive mind that opens itself to all things, in a universal sense—without prejudice or personal ego or power drives—receives, always, the bounties of divine grace in such measure as allows the satisfaction of the human cravings and the humanitarian needs that fall within the requirements of the problems confronting the entities involved. It is, simply, the immutable working of the law of Karma, which states that no sin ever goes unpunished, and no virtue remains unrewarded.

This law of balance, of cause and effect, apparently invokes its own form of metaphysical judgment. Christ was scarcely unaware of this, for he put it most plainly: "As ye sow, so shall ye reap." And: "Cast your bread upon the waters, and it shall return tenfold." Is this not the exact mirror image of what is written in the teachings of the Indian masters?

Courage—above all—was desperately needed to start the rescue operation for these terrified and mortally stricken human beings. Issels, Gerson, and Leroi acknowledged this beyond any doubt as a cardinal imperative of their therapeutic endeavor. Its essence was no more than the awakening of truth in the patient on all levels, i.e., truth about his condition, about himself, about the therapy, and about the world in which he must live and function.

For imparting courage, Dr. Issels issued a ringing challenge to the patients to go climb a mountain. He enlisted them in his fighting ranks, and placed weapons in their hands with which they could participate in the struggle by becoming his soldiers and partners. Dr. Max Gerson would hold a patient's hand closely in his, and earnestly convey that, always, there was hope, and that he would do his best. "Do not be afraid. I am in this fight together with you. I have confidence in my treatment. Come, let us begin." As for Dr. Leroi, to the patients she was a living Madonna, and, when she smiled, it was a smile as brilliant as five stars in the firmament. "Trust in God, and trust in us. There is good hope for your improvement, and perhaps for your complete recovery. With us, you are like with your own family. We will take good care of you." And again—the same smile.

Implicit in these simple interpersonal exchanges was a communion of the spirit, of mutual belonging. By the consummation of the partnership in this common struggle, the physicians joined the ranks of the wounded. This compact marked the beginning of the long road back. "We are joined in this together" was the pledge to the patient by his doctor and friend. What more could be asked?

The exemplary humanism and nobility of these three standard-bearers is remindful of a touching poem, "Abou Ben Adhem," by James H. L. Hunt, in which a haloed angel appears to Abou Ben Adhem in a dream. She carries a "Book of Gold" in which are recorded "the names of those who love the Lord." He asks whether his name is one of them. "Nay, not so," replies the angel. Abou—a bold soul—and hardly to be discouraged, "spoke more low, but cheerily still; and said: 'I pray thee, then, write me down as one who loves his fellow men.'" The angel writes, and vanishes. "She came again the next night, in a great wakening light," and, lo, when she shows Abou the names of those the Lord loves best, behold "Ben Adhem's name led all the rest."

19

Natural Hygiene

We have now reached the point where we have pretty much covered the basic issues that confront the medical practitioner and the research scientist in the field of cancer. Because of the depth and range of the subject, with its disheartening propensity for geometrical expansion, there remains always something more that could be added. We feel, however, that we have touched the important bases with the modern-day approaches to the treatment of the terminally ill patient, and also the effectiveness or lack of effectiveness attending these efforts. We must leave it to others to venture further into deeper probes of those areas of research and therapy that may be suggested by our study.

With respect to the sobering statistics, however, nothing has changed in the results being achieved today by orthodox medical practice. The grim figures rather indicate a worsening of the present one-in-four rate of cancer deaths. In *Natural Food News* for July 1978, Dr. Linus Pauling, twice-honored Nobel Prize winner, reiterated what is common knowledge and fact in the medical establishment: "Despite the expenditure of billions of dollars on cancer research, there has been during the last twenty-five years essentially no decrease in the incidence of cancer or increase in the average time of survival *after the patient is diagnosed as having cancer.*" Clearly, then, the introduction of traditional medical therapeutics, with minor exceptions, cannot influence the course of the brutal statistics after diagnosis.

The morbid psychological component is likewise distressing, as our society continues visibly infected with the cancer fear syndrome, being helped, regrettably, by the culpable media and, particularly of late, by the raucous tabloids. More recently, these have proliferated abominably at supermarket counters, and chronically oppress one with the questionable fragrance of sick headlines, many of them heralding new cancer cures. This banal press continues to hail research work in the highly experimental stage as the giant step forward toward the ultimate solution—if not the ultimate solution itself. In toting up the frequency and number of these flagrantly publicized panaceas, one can hardly avoid concluding that our arsenal of cancer remedies has now reached the medical equivalent

222

of atomic overkill. It is chancy to contemplate that an impressionable reader might be innocently encouraged to venture a slight case of cancer— just to savor the exciting experience of watching it go away!

Reverting from the bottom line, from which we must begin, the incisive underlying reality remains: that the blessed human condition starts with good health; that, unhappily, for those fated for chronic and terminal disease—for whatever reasons and causes—it moves inexorably onto the plane of occasional illness—the early nonsymptomatic stages; then recurring disease problems; then the clinically observable chronic disease state; and, finally, the terminal condition.

It follows that, if we could maintain inviolate the pristine condition, that blessed state of good health with which we normally start, might we not avoid the pitfalls of disease altogether? Many would say this is impossible—given the circumstances of our highly polluted and stressful environment today. This may be true for some who have neither the will nor the control to alter their circumstance, but, for those willing to make the requisite effort, it is entirely feasible, and, needless to say, a highly desirable objective.

In this chapter we will introduce and discuss the role of a relatively new discipline in the spectrum of health, which is now in a dynamic stage of ferment, and which dramatically manifests itself to all points and sectors in the continuum, playing a vital role throughout. But, before venturing our journey to this lookout point, let us very briefly review the nature and general character of medical practice today:

It is known more commonly as "crisis" medicine, as differentiated from "preventive" medicine. Simply put, it is the care of the patient *after* he is sick, and not at all the prevention of the disease condition. With minor exceptions, the virtually complete omission of meaningful nutrition as a course of study from the curricula of medical universities is a clear point of reference. Only about a dozen of the nation's hundred and twenty medical schools have full departments of nutrition, and the average medical student learns little or nothing about how to feed a normal human being to maintain good health. In *Nutrition Today* (March/April 1974), Dr. Charles E. Butterworth, Chairman of the AMA Council on Foods and Nutrition (1973 and 1974), says:

> I am convinced that iatrogenic malnutrition has become a significant factor in determining the outcome of illness for many patients. Since 'iatrogenic' is merely a euphemism for 'physician-induced,' perhaps it would be better to speak forthrightly and refer to the condition as 'physician-induced malnutrition.' I suspect as a matter of fact that one of the largest pockets of unrecognized malnutrition in America, and Canada, too, exists—not in the rural slums or urban ghettos—but in the private rooms and wards of big city hospitals. . . . I believe that we are beginning to see the inevitable consequences of the neglect of

nutrition education in our medical schools. . . . It is well known, for example, that malnutrition interferes with wound healing and increases susceptibility to infection. It thus becomes imperative to ensure that preventable malnutrition does not contribute to the mortality, morbidity, and prolonged bed-occupancy rates of our hospital population. So it's time to swing open the door and have a look at this skeleton in the hospital closet. . . . I am not speaking of any one hospital. . . . I have had the opportunity to visit a number of hospitals, and to discuss the situation with many physicians and nutrition scientists. As a result, I am convinced that the problem of hospital malnutrition is serious and nationwide.

One hospital case involving major heart surgery, as described by Dr. Butterworth, attributes the patient's death, on the eighty-third post-operative day, to failure to institute nutritional reinforcement procedures. He states:

> This man probably represents a classic case of iatrogenic, or perhaps more accurately called hospital-staff-induced, protein-calorie malnutrition which resulted in terminal starvation. It is well established, but not adequately appreciated, that such patients withstand infection and injury poorly. For example, Nevin S. Scrimshaw at M.I.T. and others have shown clearly that minor infections, even measles, can readily kill a malnourished child, although the true cause of death, malnutrition, seldom appears on the record or in the statistics of such cases.

With respect to the dietary regime of Dr. Max Gerson, as we have seen, it is crystal-clear. The healthy person, as he wishes, can choose to follow the main tenets of the Gerson program closely, or modify it, say, to the same extent as a recovering, or recovered, cancer patient would, in order to assure continuing good health. With one strict caution: Only a medical doctor (or practitioner of equivalent competence in the physiological and biological sciences) with a strong nutritional commitment, should closely supervise the patient. This is an imperative, but should pose no obstacle to a determined seeker after good health. It requires only the will to do it.

As for the therapeutic modality used by Dr. Leroi of the Lukas-Klinik, here, too, the definitive nutritional program, as well as the adjunctive physiological and spiritual regime, can likewise provide an easy-to-follow example that will maintain good health under normal conditions. Certain of the important diagnostic methods and tests used by the Lukas-Klinik can be adopted to confirm the condition of good health, or, in the adverse case, perhaps uncover the latent preclinical, or premalignant condition. In this latter eventuality, the Lukas-Klinik has developed a special course of treatment that can help restore the body to its original state of good health and well-being. So it is clear that appropriate means are available, in relatively uncomplicated form, for the maintenance and restoration of good health.

As for the regime of Dr. Issels, his therapy is more aggressively concentrated upon the elimination of the visible tumor and the viable tumor sites—with the simultaneous application of an immunological regime, using, predominantly, medical therapeutics such as vaccines, autogens, fever therapy, and ultraviolet irradiation. Dr. Issels also places heavy emphasis upon the necessity for an optimal nutritional program, although he has not elaborated this part of his modality to the same fine point as Drs. Leroi and Gerson.

The individual with a normal sense of responsibility for his family and society will make good health an important focal point of his attention. Can it be doubted that the enjoyment of life, and the satisfactory performance of one's filial duties and obligations, are integrally equated with well-being, whereas a breakdown in health compromises utterly the adequate fulfillment of all personal and social mores? Mental anguish, physical pain, and bedridden helplessness are the inevitable and piteous consequences for a patient in the last throes of a terminal illness. Unless one is bent upon self-destruction, is there truly any other way to go but in the direction of good health practice, preferably preventive in nature?

If we could somehow detach such bright stars as Issels, Gerson, and Leroi from their demanding clinical work, and move their rich talents into channels for the prevention of disease, we could, beyond doubt, look for a host of collective miracles. Yet, withal, from the very soil they have been cultivating in clinical practice, a rich inheritance has emerged. Brick by brick, the laborious day-to-day work experience has built a structure of reinforced steel and concrete that illuminates the true dimensions of the healing landscape. It has risen like the phoenix from the ashes of day-to-day struggles and disappointments, successes and failures.

"To every thing there is a season, and a time for every purpose under the heaven." The divine flame of the intuitive process at work has touched and germinated in the creative minds of many new and bold practitioners, revealing new truths to these outward-reaching human beings. A fundamentally preventive doctrine was the natural outcome. We can happily report that there were a host of such bright minds who did, in the lexicon of the healing arts, break through the shell of their structured academic backgrounds and training, and of the hard-and-fast drug regimes. These bold frontiersmen kept sending out signals that echoed faintly through the corridors of medical history, finally setting their feet firmly upon the stage of the twentieth century to confront the full-blown atomic age, and, incidentally, the Age of Aquarius, when great things are presaged and heralded in the Book of Life concerning the destiny of man.

Amid the cacophony of mare nostrums filling the air with their ear-shattering clamor, the modest notes of these low-keyed savants went relatively unnoticed, except for a few close observers in the healing sciences. In these latter days, however, a potpourri of devotees has ventured more boldly upon the brightly lit stage, unfurling its banners in a rousing call to arms. Transcending the frozen clutch of a medieval medical hierarchy, which held fast many untold secrets, this group of pioneers brought a new-age consciousness into reality, and placed the missing cornerstone of the lopsided structure squarely in place. As the diadem sits in the royal crown, it sat in perfect balance astraddle the main gate of health, its proper regal position in the timeless continuum.

They are men little known to the general public, and less liked, heralded, or remembered by the practitioners of traditional medicine, but surely in the archives of medical history their names should grace a special Hall of Fame. Their spoors can be detected and traced by the meticulous scholar. Most were physicians with excellent credentials, who at some point in their successful careers observed the gross limitations of their own medical school education.

As they stood bewildered at the bedsides of their sick and dying patients (despite all the nostrums applied from their awesome armamentarium), they were unconsciously stirred into reexamining the disciplines they had learned in their universities. In this school of real life experience, doubts and fears began to creep in.

At first, faint wrinkles of puzzlement furrowed their brows as they observed highly touted nostrums and methods fail to work. Slowly, questions rankled their minds, and remained unanswered, as they feverishly combed through their medical textbooks and pharmacopoeia. The sensitive, searching ones were touched first by doubt, then by fear and consternation, and, finally, for the rare few we are talking about, stirred into active rebellion against the unfeeling, hardcore Establishment.

It was impossible for them to avoid noting the fundamental contradiction: that there was an inherent violence in their drug-saturated regimes that violated the harmony of Nature. Shudders of pain and anguish—and often of death—shook them daily to their roots. Their patients literally begged for a more gentle touch, a better taste on the tongue, a lesser torment of their bodies, and a more compassionate attitude toward their affliction. In an agony of unendurable suffering, they raised their piteous cries to the very heavens: "God be merciful! God be merciful! There must be a better way."

And there was. Working within the framework of the healing sciences, a handful of bold hearts slowly evolved a body of knowledge that today stands as the keystone of the arch. The science they developed and refined is known as Natural Hygiene. It fleshes out the structure of all the health disciplines, and gives to them a wholeness that thunders the gospel of truth in healing.

Natural Hygiene effectuates a union of nature and man in the health sciences without clash or dissonance. As we shall see, it insinuates itself into every sector of the healing spectrum, from health to terminal disease, in perfect harmony with the natural growth forces and influences. It does not stand apart mocking orthodox medicine, or any of the diverse and sometimes closely allied nature-cure methods. Nevertheless, Natural Hygiene stands clearly on its own axis and in its own space—with a highly defensible philosophy, a scientifically supportable theory, and a very real and specific body of practice.

It will be easily seen, too, from its exciting history, how the science of Natural Hygiene blends in perfect harmony with the orchestration of the threefold paths of Issels, Gerson, and Leroi.

GENESIS

In America, perhaps a dozen men and women, all told, are responsible for having closely husbanded and nurtured "the idea whose time had come." It was no sudden awakening such as the sledgehammer blow that struck Paul on the road to Damascus, with its great explosion of light that blinded his eyes and bore a pounding voice to his ears. It was rather more a laborious accumulation of traumatic experiences, in the grinding day-to-day confrontations with the sick and the ailing. And, sometimes, the heartbreaking deaths—as the physician stood dumbly by, with saddened mien, mumbling meaningless excuses and regrets. Out of much helplessness and tragedy, noting the failures as against the successes, a handful of medical doctors, with a sensitivity to human suffering and a certain measure of wisdom, were horrified at the game of Russian roulette they were actually playing.

These few had ventured into the medical profession truly believing that their schooling and training would allow them to minister to the sick—to bring light, joy, and health to their charges. Some, in fancy, might have even imagined themselves role-playing God, indulging little miracles, routinely, at the patient's bedside. Only it wasn't always quite like that. Just as often, those patients whom they attended, worsened; some remained chronically ill; and many even died. Ultimately, the hard fact of medical fallibility penetrated the open mind and the understanding heart.

For most, it was a slow process of awakening. Dr. Isaac Jennings (1788-1874) spent twenty years in the drugging, blistering, purging, and bleeding practices of those times before changing his course. Dr. Russell Thacker Trall (1812-1877), on the other hand, almost from the start of his medical career, had strong doubts regarding the rules of practice as taught in the standard textbooks. These, and other honest souls, did not enter medicine for money, or even for fame—neither prospect being a strong probability in those days of the harassed general practitioner and country doctor. However, the last thing they would have chosen voluntarily was a job as a dealer in a game of chance where the wagers were often as high as death. It was a grim, grossly unfair game, to boot, because, although the dealer himself played—and was always in full control of the hand—he never laid a chip of his own on the table. Nor did he undertake any risks; whereas the other participants—the sick and the wounded—played always "showdown," subject to the remorseless consequences of the dealer's selection of the cards, and the playing out of every hand for each and every one of them. They had no choice but to bank upon the dealer's integrity and competence, staking their very lives on the outcome of the play, which, in effect, they could neither control nor influence.

Most of these devoted pioneer doctors and practitioners we shall discuss worked by trial and error, finally arriving at some roughhewn kind of order in their conceptualizations and methods, rather than a cohesive scientific system. Yet they were led by sheer drive and determination in the right direction.

We are speaking of that discordant era of the eighteenth and nineteenth centuries, perched on the brink of the atomic age. Medicine suffered severely from a questionable inheritance of the Middle Ages—when the pharmacopoeia of seventeenth-century London still included such healing remedies as bat's blood, animal dung, and moss from the skulls of criminals hanged by moonlight.

Sixty million people died of smallpox in Europe in the eighteenth century; childbirth fever killed tens of thousands of mothers; and tuberculosis was rampant, striking down hundreds of thousands, including such notables as Chopin in Paris, Elizabeth Barrett Browning in Florence, and Keats en route to Pisa.

Bacteriological and microchemical analyses were in their infancy; the complex modern diagnostic methods such as electroencephalography, microspectrophotometry and cardiac catheterization, unknown. Anatomical methods such as frozen sections, cinematography, and vascular injections barely discernible in the future, and even simple anesthesia, with chloroform, came only in the middle of the nineteenth century, introduced by the Edinburgh obstetrician, James Young Simpson. Biochemistry came later, too, with the development of vaccinations and the discovery of hormones, electrolytes, and vitamins—and, in the offing, in the areas of sophisticated surgical techniques and adjuvant technology in all the specialities, an armamentarium of tools and equipment to boggle the mind; with chemotherapeutic approaches to acute and chronic disease hardly yet a glimmer in the researcher's eye, as he stood poised on the very edge of the onrushing age of technology.

It therefore fell to those who later came on the scene to take the observations and findings, the pamphlets and the books of their progenitors, and sort and process this data, integrating and organizing it with the massive input of new-age knowledge into the science of health that later became known as Natural Hygiene.

According to Dr. Herbert M. Shelton, today's Dean of Natural Hygiene, Dr. Isaac Jennings (1788-1874), Sylvester Graham (1794-1851), and Dr. Russell Thacker Trall (1812-1877), were the three leaders who launched the National Hygiene movement in America. Shelton quickly adds, however, that "far from being alone in the creation of the modern system of Natural Hygiene, these three men . . . have contributed most to our understanding of this field of knowledge and art."

They had much in common. Above all, they shared that central area of agreement that disease was systemic, and that the human organism was a total system, not a disorganized assortment of haphazard and disparate parts to be viewed or treated separately. They can be said to also have been the front-runners of the rampaging health movement in America today. The Natural Hygienists, however, and most notably Dr. Shelton, have taken Jennings, Graham, Trall, and other notables more closely to their bosoms, salvaged their names from the obscure pages of history, recognized their valor, and welded their philosophical premises and scientific truths into a modern-day viable doctrine and practice.

PIONEERING NATURAL HYGIENISTS

BREAD AND WATER: DR. ISAAC JENNINGS (1788-1874)

Dr. Isaac Jennings, the point man of the Natural Hygiene movement, would be cordially welcomed into the Ganzheitstherapie school of today. His belief in the principle of totality was founded on empirical experience and encompassed also the essential spiritual ingredient in its conceptualization. "None who believe in the existence of a Supreme Creator," he wrote, "and are in the habit of observing the exact order and harmony that prevail in all the material substances and bodies around them, will question that their own bodies, which are so 'fearfully and wonderfully made' are constituted in accordance with fixed principles and that ordinarily, at least, all the vital machinery of their physical systems is controlled by express law."

Depletion of the vital energies, he believed, was caused by dietetic errors, including drinking of tea, coffee and alcohol; also excessive exertion, sexual excesses, insufficient rest and sleep, and emotional strains.

After twenty years as a practitioner of traditional medicine, he came around full-circle, convinced by hard experience that Nature knew best, and that she had invested the body with remarkable capabilities for rehabilitating itself, provided she was either left alone, altogether, or assisted in the pinches—not by vile-smelling, vile-tasting, and equally ineffective nostrums, but with materials of her own making, namely, simple foods in moderate quantity—like fresh fruits and vegetables, pure water, fresh air, sunshine, and adequate rest and sleep. He learned that outwardly alarming symptoms like fever, chills, vomiting and other manifestations were simply Nature's response to disease; that she should not be abused or thwarted in this effort, but rather aided in her own way to reject the oppressive intruder.

Dr. Robert Walter (1841-1921), another member of the growing hygienic community, underlined Dr. Jennings basic postulates: "Natural Hygiene Science," he explained, " 'cures' sick people by removing the cause of disease. It removes the disease by removing the necessity of it. It believes Nature is right, and hence does not seek to thwart her operations. It declares that disease is a natural process of purification, and should not be stopped, but aided. Its remedies are Nature's health preservatives. Obedience to Nature is its greatest panacea. Air, light, food, water, exercise, rest, and sleep in such a manner and degree as Nature can use, are its curatives. Remove the cause, and the effect will cease. This is Natural Hygiene Science."

In this context it should be remembered that the physician of that era was almost invariably a general practitioner, and just as often, in fact, a country doctor—expected to saddle up his horse and be ready to ride at a moment's notice. These were, more often than not, emergency situations, because his charges did not lightly call upon the overtaxed physician of those days. Neither rain, sleet, nor gloom of night could prevent these rough-and-ready healers from responding to a patient's needs. Day and night were all the same; crises did not wait, and neither did the occasional childbirth, because the baby normally made its entrance quite unconcerned with the doctor's office hours.

Dr. Isaac Jennings could easily file his decent claim to fame as a frontiersman for the Natural Hygiene system. But his most striking contribution was a revolutionary and seemingly foolhardy experiment: actual clinical testing (of sorts) on a massive scale. Disenchanted with the dreary results of orthodox practice, he decided on a master stroke that in today's hard-crusted medical community could have sent him straight to the wall. His fantastic brainchild made him—beyond doubt—if not the first, then certainly the greatest exponent and superb master of the art of placebo treatment in the history of medicine, a scheme he developed into a fine art—and kept in total secrecy for more than fifteen years. And—not surprisingly—it worked.

Jennings—surely a man for all seasons—decided on a bold thrust—

the kind that makes kings, heroes—or martyrs. One day, he simply emptied his saddlebags of nostrums for purging, lancets and cups for bleeding, plasters for blistering, and sundry other diverse and noxious powders and draughts. His stout heart and resolution were strengthened by recollections of twenty years at pain-wracked bedsides where he, like the other practitioners, had exhorted every orifice of that quivering body, and every square inch of skin, to produce copious quantities of blood, sweat, and tears, or die in the attempt—which, not surprisingly, many of them did. One notable example: General George Washington. In 1799, Washington, still vigorous at sixty-seven, was bled four times between dawn and midday, a total of probably two and a half quarts, for his severe throat infection, and died the same night!

Jennings filled one of his bags with an assortment of innocuous bread pills; the other with a variety of powders made of wheat flour, which he scented and colored; and placed in his pockets a quantity of vials filled with pure, soft water of various hues. For more than fifteen years, this was to be his "medicine."

As reported by his friend and admirer Russell Thacker Trall, "With these potencies in the healing art, he went forth 'conquering and to conquer.' Disease vanished before him with a promptness unknown before. His fame spread far and wide. His business extended over a large territory. It was said about him that no other physician could live at the trade of pill-peddling in that place."

Jennings must have been a consummate actor—certainly a master psychologist. He would dispense a box of bread pills with explicit directions as to when and how they should be taken, and at the same time he would counsel his patients on sound principles of diet and hygiene. Finally, in 1853, after fifteen to twenty years of the bread pills and pure water practice, Jennings could contain himself no longer, deciding to break the "glad tidings" to his medical brethren and to his community!

The first expectable reaction of the medical establishment was consternation, then bedlam—and within a short time wrath and fierce criticism of this rebel who had broken all the rules of correct medical conduct. Some of his own patients denounced him as an impostor, accusing him of abominable deception, and even complained bitterly that he had charged them for "medicines" they had not received. However, there were a host of others with a deep sense of gratitude, despite the ruse, who told Jennings: "If you can cure our diseases without medicine, then you are the doctor for us."

Despite all, Jennings carried on his "let alone" drugless practice, as he called it, for another twenty years before retiring. Although not a crusader, he accrued many converts among the professionals of his time, who were impressed with his results and decided to follow the Biblical injunction to go out and do likewise!

REBEL WITH A CAUSE: DR. RUSSELL THACKER TRALL (1812-1877)

Dr. Russell Thacker Trall and Sylvester Graham were two of Dr. Jennings's ardent contemporaries and allies. They joined hands in a dietary crusade that opened the door wide on vegetarianism, setting the stage for today's thrust of the new-age health groups by encouraging the use of fresh fruits and vegetables—as against animal proteins and by-products—and proscribing the use of processed and denaturalized foods, white bread, tobacco, and alcohol. Trall was considered by his contemporaries as the "father" of the hygienic system, having discovered its basic principles and developed its philosophical framework. A writer in the *Herald of Health* in January 1865 said about Trall: "While others have done much to agitate the public mind and develop great truths in the healing art, it was left to him to solve the great primary problems, which must underlie all medical systems, and to base a theory of medical science and a system of the Healing Art on the laws of nature themselves. Trall traced medical problems back to their starting point and thereby discovered their harmony or disharmony with universal and unalterable law. In this manner, he has been enabled to explain the nature of disease, the effects of remedies, the doctrine of vitality, and the law or conditions of cure."

Both Graham and Trall reduced the dietary regimes to a nutritional science. In 1853, Trall published his *Hydropathic Cook Book,* a classic work on food and diet. His poignant words, echoing across a time gap of a hundred and twenty-five years, carry a thundering indictment of a hoary medical establishment that appears to have learned very little from history, and is therefore doomed to repeat it: "However strange may seem the assertion," he said, "it is nevertheless true that neither health nor the philosophy of diet are taught in the medical schools, nor explained in their books, nor much regarded in the prescriptions of their physicians. Physicians, generally, are as profoundly ignorant of the whole subject as are the great masses of people."

In our own time the scene and the personalities have changed, but not the script. As mentioned previously, only about a dozen of the nation's one hundred and twenty medical schools today have full departments of nutrition, and the average medical student learns little or nothing about how to feed a normal human being to maintain good health. In *Nutrition Today* (March/April 1974), Dr. Charles E. Butterworth, Chairman of the AMA Council on Foods and Nutrition (1973 and 1974), says:

> I am convinced that iatrogenic malnutrition has become a significant factor in determining the outcome of illness for many patient. . . . I suspect as a matter of fact that one of the largest pockets of unrecognized malnutrition in America, and Canada, too, exists—not

in the rural slums or urban ghettos—but in the private rooms and
wards of big city hospitals.

Voice in the Wilderness

In February 1862, at the Smithsonian Institution, Washington, D.C.,
Dr. Russell Thacker Trall made a most extraordinary appearance before
a superelite audience of members of Congress, military officers, Army
surgeons, physicians of different schools, scientists, writers, and judges.
It was an assembly of the most prominent and progressive people in
the city. From 8:00 to 10:30 P.M., he delivered to this blue-ribbon
group, a spellbinding two-and-a-half-hour, nonstop oration of Churchill-
ian temper and proportions. His primary concern was to call attention
to the miserable plight of soldiers of the Union Army who were dying
by the thousands of typhoid fever, pneumonia, measles and dysentery,
which diseases were exacting a greater toll than the battlefield itself.
A few highlights from this highly provocative and challenging message
will illustrate its import:

"The subject of the best or most successful treatment of the diseases
of our officers and soldiers in the field being of national importance, it
seemed to me that I could present the merits of our school versus the
drug school, in high places, so as to be heard by the dignitaries of the
land, and through them by the civilized world.

"The soldiers of our camps and hospitals are dying off fast of typhoid
fever, pneumonia, measles, dysentery, etc., and quite unnecessarily. I
know that the application of our system of Hygienic medication would
save most of their lives. I am well advised that there are surgeons of
our school in the army who give no drug medicine in these diseases, and
who lose no patients, and I have been in correspondence with nurses
who attended our school, and who are saving the lives of all the sick
soldiers in their hands, by putting aside the drugs, and nursing them
properly.

"I have myself, during the sixteen years that I have practiced the
Hygienic Medical System, treated all forms and hundreds of cases of
these diseases, and have not lost a single patient. And the same is true
of scarlet and other fevers. And several of the graduates of my school
have treated these cases for years, and none of them, so far as I know
or have heard, have ever lost a patient when they were called in the
first instance, and no medicine whatever had been given.

"I have visited the camps and hospitals of our armies in this vicinity,
and I have learned—just what I knew before. One of the surgeons told
me yesterday that his regiment was the most healthy one in the department. HE GIVES NO MEDICINE, and his associates almost none.
They have had several cases of dysentery to treat, and have lost none.

"I have publicly announced that the system of Hygienic Medication,
which I teach and practice, and which I claim to be the True System of

the Healing Art, would, if applied to the treatment of typhoid fevers, pneumonia, measles and dysentery, so prevalent in our camps and hospitals, save to our country the lives of thousands of our officers and soldiers, and to our treasury millions of money.

"I fear there is too much truth in the statement of Professor B. F. Baker, M.D., of the New York Medical College: 'The remedies which are administered for the cure of measles, scarlet fever, and other self-limited diseases, KILL FAR MORE THAN THOSE DISEASES DO!'

"During a recent tour to the West, I have seen the graduates or practitioners of our school, who reside in Peoria and Aurora, Illinois, Iowa City, Wabash and Huntington, Indiana, and Dayton, Ohio, all of whom give the same testimony. Deaths of these diseases are frequent all around them, but none of them have yet lost a patient.

"Professor Austin Flint, M.D., of the New York Medical College, and physician to one of the large hospitals of our city, said a few weeks since, in a clinical lecture to his class of medical students, that, in treating pneumonia in the hospitals, he did not give any medicine at all.

"Professor B. E. Parker, of the New York Medical College said, not long since, to a medical class: 'I have recently given no medicine in the treatment of measles and scarlet fever, and I have had excellent success.'

"Dr. Snow, health officer of Providence, R. I., two years ago, reported for the information of his professional brethren, through the Boston Medical and Surgical Journal that he had treated all the cases of smallpox which had prevailed endemically in that city, WITHOUT A PARTICLE OF MEDICINE, and that all the cases—some of which were very grave—recovered."

Dr. Trall continued in his talk to make a strong case for his Hygienic school and system of practice as against prevailing medical modes. He then cited from medical journals and from an endless roster of medical critics of quite impeccable credentials some of the grave weaknesses and failures of common medical practice:

From the Dublin Medical Journal:

"Assuredly the uncertain and most unsatisfactory art that we call medical science, is no science at all, but a jumble of inconsistent opinion; of conclusions hastily and often incorrectly drawn; of facts misunderstood or perverted; of comparisons without analogy; of hypotheses without reason, and theories not only useless, but dangerous."

Dr. Ramage, Fellow of the Royal College, London:

"It cannot be denied that the present system of medicine is a burning shame to its professors, if indeed a series of vague and uncertain incongruities deserves to be called by that name. How rarely do our medicines do good! How often do they make our patients really worse! I fearlessly assert that in most cases the sufferer would be safer without a physician than with one. I have seen enough of the malpractice of my professional brethren to warrant the strong language I employ."

Professor Jamieson of Edinburgh:

"The present practice of medicine is a reproach to the name of Science, while its professors give evidence of an almost total ignorance of the nature and proper treatment of disease. Nine times out of ten, our miscalled remedies are absolutely injurious to our patients, suffering under disease of whose real character and cause we are most culpably ignorant."

Sir John Forbes, M.D.:

"Some patients get well with the aid of medicines; more without it; and still more in spite of it."

Although Trall's impassioned address left many with ears burning, he had no noticeable effect on the medical community of his time. It was a good try, but nothing changed. History again was doomed to repeat itself!

It is not our intention here, nor is it desirable, to produce a compendium of all who may have contributed to the process that ultimately evolved into the science of Natural Hygiene. Such an effort would not only exceed limitations of space, but violate the thematic imperative of our treatise, which seeks to achieve as clear and relevant a focus as possible on the central issue—terminal cancer—and what we can do about it within a work of manageable proportions. We shall therefore now touch on a few more key figures in the early evolutionary period, with apologies in advance for errors of judgment in the selective process, and then move along briskly to the active ferment on the current scene.

THOMAS LOW NICHOLS, M.D. (1815-1901)

On September 15, 1851, Dr. Thomas Low Nichols, assisted by his devoted wife, Mary Gove, opened "The American Hydropathic Institute" in New York City, a "medical school for the instruction of qualified persons of both sexes in all branches of a thorough medical education, including the principles and practices of Water Cure, in acute or chronic disease, surgery, and obstetrics." It was the first such school in America, and the world's first drugless college.

Dr. Nichols's curriculum included one component that was to become—perhaps unsuspected—the most dominant factor in the Natural Hygiene modality of our times: this was the use of fasting as a healing measure, i.e., complete abstention from food—drinking only pure water. "What is well for the well man," he wrote, "is not always well for the sick. It is well for the well man to eat, drink, take exercise, labor, and partake of all enjoyments. But the best thing for the sick man may be to entirely stop eating, and to rest mind and body. The effort to digest food, to take exercise, and to 'keep up' is a cause of exhaustion. Fasting, or absolute rest to the stomach, is one of the simplest means of cure, in both acute and dyspeptic diseases. No food, not one atom of any kind should ever be taken in any case of acute disease, until it is cured. Fasting and drinking of water is all that is needed for the digestive apparatus. And in all chronic diseases, which are dependent upon or complicated with dyspepsia, the whole digestive system needs rest, absolute rest, more than anything else. Let such a patient eat nothing; and drink water for three weeks and it will go farther to secure a cure than months in the most active treatment."

Dr. Isaac Jennings, Sylvester Graham, Dr. E. A. Kittredge, and many others, likewise placed great emphasis upon fasting patients as part of their healing regimes, with Dr. Kittredge employing it most intensively in the treatment of chronic diseases. All told, however, they did not give it the same importance as does today's Hygienic practitioner. Fasting was later incorporated by Dr. Herbert M. Shelton as the primary component of the Natural Hygiene modality, and short or extended fasts —some for as long as thirty or forty days—are routinely used today by every Natural Hygiene practitioner as the cornerstone of his healing regime. Fasting—it might be added—is an important part of the regimes of almost every biological clinic in Europe. Although it cannot be said, absolutely, that it is the ultimate constituent of the Hygienic art, nevertheless the Hygienists depend so much upon it that it would be fair to say that Natural Hygiene, as it is practiced in its pure form today, would not be the same without it.

MARY GOVE AND DR. AUGUSTA FAIRCHILD

Mary Gove, Dr. Nichols's devoted wife and helpmate, lectured widely in many cities. With two such freethinkers on the same team, it is not surprising that she also distinguished herself as one of the leading activists in the struggle for women's rights.

The establishment of Dr. Nichols's school proved a double-barreled shot in the arm to the ongoing social revolution: On one front, it was the first such school in America—and the *world's first drugless college*— and, on the other, it was the first time that a chartered medical university admitted female students into its classrooms. In a totally male-dominated society, practicing physicians would not even accept them as apprentices. However, Dr. Nichols (as well as Dr. Trall) opened their classes to women, and graduated them with a degree of Doctor of Medicine.

Many bold and bright women leaped enthusiastically into this breach, enrolling in the new medical schools. Upon graduation, they were eagerly received by the people, although given a less than rousing welcome by their male peers. Dr. Augusta Fairchild, one of the earlier women physicians, graphically describes the grim scene: "Comets were once looked upon as omens of war. Female doctors may be viewed in very much the same light, for wherever they have made their appearance, there has been a general uprising of the people to welcome them—but a most vigorous attempt of the *regular* masculine dignitaries of the 'profession' to quell the 'insurrection' has been the result."

As a leader of the women's contingent, Dr. Fairchild sensed a tide that was at its flood, and reacted in kind to male persecution: "Are female doctors acceptable?" she asked. "Do people respond to them?" Both of these questions she answered in the affirmative: "Yes, there is a great demand for them. Sick sisters are everywhere. Young girls are sick; they apply to a male physician; he gives drugs, which fasten her name in his books as a life-patient. From year to year she drags through girlhood and if she is strong enough to live in spite of her 'remedies,' she enters with a broken down constitution upon womanhood.

"A woman doctor is naturally a Hygienist. Some were educated at drug schools, but they do not imbibe the poisons—they don't believe in the drug practice, for they don't follow it in their treatment. They know and see that the Hygienic treatment is most successful; it is more in accordance with nature. It is true. So they practice it—and teach it—and wherever Hygiene is taught, there druggery receives a death blow. Assentions to the cause of Hygienic medication are being made constantly and we may expect more, for in these days, people think, and thinking will come to the truth." She adds, re the woman doctor, "Her suffering sisters welcome her with delight and will not let her go till she has repeated to them of how the precious bloom of health may be restored to them."

In the April 1853 issue of *Nichols's Journal,* Mary Gove describes a grim experience: "I acknowledge I have been mobbed on account of my dress. Fourteen years ago several persons determined to tar and feather me if I dared to lecture in a certain small city. I thought I was needed there, and I went with solemn conviction; and God gave me favor with the people. I outlived all this ignorance. Still it is true that prejudice was bitter and cruel in those days. . . . Years have greatly mended the manner of the mobs, but more than one scamp has felt the weight of my husband's cane in this city."

This article contained a piteous plaint for succor from woman's grievous predicament: "Women have so long acted, and almost existed by leave granted by the majority, that they have little idea of independent action. The public puts its mold upon us, and we come out as nearly alike as peas. Our wrists and feet just so small and delicate; our minds just so dull and stupid; our bodies bagged; and our whole lives belittled into feminine propriety. Mind, health, beauty and happiness are all sacrificed to the processes of mold; but then, woman has the comfort of keeping in her sphere, till her brief and terrible misery is over and she dies out of it. My remedy for all this slavery of women is for her to begin to judge and act for herself. God made her for herself, as much as man was made for himself. She is not to be the victim of man, or false public opinion."

Mary Gove here used an idiom that we may find quaint today, but it nonetheless gives one pause, to reflect that her cry for help went largely unheeded—and cast its imploring shadow well into the loins of the twentieth century.

THE UNIVERSAL CAUSE: DR. JOHN H. TILDEN (1851-1940)

Dr. John H. Tilden practiced orthodox medicine for thirty-five years before he lost faith in drugs. He developed a theory that there was a definite relationship between the body's loss of vital reserves and the accumulation of waste products in the system. He called this lowering of resistance "deficiency of forces," or enervation. Tilden was unequivocally convinced that he had discovered *the* giant truth about disease: that toxemia was its universal cause. He then proceeded boldly to define and explain it:

"Toxemia means poisoned by toxins taken into the body, or by one's own waste products—retained metabolic waste—brought about by inefficient elimination; and faulty elimination is caused by enervation—a weakened state of the body—lost resistance. The body is strong or weak, as the cause may be, depending entirely upon whether the nerve energy is strong or weak. And it should be remembered that the functions of the body are carried out well or badly according to the amount of energy generated. It should be known that without nerve energy not an organ of the body—a gland or muscle—can perform its function. . . . For the human body to function normally—for the physiological processes to be carried on in an ideal way—just the proper amount of nerve energy must be generated. This means that waste and repair are adjusted to ordinary needs, and that for these needs sufficient energy is generated to carry on the work. But no provision can be made for the supply of more energy for extraordinary demands such as are experienced in civilized life. Work, worry, and the pleasure-seeking peculiar to civilization draw heavily on the capital stock of nerve energy. The consequence is that everyone is in a more or less enervated state. This weakened state, this state of used-up nerve energy, shows itself in imperfect elimination— the inability of the organism to rid itself of waste products. The longer toxemia exists, the less nerve energy or resistance there is. Hence those with the least resistance are the first to go down under strain, let that be physical exertion, excitement, self-abuse or overindulgence of the appetites or passions, weather conditions, or any influence requiring nerve energy to resist.

"For thirty-five years," he said, "I practiced the science of medicine. During most of that time I did not know why people were sick, why they got well, nor why they died. When visiting the sick, and treating them in the most approved style, I had no idea of how I should find them at the next call. I did not know if the disease would end soon or late. I did not know if it would take on a severe form, or quickly run its course. I did not know whether or not there would be complications. In fact, I did not know anything that would make me comfortable regarding the outcome of the disease; and, of course, I could not say anything of a real comforting nature to my patients or their friends. I had the usual stock-in-trade subterfuges and little nothings that are worked off on a confiding public by the profession everywhere. Here is one: 'If no complications arise, the patient will recover.'

"Was my experience unique? Was it peculiarly my own? Not by any means. My experience in those days was an exact duplicate of the experience of the best, as well as the worst, physicians today. I defy the so-called best practitioners of this or any other country to undertake to prove that what I am saying is not true. Not one of the best practitioners can tell from one day to another how his patients will be. Not one can truthfully say that there is not an element in every case that is not known to him, and not knowable. Not one can say with any certainty that the drug he prescribes will have the action he hopes to experience. Not one can tell, after the first twenty-four hours of medication, whether the symptoms presenting themselves are those of disease proper or due to drugs. Not one can tell after the disease has been under treatment for a day or two, whether his patient is suffering from disease free from drug action, food poisoning, deranged emotions, or mental depression.

"To sum up: No doctor, from the professor in college to those in the rear rank, knows anything definite about his patients after the first day's drugging. Every honest doctor will admit that there is an unknown quantity about every case he treats which forces him to guess if asked to give his opinion. This wholesome guesswork is made necessary because the whole scheme of theory and practice is an unorganized mass of theory, science, empiricism and superstition. Every disease is looked upon as an individuality; each disease—name—has a special germ created to cause it. Nonsense! This is no more truth than that words are made up of letters independent of the alphabet. As truly as every word must go back to the alphabet for its letter elements, every disease must go back to toxemia, and the causes of toxemia, for its initial elements.

"The toxin theory of the healing art is grounded on the truth that toxemia is the basic source of all diseases. So sure and certain is this truth that I do not hesitate to say that it is by far the most satisfactory theory that has been advanced in all the history of medicine. It is a scientific system that covers the whole field of cause and effect—a system that synthesizes with all knowledge, hence a true philosophy."

Although there was an abundant glitter of truth among the rough gems that reflected from Dr. Tilden's impassioned pen, the unpolished stones were still obscured by the veils of the time continuum, which shrouded the future. He, like many others, was looking through a glass darkly, especially unable to nail down his concepts and convictions with absolute scientific proof. Only the incisive technology of the obtruding twentieth century made it possible for those who came later to hold up to a brighter light and sharper focus Tilden's understandably broad-layered conclusions and importunities.

Some of the best-known figures on the medical scene today—many of them Nobel Prize laureates, like Dr. Otto H. Warburg (1931), Dr. Linus C. Pauling (twice so honored—1954 and 1963), and Dr. Albert Szent-Gyorgyi (1937)—have, through their brilliant research, helped validate Dr. John Tilden's basic postulates. Their relevant research areas have been in the nature and mode of action of the respiratory enzyme (Warburg), the nature of the chemical bond and its application to the elucidation of the structure of complex substances (Pauling), and discoveries in connection with the biological combustion processes related to cellular respiration (Szent-Gyorgyi).

Disease is an expression of unfavorable factors affecting the biological activity and life of the organism, so that the interaction with the body of its external and internal metabolisms is of paramount concern, and can be observed centering ultimately in the body's activity on the cellular level, because the cell is the basic building block of all living things.

Other notables who have addressed their treatment modalities to this important area of concern should be mentioned: Issels, Gerson, and Leroi with their impressive use of assorted nutritional and medical therapeutic agents and methods providing oxidizing enzymes and detoxification regimes; Dr. Kazuhiko Asai with his synthesis and use of the oxidizing element germanium; Dr. Takeshi Kuyama, employing hyperbaric (pressurized) oxygen to assist damaged cells in the utilization of oxygen; the controversial Dr. William Frederick Koch with his dramatic use in all disease states of glyoxylide—an oxidizing catalyst that he discovered; Dr. Robert C. Olney, applying ultraviolet blood irradiation treatment, together with an oxidation catalyst—and a host of others, all lending credibility to Dr. Tilden's toxemia theory.

Each of these physicians and research scientists started from a slightly different intersecting point in the biological continuum, but all, as will be seen, ultimately achieved a consensus on the basic cause of all disease, having traced their painful way back from the body's outward, symptomatic manifestations, to the cellular level, where it was possible to confirm, empirically, the influence of biochemical environmental factors—as well as the psychic stress components—upon the state of the living organism.

If Tilden had had access to the electron microscope, X rays, and cyclotrons; to the explosive knowledge, techniques, and instrumentation of twentieth-century biochemistry; to isotope diagnostics and therapies, and the countless other breakthroughs in every medical discipline of this atomic age, it is fair to say that he would doubtless have been able to offer a far more scientific and cogent case to support his sometimes generalized, although intuitively accurate, assessment of the problem. Yet if he had done nothing more than light a candle, it would have been enough to entitle him to some share of the plaudits won by those who came later. As it was, his toxemia concept, was, in fact, a Rosetta stone pointing the way.

Insofar as Natural Hygiene is concerned, it accepts, without reservation, John H. Tilden's fundamental hypothesis that the underlying cause of all disease is toxemia—a gradual poisoning of the body resulting from the poisoning of our air, food, and water—our "external metabolism," as Dr. Max Gerson called it.

THE SHELTON STORY

The grand old man of the Natural Hygiene movement today, and its acknowledged godhead, is Dr. Herbert M. Shelton, D.C., D.N. Over the years, he acquired a respectable number of zealous followers, but only one apostle—Rafael J. Cheatham, of the Shangri-La Natural Hygiene Institute, Bonita Springs, Florida—about whom more later.

Dr. Shelton, to use an Eastern designation, is a Karma Yogin, a pick-and-shovel worker, the devotee who indefatigably mined the rough stones, gave them form and polish, and finally fixed them into a brilliant Natural Hygiene setting. He eloquently underlines the Law of Karma—cause and effect—as it operates within this science: "In the natural order of things," Dr. Shelton writes, "there is no escaping from the consequences of our acts. Hence, Hygiene teaches and insists upon the principle that before health can be regained, there must be entire conformity to Hygienic law.

"Unlike the curing systems, Hygiene holds out to no person, immunity from the consequences of actions and modes of living that violate or are in conflict with the laws of being. It does not tell the sick that they may continue to live in violation of these laws and still, by some magic potency, recover from the consequences. But it does point to the fact that living organisms are so constructed and endowed as to be able to repair their damages and restore their functions when the violations of biologic law are discontinued. In place of the systems of healing that now commend the blind patronage of the sick, we offer a simple, plain, easy-to-understand system of mind-body care, with nature as its guarantee, the cardinal principle of which is that nature works for the restoration of health by the same means and processes, in kind, by which she works for the preservation of health. . . . Hygienic care is not directed to the cure of disease, but works to provide the most favorable conditions for the efficient operation of the body's own healing processes. We recognize the so-called disease as an effort to resist and expel morbid causes and repair damages, not as an enemy to be cast out or killed."

Dr. Shelton's whole life and his inexhaustible energies (he is now in his eighties) have been applied with the fanatical zeal of a crusader to the cause of Natural Hygiene. As he so well puts it, in answering a question posed in a recent interview: "My major contribution to the Hygienic movement has been that of resuscitating a movement that was almost dead. Almost alone at the start, I fanned its glowing embers into a fierce flame. In doing this, I had to *resurrect* men and women who had been buried beneath an avalanche of palliatives and cures, and revitalize principles that had been forgotten. At the same time I had to repopularize a literature that was being allowed to slip unobservedly over the precipice into oblivion. Today, thanks to my untiring effort— and the efforts of those who joined me in the work—men that were dead, live again, principles that were forgotten have been refurbished, and a whole literature has been salvaged."

Without the Herculean efforts of this staunch historian and modern scribe, the names of men like Jennings, Graham, Tilden, and Trall would long ago have been scattered like dust before the uncaring winds of time. Shelton openly acknowledges that, in making his discoveries, he, like Newton, rode "piggyback on the shoulders of colossi." He diligently researched, assimilated, and synthesized the vast storehouse of knowledge and wisdom of the pioneers in natural health. From voluminous sources of unorganized data—from thousands of books, lectures, papers and tracts—he painfully culled the precious nuggets, and published well over forty books and booklets, producing, in effect, a New Testament of Natural Hygiene. In this area of the natural sciences and natural healing, one is tempted to equate in metaphorical terms, his Hygienic Gospel with the Biblical Gospel of Luke, the Great Physician!

The first thrust giving practical expression to Shelton's ideas and ambitions was the opening of "Dr. Shelton's Health School" in San Antonio, Texas, on September 1, 1928, a quite momentous date in the annals of the movement, because the school was to become the central focus of his activities until the founding of the American Natural Hygiene Society some twenty years later. The title of "school," however, must be classed as something of a misnomer, chosen for expediency's sake, as are the euphemisms of "students" and "guests" applied to those who register there. The Health School is, in fact, an institute where people go—primarily to fast—for weight loss, or to recover from assorted aches and pains, as well as from chronic disease problems. The regrettable although necessary semantics is due to the hazard of legal confrontation with the medical Establishment, which dogs the steps of all who dare to practice Natural Hygiene methods. The watchdogs of the AMA appear on a twenty-four-hour alert to prevent trespassing on their sacrosanct premises. And the ultimate in transgressions? Practicing medicine without a license!

Twenty years after the opening of the Shelton Health School, Shelton was instrumental in founding the American Natural Hygiene Society (ANHS), on April 1, 1948, and was elected its first President. There began a period of growth through membership and affiliation by a number of dedicated supporters and practitioners. On the Hygienic roster of sometime fully confirmed, simon-pure adherents and practitioners have appeared such names as Christopher Gian-Cursio, D.C., William L. Esser, N.D., D.C., Keki Sidhwa, N.D., D.O., David J. Scott, D.C., Alec Burton, D.O., Robert R. Gross, D.C., John M. Brosious, N.D., D.C., and Virginia Vetrano, D.C., Dr. Shelton's lifelong associate and greatest aide, presently managing the Health School in Texas. As noted, almost all of them have degrees in Chiropractic, and some additionally in Naturopathy—sometimes referred to on the Continent as "Nature-Cure."

If Dr. Shelton were asked today to set forth the basic ideas and the rules of practice of the science of Natural Hygiene, his response would be today exactly what it was when the organization was first formed thirty years ago; the underlying principles, with minor exceptions, are easily recognized as containing the essence of the philosophical configuration, the fundamental truths and practices of Hygiene's venerable forebears.

The American Natural Hygiene Society was well conceived and timely. It rushed into a yawning vacuum in the healing community, and it was Dr. Herbert M. Shelton, the lionhearted, who, virtually single-handed, erected this upstart new-dimensional structure in the midst of the healing complex. It flashed like a rebellious comet across a burgeoning technological macrocosm of the twentieth century, eschewing mechanistics in medicine, and opting rather for a nature-oriented totality that excluded every drug, herb, and potion. Shelton's seemingly simplistic back-to-nature idea was all the more praiseworthy because it was conceived, nurtured, and flowered in the very bowels of a technological society where the machine was king, and where Nature was being treated like a retarded child. Here was a new breed of prodigal son, returning—not empty-handed and hopelessly shattered by his long sojourn in alien lands, but rather as a battle-scarred philosopher, rife with seemingly primitive ideas, boldly claiming honor in his own country—and challenging a self-centered materialistic society whose gods were sophisticated second- and third-generation calculators and computers. In a way, Shelton resembled Stone Age man, insisting upon his primitive culture as a superior way of life, daring to confront the egomania of euphoric bio-chemists in their awesome laboratories, hyped-up engineers at their innovative drawing boards, and gimlet-eyed galactic scientists staring tight-lipped at multicolored lights on their signal panels as they awaited the final countdown that would send a spaceship to the moon, Jupiter, or Mars.

What a moving picture Shelton makes, furrowing the bare soil with his naked feet—with a handful of fruits and a few nuts in his hands—fronting the monolith—the mechanized monsters that tower above his puny figure—and defying them to accept his naked challenge!

Dr. Shelton must be credited with having established an early foot-hold, and with playing a leading role in culturing the soil that fed the tiny rootlets of the embryonic health movement, which has today blos-somed into a proliferation of national organizations, societies, and com-munities of transcending proportions and influence. His was backbreaking pioneering that called for total devotion and sacrifice, drone work—dig-ging into moldy archives and dusty library corners to extract occasional kernels of wisdom, morsels of value, and building them into an organized and convincingly rational science, where it stands, baleful and unashamed, challenging medical orthodoxy on its own terrain.

As the maximum Hygienist, Shelton is best pictured and loved by his adherents in the role of a modern-day Sir Lancelot. An aura of romance and drama surrounds him as he enters the joust; the lovely "Lady Hygiene" is his Queen Guinevere; and he responds to the thunder of the trumpets, and the tumultuous cries and shouts of the galleries, which rise to their highest crescendo as he takes his place in the lists, drops his visor, and tilts his lance against the monstrous forces of evil—notoriously the much-maligned medical Establishment. This is Shelton at his best, emotionally committed, and wearing the colors of his favorite lady as he flings all caution to the winds and spurs his gallant horse to the clash of combat!

This is not a game of chance, where the enemy is accidentally chosen. No! Shelton's hard-nosed, uncompromising attitude may be blamed for his lack of popular acclaim by the medical community, but it has its formidable and highly defensible base. Shelton has observed thousands who have fled the disheartening assaults of medical orthodoxy, and knows from empirical experience how easily so many have been rescued from severe afflictions and chronic disease by simple Hygienic measures. Therefore, for him—a dedicated healer—every day is a time to try men's souls, as he sadly observes these medical casualties. It is difficult to fault this kind of angry man.

Some movements have their Paul—the Evangelist who carries the message of the prophet throughout the land, shouting the good news from the housetops. Others nobly serve their cause by example—and by their writings. It seems that Shelton, in the early years, combined both these talents prodigiously, but later became mired down in his almost exclusive commitment to his guests at the institute, and to his writing—withdrawing from an active leadership role in the Society. As a result, the ANHS was diverted from what should have been its major objective: the establishment of a bona fide educational institute with appropriate curriculum and accreditation. Such a thrust, pursued with skill and determination, would have enabled it to achieve some kind of acceptable professional status, avoiding the unpleasant and continuing clashes with medical orthodoxy.

However, it is a regrettable commentary upon the American Natural Hygiene Society that its leadership began to suffer from a lack of vision and foresight in its organizational planning. Shelton certainly recognized the key necessity, the paramount importance of a center of learning, and envisioned, at the start, that his "Dr. Shelton's Health School" would evolve into such an institution. Unfortunately, he was caught up in the press of tending sick patients and, additionally, could not abate his own frenetic writing pace in getting the Hygienic literature out into the public marketplace. So his noteworthy dream of an accredited university just bumbled along, with mountains of empty rhetoric accumulating within and without the Society, but little concrete action resulted. Ergo, rather than achieving an adaptation to its hostile environment—as in the natural process of evolution—this strange new creature emerged, figuratively, from its primeval bed, and apparently decided that, because it could not adapt, it would transmute. And, in the process, it became a most confusing hybrid, sometimes tending more to repel than attract.

The paramount necessity of the Hygienic movement to gain credibility and acceptance, and to establish professional status and legality within the parameters of the medical community—no matter how diminutive might be its initial foothold—died on the vine. It would have been no easy task in any event, but neither was the harrowing gauntlet originally run by such disciplines as homeopathy, osteopathy, and chiropractic; but all these finally received acceptance within the traditional medical framework. Without legal status, Dr. Shelton and others practicing Hygiene were daily looking into the open end of a gun barrel. And the reality of the hazard is that, almost without exception, every Hygienic practitioner has suffered this hot pursuit, and at one time or another been unhappily involved in lawsuits, the most recent such action, ironically enough, involving the Dean of the movement himself, Herbert M. Shelton.

Lacking legal recognition, and apparently prompted by the necessity for survival of its handful of practitioners, the movement spawned—unfortunately—a language of its own, employing such semantics as calling patients "guests" and "students"; it proscribed such words as "treatment," "healing," and "cure" from application to the practitioner's therapeutic activity, establishing a patois that often baffled the tongue in dialogue, as it tried to formulate simple ideas in the conduct of normal communication. This backlash served only to confuse and irritate foe and friend alike.

A brief excerpt from Shelton's writings may give some indication of the problem: "Hygienists do not *treat* disease. From its origin Hygienists have agreed that disease should not be *treated*. They have repudiated the idea that disease should be *cured*. They have asserted that *disease is a curative process.* They do not seek to CURE the CURE." (Our italics.)

Much of the semantics may be reasonably attributed to the inherent nature of the concepts, yet, even here, a sympathizer might fault them for overpressing, for attempting an isolating parochialism rather than seeking that elastic base of an already extant, common terminology that conveyed familiar symbols and patterns and that allowed easy communication with other like-minded peoples, organizations, and groups—and even those in the medical community who did not at all deny the body's own healing potential.

The point is that this hairsplitting contentiousness is a disconcerting dialectic, favoring the growth of a cult, rather than an ongoing dynamic philosophy and science in an expanding state of flux. Its immediate tendency and effect were to wall off Natural Hygiene from its natural allies such as nutritionists, vegetarians, naturopaths, herbalists, macrobiologists, organic gardeners, and farming groups and communities; and, yes, even chiropractors and osteopaths, who also incorporate in their holistic approach many basic principles of Natural Hygiene.

All this has proven self-defeating. The Natural Hygiene movement has thereby failed to achieve a meaningful relationship with the many groups and movements whose sympathetic cooperation could enrich the Society and its membership, and greatly accelerate its growth. Mute testimony to its failure are the unhappy statistics: Today, after thirty years, the Society can boast of no more than thirty-five hundred adherents and perhaps ten so-called practitioners in the entire world! It is also relevant to note that the Society has yet to enlist a single medical doctor who totally accepts its principles and practice, although there are a handful who acknowledge its values and occasionally may appear as guest lecturers at its annual conventions.

Dr. Shelton himself belatedly admits that "the growth of the Society has been disappointingly slow, and its influence has not been as great as was hoped. It has reached a point in its development where all of this should be changed. I think we can look forward to greater growth and a widening and intensive increase in its influence."

Dr. Shelton is referring here to the recent election of a new President, Mark A. Huberman, a feisty young attorney who has been spoon-fed from birth on a Hygienic regimen—never having even once tasted cooked food—and who is completely sold on its benefits. Throwing himself passionately into his new job, Huberman is trying to energize the movement with a transformed and exciting journal, *Health Science,* and with a broader perspective that may, it is hoped, loosen up the Society's arthritic joints, and break the archaic chains of sectarianism that characterize it today. Huberman seems alert to the order of priorities and will, it is hoped, placed this item of an accredited educational institute at the top of the Society's agenda.

It is entirely foreseeable that, working cooperatively within a viable community that shares common interests, by using an ecumenical approach, so to speak, Natural Hygiene could gain wider public approval for its fundamentally sound principles and practices, and clarify its present muddied image.

DANCE OF THE ANGELS

There is one sector of Natural Hygiene—food selection and food combining—as developed by Dr. Shelton, that warrants our close attention before moving to the story of Rafael J. Cheatham—the most dynamic personality to illuminate the current scene.

As Dr. Max Gerson dramatically proved, nutrition is, literally, the ultimate weapon. Because the system of food selection and food combining rates high in its program, it is imperative to examine the Natural Hygiene position, which presents certain controversial aspects, in order to avoid a distortion of values that may result in a faulty perception of the whole.

Here are the Natural Hygiene "No-No's" of *food selection:*

1. no animal proteins or animal by-products such as eggs, milk, butter, buttermilk, cheese, or yogurt
2. no cooked foods
3. no fruit, vegetable, or other juices; no grains, cereals, honey
4. no vitamins, minerals, or food supplements
5. no herbs in any form, medicinal, teas, or other
6. no hot or irritating foods that contain mustard oil, or other irritants, such as onions, garlic, leeks, chives, shallots, radishes, and watercress.

The other side of the food modality deals with *food combining,* also a Dr. Shelton offspring. This, too, has for so long saturated the literature of Natural Hygiene that it has come to be accepted as gospel—and is erroneously attributed by most followers to the same historic backgrounders and sources upon which Dr. Shelton relies for his other teachings. He makes his case for food combining in his popularized booklet "Food Combining Made Easy." For those interested in a more elaborate dissertation of his hypotheses, this can be found in a larger work, *Orthotrophy,* which is the first volume of *The Hygienic System.*

We shall first cite an extract taken from "Food Combining Made Easy," which will serve as an indicator of Shelton's generalized direction on this subject: "I want to differentiate between natural food combinations and the haphazard combinations commonly eaten. The human digestive tract is adapted to the digestion of natural combinations, but it is certainly not adapted to the digestion of the haphazard and indiscriminate combinations that are eaten in civilized life today. Natural combinations offer but little difficulty to the digestive system; but, it is one thing to eat one food, however complex in nature; it is quite another thing to eat two foods of 'opposite character.' The digestive juices may be readily adapted to one food, such as cereals, that is, a protein-starch combination; they cannot be well adapted to two foods, such as bread and cheese. . . . From medical sources, as well as from the camp-followers of medicine in the other schools of so-called healing, and the dietetic camp-followers of allopathy, certain objections are made to the practice of avoiding certain food combinations and eating others. These objections are all based on the assumption that the human stomach is equipped to easily and efficiently digest any and all possible combinations of foods which may be introduced into it. Very little special attention will be devoted to meeting these objections, as the facts presented in this little book constitute sufficient reply to the objections."

The Natural Hygiene food combining system divides foods into the following six broad classifications:

> *Proteins:* most nuts, *dry beans and peas, *peanuts, soybeans and avocados
> *Carbohydrates:* *dry beans and peas, *peanuts, chestnuts, squash, pumpkin, cauliflower, beets, carrots, and so forth
> *Green vegetables:* lettuce, celery, endive, cabbage, broccoli, brussels sprouts, spinach, chard, okra, chicory, kale, eggplant, cucumbers, green beans, and sweet peppers
> *Sweet fruits:* bananas, dates, figs, raisins, prunes, persimmons
> *Subacid fruits:* fresh figs, pears, sweet cherries, papaya, sweet apples and peaches, apricots, huckleberries, and mangos
> *Acid fruits:* oranges, grapefruit, lemons and limes, pineapples, apples, peaches, plums, and grapes (except the Tomson and muscat variety—considered in the sweet fruits category).

As for the simple "Do's" and "Don'ts":

Either proteins or starches are considered a good combination with green vegetables, but not with each other.

*These are classified as both proteins and carbohydrates.

Fruits and green vegetables make a poor combination, so they are not recommended; likewise, proteins or carbohydrates with fruits.

As for the fruit family itself, combinations of sweet and subacid fruits, or subacid with acid fruits are considered only fair, whereas acid and sweet fruits are definitely not recommended.

On the face of it, these combinations would appear reasonable, and yet there is always the nagging question as to whether a balanced meal or diet can be realized from rigid adherence to such a regime, especially when it is considered that all animal proteins and by-products, e.g., milk, butter, cheese and eggs; cereals and grains, vitamins, minerals and supplements are ostracized from this diet.

Few of the old naturopaths or Hygienists held for the rigidity that seems to characterize today's Hygienic food regime, especially their stringent list of prohibitions. Dr. J. H. Tilden, for example, while agreeing with the general food classifications that decried mixing of starches with meats, or with sugars—or having more than one kind of protein at a meal—nevertheless allowed meats, simply prepared, i.e., "properly stewed, roasted, or broiled." Poultry, fish, and milk were also acceptable in his diet. He recognized the place of cooked food in the diet of modern man. Tilden, therefore, stood on more rational ground when he said: "It is my opinion that there is a place for all foods; and, as meat, milk, and other animal foods are easier for digestion than the grains, it shall be my endeavor to point out, as nearly as I can, the place that animal foods should occupy in a well-balanced dietary system."

Dr. Russell Thacker Trall was likewise partial to allowing meats from herbivores, like beef and mutton; also poultry, eggs, and grains. No fetish was made regarding outlawing onions, leeks, garlic, or shallots from the diet. Harry Benjamin, N.D., in *Everybody's Guide to Nature Cure,* endorsed a fruit and milk diet, considering milk as a complete food; permitted cooked foods, grains, cheese, and eggs; and encouraged, also, "other forms of natural treatment such as hydrotherapy, massage, and spinal manipulation" (which therapeutic methods, incidentally, are anathema to the Hygienic System!).

Otto Carque, one of the most eminent of earlier writers in this area, like all the others, heartily endorsed the integral parts of the Hygienic system, such as the exercise regime and the need for pure water, rest, sunshine, poise, and peace of mind. He felt, however, that no narrow set of "proximates," as he called them, which excluded any valuable nutritional constituent from a completely balanced diet, could adequately sustain the vital forces of the organism. He was here actually expounding the principle of totality. Carque was adamantly opposed to meat eating, and, though not recommending eggs, milk, cereals, and legumes—which latter he considered acid-producing—he nevertheless allowed their inclusion in human nutrition, in moderation, emphasizing that their value would be appreciably increased by proper combining, especially with green leafy vegetables.

He appears one of those rare sages who recognized that man had developed certain habits over the thirty thousand years since the discovery of fire and cooking. Theoretically he could agree that a totally raw food diet had its merits, but "the change in diet should be made gradually and intelligently considering our state of health and the conditions under which we have to live at present. By subsisting for many centuries largely on cooked foods, and deprived of the necessary out-of-door exercise, the digestive organs of civilized man have become more or less weakened, so that in many cases he cannot suddenly change to a diet of uncooked foods, especially cereals, fibrous and starchy vegetables, without much inconvenience. We just begin with discarding all denatured products and prepare our foods without depriving them of the essential organic salts. There is no doubt that cooking, especially if prolonged, renders all food less valuable. But we should remember that the majority of persons, owing to their imperfect teeth, cannot thoroughly masticate many raw foods, and their digestive juices are not strong enough to extract adequate nourishment therefrom."

Lastly, we cite one of the great historians and broad-ranging scholars of modern times, Edmond Bordeaux Szekely, who sagely writes, in *The Book of Living Foods,* that past civilizations "were strongly rooted in an agricultural society whose citizens ate the simplest of natural foods. The two that come to mind first, ancient Greece and Rome, faced deterioration only when exotic imported foods began to be popular—in its early years of splendor, the staples of the Greek diet were figs and milk, while the fantastic stamina of the Roman warrior was attributed to whole-wheat bread and onions. The main food of the Mongols, who, led by Ghenghis Khan, conquered all of Asia and most of Europe, was sour milk. There was nothing magical in any of these foods; they simply ate what was most readily available, in its crude, natural state. The Romans, Greeks and Mongols were not nutritional experts; they only ate what nature provided and did not change it in any way, thereby assuring the maximum vitamin, mineral and enzyme content."

To summarize: While agreeing broadly with certain rational dietary laws concerning allowable food combinations, Shelton, even here, is quite unbending. He compounds the problem further by his contentious stance in exorcising a large and important group of normally acceptable and nutritionally valuable foods, food products and supplements, which is altogether unhappily reminiscent of the classical doctrinal debates by medieval theologians who were at one time locked in mortal combat over exasperating trivia such as how many angels could dance on the point of a needle!

Serious nutritional deficiencies may result in functional weaknesses and/or life-threatening failures of certain organs, which may necessitate the administration of oxidizing enzymes, juices, protein components, vitamins, and supplements, or other nutrient and medicative therapeutics during the crisis and recuperative period. Most practitioners, even those wholly nutritionally oriented, would not gainsay this, and thus the violent objection of the Hygienic system to such input is viewed by most with a jaundiced eye, and may, unhappily be classed as arising out of ignorance or fanaticism.

As outlined in the foregoing, our examination of the dietary regimes suggested by virtually all of the early pioneers, like Tilden, Trall, Carque, and many others in the "Natural Hygiene" or "Nature Cure" groups, reveals a generally simple fare. There is no belaboring of the problems of angels, no radical beleaguering of traditional modes—except to eliminate synthetic products, processed and adulterated foods, irritating peppers and spices, flamboyant desserts such as rich pies and pastries, coffee, tea, tobacco, and alcohol. In other words, a strong accent is placed upon plain, natural foods without stringent restrictions otherwise, usually admitting meats, poultry, milk, and cheese, in moderation, into the normal diet.

Although Shelton here and there cites authority for his broad-ranging absolutes, most are fragmentary, and few of his references can qualify as acceptable scientific research studies. It becomes clear, therefore, that, despite particulated support in the medical literature of food and diet, we can take him at his word in the following—that his conclusions in this area are primarily subjective:

"More than thirty-one years spent in feeding and caring for the young and the old, the well and the sick, male and female, rich and poor, educated and ignorant, nearly twenty-five years of this spent in institutional practice, the balance in office practice, certainly entitle me to speak with some authority on the subject."

The "institutional practice" refers to his own "Dr. Shelton Health School," and, because the Natural Hygiene therapeutic program employs no tests, no diagnostics, no laboratory controls of any kind, and maintains no follow-up of guests or patients, it is fair to conclude that Shelton's position is centered fully upon highly subjective personal observation, permitting little, if any, scientific validation.

To repeat, insofar as the broad contours of the hypotheses re food combining are concerned, as already mentioned, it is doubtful that any properly accredited dietitian, nutritionist, or nutritionally oriented doctor would raise violent objections, but, compounded by the stringent exclusions of foods and food components, it assumes, regrettably, the proportions of an "un-natural" and extremist dietary system.

It goes without saying that a more elaborate refinement of dietary modes might easily have been achieved by the frontiersmen of the movement, if they had ceased a bit from their arduous caseload and applied themselves to such specific studies, but it is doubtful that even their more substantial research would have led to any major deviations from the general dietary principles and modes they subscribed to.

Nevertheless, Shelton chose to view this absence of minute prescription as an error of omission, and reacted with a vengeance, by rushing into the vacuum with a zealousness that might have raised an eyebrow— if not a furrow of consternation—on Trall's resplendent forehead.

It may be conjectured that Shelton's fillip into this highly controversial area was triggered by a burning desire to depart from his wholly admirable role as historian, scribe, and tutor, and to insert his personal imprint to enrich, and perhaps enlarge, the parameters roughly outlined by the early pioneers—a quite understandable ambition. Regrettably, he doesn't quite pull it off, but rather seems to have created and codified a dogma of food strictures that must strike some as an alarming mystique. This needs to be clearly identified and rationalized within the context of the whole, so that its weaknesses do not distort or invalidate the major outlines of the altogether sound principles and practices of Natural Hygiene.

Although seemingly out of context with the subject of food combining and food selection, nevertheless at this point in our discussion it appears appropriate to mention one another remaining and highly controversial sector of the Hygienic modality that perpetually surfaces to confound its devotees because of its open challenge to the mass of the healing community worldwide—and that is their violent objections to the use of any type of physiological stimulation or manipulation of the body, such as hydrotherapy, massage, acupuncture, shiatsu, packs, reflexology—yes, even chiropractic or osteopathy. It is this *idée fixe* that plagues even the loyal adherents and gives rise to occasional tremors of inner turmoil and misgivings.

It has been necessary to discuss these Hygienic views in the controversial areas, because they are part of the fulcrum of Natural Hygiene's wheel of health, but more particularly because it is mainly here that most homogenous health groups have felt a frustrating rigidity and estrangement, and where, also, the slings and arrows of the enemy camp have been used with most telling effect. More than anything else, it is these austerities that have insinuated themselves into the Hygienic litany, setting them apart from their brethren—the new-age health-oriented groups—and—most decidedly—from the medical community.

Having provided this candid view of the "holes in the net," it is hoped that the matter has been given its proportion, so that the faults discussed will not flaw the main theme and premises, or detract from the magnitude of Hygiene's essentially sound health-giving principles.

20

Shangri-La

Dr. Herbert M. Shelton dreamed of a Natural Hygiene Shangri-La, and James Hilton imagined it, in his famous classic *Lost Horizon*; but it was Rafael J. Cheatham who materialized the dream and nurtured it into reality. As a modern-day apostle and supreme exponent of the Natural Hygiene system, Mr. Cheatham created his own Shangri-La in the sleepy waterstop town of Bonita Springs—on the Gulf Coast of Florida. It was not a fabled community hidden in the fastnesses of a remote, mist-shrouded Valley of Eden, amid the towering peaks of the mighty Himalayas, but an earthly paradise, where he practiced, preached, and lived Natural Hygiene. But now, let Mr. Cheatham himself—or "R.J." as he was familiarly known—tell his own revealing and dramatic story. It begins with his confrontation with an insidious killer.

R. J. CHEATHAM

I recovered from cancer and I should like to tell you how it happened: April 14, 1948—a day I will always remember . . . I had gone to a hospital for an examination of what I had considered to be a minor problem. It was a lump on my right chest, which had developed into an open running sore. After an extensive examination, X rays, and a biopsy, the physicians came forth with a diagnosis of malignant melanoma or cancer on the right chest area. They recommended an immediate operation.

THE OPERATION

It had never occurred to me that I should question the physician's diagnosis, so we proceeded to make arrangements for admission to the hospital the following day. The operation was performed at the Hines Veterans Administration Hospital in Hines, Illinois, a suburb of Chicago. I was in the operating room for over five hours and the surgeons removed

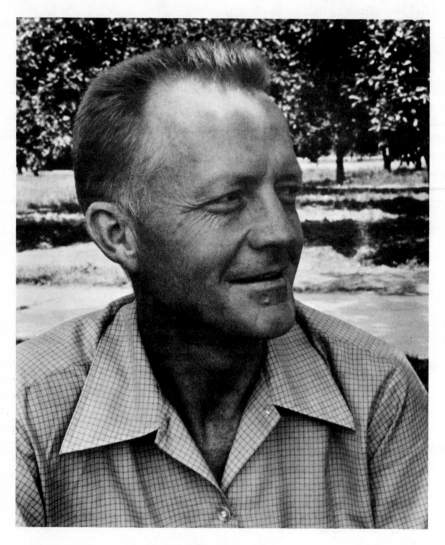

Rafael J. Cheatham

the entire surface of the right side of my chest, leaving the bones covered with only a little skin and a scar seventeen inches long. The next three months I spent in the hospital recuperating from the operation and trying to regain my health by following the orthodox procedures. Every few hours I received a shot of penicillin and on alternate hours a pill or some other type of medication. Interspersed with the medications were the typical hospital meals. Finally, on July 30, 1948, I was released from the hospital with instructions to eat a "well-balanced diet" and a warning from the Chief Surgeon that I should not expose my body to the sunshine under any circumstances.

SEARCH FOR TRUTH

It was while recuperating in the hospital that I found time to think about my cancer condition and its causes. I began to question the physicians, surgeons, nurses, and other patients. After considerable questioning, I found that mine had been a very serious condition, the chances of recovering from the operation about fifty-fifty and, further, that the maximum life expectancy after such an operation was only about five years.

I then tried to find out what the cause was and what I could do to prevent any further problems. The answers I received from the physicians and surgeons did not seem to satisfy me, and I found myself embarked upon a search to find an answer that would satisfy my now curious mind and possibly save my life.

During the next two years I ran the gamut of practically all of the so-called "healing professions." I took their prescribed medicines, pills, shots, drugs, and accepted their treatments of massage, adjustments, vibrations, X rays, colonics, and a host of other "cures." In spite of being continually "cured" by all this medical science, my condition did not actually seem to improve. To the contrary, when I returned to the hospital for routine examinations, the surgeons found more lumps and began to operate again to remove sections for biopsy or examining purposes. Hearing of the third death among my cancer-ridden hospital roommates did not improve my mental outlook. To make matters worse, one insurance company canceled my life insurance, and other companies flatly refused to provide me with any insurance at any price. Reflecting on the past, and the obvious inability of the orthodox methods to help my condition, I lost confidence in all the physicians and their efforts to "cure" me.

About this time (1950), I began to frequent the health food stores, where I purchased their various products as well as magazines and books. Any book I could find on the subject of health improvement was studied thoroughly from cover to cover. Every health lecturer who came to town found me in attendance to listen, to buy his products and books, to take his courses, and to ask questions. As time went by I became familiar with most of the people speaking on health improvement, and I knew what their point of view was. Fortunately, from each of these I was able to glean a little truth and I put into practice the ideas that made sense to me.

NATURAL HYGIENE

One evening I noticed an advertisement in the newspaper about a lecturer who was going to speak on the subject of how to improve health through Natural Hygiene. This was something new to me, so I made it a point to be at the meeting, if for no other purpose than to determine what he had to sell and what his point of view was. I had been through the mill and by this time was a true skeptic. But the principles of Natural Hygiene, or the laws of Nature, with their simplicity, logic, and common sense, impressed me. By the time the lecture was over I felt sure that here was the answer to health and disease, to living or dying.

Having found what promised to be the answer, I purchased book after book and attended many lectures on the subject. Later I was privileged to attend one of the Annual International Conventions of the American Natural Hygiene Society. After attending the many classes and lectures given by the leading professional and lay hygienists on the many facets of Natural Hygiene, after listening to and participating in the question-and-answer periods and after talking with many people who had followed this way of life, any doubts or reservations I might have had were completely eliminated.

To put it briefly, the study of Natural Hygiene taught me that cancer, or any other disease, is not a chance thing, that disease isn't something that you accidentally catch, but is the result of definite causes. Disease is not harmful but rather the vital action of the body trying to correct itself and is actually beneficial. One should not interfere with disease by the use of palliative and suppressive drugs, medications, and treatments, but one should assist this eliminative effort of the body by complete rest and fasting if possible.

Natural Hygiene teaches that, if we want to have good health, it is necessary to eliminate the causes of poor health. It teaches that the human body must have adequate sunshine, fresh clean air, pure uncontaminated water, regular exercise, sufficient rest and sleep, bodily cleanliness, and mental and emotional poise. Further, that we must provide the body with fresh, unprocessed natural foods at the proper time, in the proper quantities, and in the proper combinations.

After the Convention, I resolved to do everything I could to help communicate the knowledge of this better way of life to the rest of the world. Becoming active as an officer of the local Detroit Chapter of the American Natural Hygiene Society probably helped me more than anything else to develop sufficient self-control and self-discipline to put into practice the hygienic principles necessary to restore my own health. Each year I have managed to get to the Annual Convention wherever it was held. It was my pleasure to be appointed Convention Manager for the 1959 International Convention, which was held in Detroit, Michigan.

THE RESULTS OF BETTER LIVING

Having told you about my experience in Natural Hygiene, let me tell you a little about the results of living this better way of life. After giving my body a chance to rehabilitate itself through fasting, working out a daily exercise program, arranging my time so that I could get plenty of rest and sleep, planning for regular sun and air baths, and correcting my diet by eliminating substances such as meat, fish, fowl, white bread, white sugar, salt, coffee, tea, soda pop, chewing gum, spices, condiments, and so forth, and substituting plenty of live foods, such as fresh succulent salads, fresh vegetables, fresh fruits and fresh nuts, I found that I was able to eliminate the eyeglasses I had worn for about ten years. When I took the test for renewing my driver's license, the examiner passed me without question. An insurance company examination found me qualified for a larger policy. My physical examinations revealed no further lumps or problems. Mrs. Cheatham and I have had four additional children since the operation. These children have been brought up from birth in this better way of life. They are all lovely children— all pictures of health—and without the "benefit" of any medications, shots, or treatments of any kind. Incidentally, our last three children were born at home, with myself in attendance for the delivery.

Perhaps most important, over twenty-five years have passed since my cancer operation. Those who were with me, in the same hospital, with similar conditions and orthodox care, have long since passed away.

A PLAN DEVELOPED

In order to pursue my new interest in Natural Hygiene, I decided to sell the successful business that I had owned and operated in Detroit, Michigan, for almost ten years, and move to Florida so that I would have a more desirable climate for myself and my family. Soon after making this decision, during 1959-60, I was privileged to serve as National President and General Manager of the American Natural Hygiene Society. I then took it upon myself to make a lecture tour of the United States to visit all the local chapters of the American Natural Hygiene Society and also the vegetarian-hygienic resorts and institutions that were in existence at that time. It was during this tour that I first began thinking of trying to locate, organize, and develop a place where these wonderful laws of Nature could be taught, lived, and practiced. I began a new search for a location at which to establish a hygienic institute. In order to prepare myself for this new work I intensified my study of Natural Hygiene, obtaining and studying every single work of Dr. Herbert M. Shelton and all the other leaders of the Hygienic movement. In addition, I took extensive courses, obtaining diplomas in Naturopathy, Homeopathic Medicine, Osteopathy Life Science, and Metaphysics.

My search for a suitable location lasted for over two years, taking me all over the United States, through Canada, the Bahama Islands, Jamaica and Mexico, until I finally found exactly what we were looking for in Bonita Springs, Florida.

We named it Shangri-La, after the fabled lost community in the Himalayas that James Hilton so enchantingly described in his classic novel *Lost Horizon*. It is the story of man's search for the unattainable, the possibility of its manifestation and the ease with which it can be destroyed. The word "Shangri-La" originated in this book, and was used to describe a haven of peace away from the cares of the world.

THE SHANGRI-LA

The Shangri-La Natural Hygiene Institute provides the best environment available for healthful living, a place where health-minded people, without restriction as to race, color or creed, can come to get away from the pace of our "civilization."

OUR OBJECTIVE

The Shangri-La is operated as—

1. a Health Institute, where people may come to learn the Natural Hygienic way of life
2. a Year-Round Resort, where health-minded folk may enjoy a real, healthful vacation
3. a Retreat, where the overweight and the underweight may come to normalize their weight through fasting and/or a corrected nutritional program
4. a Sanctuary, where those in distress with physical problems may come to get well through the discovery of the causes of their "dis-ease" and the correction of their living habits.

In short, the Shangri-La is dedicated to teaching Natural Hygiene— the Truth in matters of health and correct living. We have devised a comprehensive program whereby people may learn how to recover their health and then how to maintain it, a program based upon the science of human ecology, which is a part of Natural Hygiene. Our objective is to make information on this better way of life available for all who desire it.

THE SHANGRI-LA PROGRAM

Our primary function as an educational institute is to teach both the well and the sick how to live an orderly and healthful life—one that conforms to the laws of Nature. This is done through lectures, literature, question periods, and tape recordings. In addition, we make every effort to provide the requirements for good health for our guests. Only the very best and freshest, properly combined, natural foods are served. We have our own organic gardens and many fruit and nut trees, all being raised by strictly organic methods. Whenever we have the need to supplement our own products, we obtain organically grown foods whenever possible for our delicious vegetarian-hygienic meals.

NO CURES OFFERED

The Shangri-La is not a hospital, it is not a clinic, it is not a sanatorium, it is not a nursing home, it is not an institution dedicated to the care of illnesses or diseases; it administers no drugs, it employs no treatments, it relies on no antivital factors for the restoration of health. The thinking person will realize that wounds have healed, bones knitted, and the sick recovered from their illnesses for millennia before there were any "healing professions."

We are convinced that healing is a biological process; it is the result of the lawful and orderly workings of forces and processes intrinsic in the living organism. Here, at the Shangri-La, no effort is made to find or employ substitutes for this biological process. As Natural Hygienists, we are of the firm conviction that, for the sick person, the necessary conditions must be provided so that the operation of the natural laws produce the desired results; that we work with the laws, not against them.

NATURAL HYGIENE—THE SENSIBLE WAY OF LIFE

There are many reasons why the Hygienic way of life appeals to me, but the most important consideration is that the principles make sense. My reason tells me that this is a universe of law and order. Wherever we look in nature we find evidence of this. The stars and planets do not collide with one another, but continue their cycles along precise paths. The trees, plants, and flowers, in all their beauty and profusion, follow definite patterns or laws. For example, you can count on a daisy coming up when you plant a daisy seed, and an oak tree will inevitably spring up from a little acorn, just as will every other seed bring forth its kind. With God's creatures too, we observe order. Rarely do we find sickness or disease in animals in their wild or natural state. It makes sense to me, too, that law and order should also reign as far as the health and functions of the human body are concerned.

We know that every living organism must carry on certain basic activities or functions in order to maintain life. These basic needs are the same today as they were a thousand or a hundred thousand years ago. While man has made many superficial changes in his way of life or culture, he has not been able to, and cannot alter his organic requirements such as air, food, water, sunshine, warmth, activity, emotional tranquility, rest and sleep.

The supporting logic is self-evident: since we know that we cannot live for more than a few minutes without air or oxygen, we can establish this requirement as one of the essentials of life. We also know that man cannot live for very long without food, and so we can say that the need for food is another essential of life, and so on, with all of the other requirements of the human organism. Natural Hygiene is simply an effort to acquire a better understanding of these essentials and how we can best satisfy or provide them.

When I first approached Natural Hygiene, I did so with hesitancy and reservations, but, the more I studied the principles, and thought over the questions posed by my inquiring mind, the more sense it made to me. As my understanding developed, I began to realize that here was indeed a sensible way of life, a practical way of life, a better way of life.

BASED ON NATURAL LAW

Natural Hygiene is not just a new theory, it is not a passing fad. For almost a hundred and fifty years its founders and subsequent dedicated followers have been systematizing and defining the application of these principles. They are based on the solid bedrock of natural law and will endure as long as the laws of being exist. Simply stated, Natural Hygiene is the skillful and intelligent use of all the resources of life, to the end that we may possess better health, greater strength, the ultimate in efficiency and usefulness, higher mental attainment, and longer life.

As a science, it is brought to bear upon the well and the sick, according to the needs and capacities of the living organism under any particular set of circumstances. "Nature" embraces all existing things—the oceans and sky, the mountains, forests and deserts, plants and flowers; all the wild creatures, including the birds and the insects; and the vastnesses of far-flung galaxies with their billion worlds of planets, stars, and endless space. And "Nature" includes man. We are an integral part of the environment, and we must live in concert with it.

Our discovery of nature's laws does not mean entering a state of self-denial and slavery. On the contrary, once we know what the laws are, we can learn to cooperate with them. Take fire, for example. We learned far back in our aboriginal state that fire burns if you touch it, not to punish you, but because that it the natural law of fire. And by understanding this law we are enabled to use fire without danger, to provide warmth for our bodies and for many other purposes.

Natural Hygiene is a science concerned with the relation of living things to their environment, and with the factors that influence that environment. Man must give over trying to mold the rest of the natural world to his wishes, without understanding and respecting the laws that govern it.

This ends Mr. Cheatham's personal story.

YOU ARE CORDIALLY INVITED . . .

In an early burst of irrepressible enthusiasm, Mr. Cheatham sent a dissertation on the Hygienic system to the President of the United States —Richard M. Nixon! As might have been expected, the reply (which came from the National Cancer Institute) stated that "Institute scientists have not found any diet that can prevent cancer in man. Treatment of cancer by diet alone is not recognized as approved therapy by experts in this disease."

It is not known whether President Nixon ever read Mr. Cheatham's letter!

The NCI response (June 16, 1971) is of the "straw man" type: it ignored the totality of the program as outlined in Mr. Cheatham's letter, curiously focusing—for their pedantic shafts—upon the food component, and deliberately ignoring the holistic concept that had been presented. Undaunted, "R. J." responded with alacrity on June 21, carefully expounding on his first letter. Edited excerpts, which follow, provide a capsule summary of the Hygienic system today:

"Since you are primarily concerned with Information and Education, perhaps it might be of value if I emphasized the viewpoints of Natural Hygiene.

"I am sure you will agree that preventives of evil are far better than remedies; cheaper and easier of application, and surer in results.

"From the Natural Hygiene point of view we feel that all disease has a cause. In other words, it is not something we catch from a virus, germ, or bacteria. Certainly the environmental hazards are a major contributing factor, but fortunately the most prevalent problems are those that we can, as individuals, control, at least to a great degree. Specifically, let me list a few thoughts for your consideration:

"1. Natural Hygiene is a way of life that allows those with good health to keep it . . . those who have lost their health to regain it . . . and those who never have had good health to experience it.

"2. Natural Hygiene defines good health as having the most strength and endurance that one can build, as 'feeling good' all the time, as being efficient and useful throughout a long and happy life.

"3. The practice of Natural Hygiene includes a balance of those things usually included in any conventional health program, such as fresh air, pure water, sunshine, sleep, exercise, relaxation, and mental and emotional poise.

"4. However, Natural Hygiene departs from the conventional by (a) advocating a diet made up exclusively of fruits, nuts and green leafy vegetables, organically grown and eaten raw; (b) rejecting as harmful all medicines, treatments, and cures customarily employed in dealing with illness; (c) suggesting fasting (total abstinence from all food except water) as an essential practice in most sickness and disease.

"5. Natural Hygiene bases its position in regard to diet on two principles: (a) Man is acknowledged to be the highest form of life on this earth. In terms of his physical body he belongs to the order of Primates, which includes monkeys and apes. These tend to live almost exclusively upon fruits, nuts and green leafy vegetables, which they consume in the natural, raw state. Man is also in a class known as mammals, which are warm-blooded, hair-covered, live-bearing, and milk-producing. Dogs, cats, and bears are meat eaters. Cows, horses, sheep, deer, camels and goats are grain, grass and cereal eaters. Pigs and other swine are scavengers and eat almost anything. (b) Cooking and processing destroy and degrade nutritional values in foods. The conclusion reached, therefore, is that the natural food of man is considered to be fruits, nuts and seeds, and green leafy vegetables, eaten raw.

"6. Natural Hygiene abhors the use of tobacco, alcohol, coffee, tea, drugs, narcotics, and any other substances or indulgences that disturb the physiological and psychological equilibrium. It likewise rejects medicaments, inoculations, vaccines, X rays, blood transfusions, vitamin pills, food supplements, and all other 'treatments' as being of any use in restoring the body to a state of health. It views so-called therapeutic agents and methods as interfering with, and detrimental to life and health.

"7. As alternatives, Natural Hygiene offers supervised bed rest and fasting in a calm, quiet environment as the most effective, efficient, sensible means of dealing with most illness and disease.

"8. It is obvious and provable that healing (getting well) is a normal activity of the body. When you burn, bruise or cut yourself, or when a surgeon operates or sets a broken bone, it is the body that heals itself. Not the salve, bandage, Merthiolate, stitches, cast, or the surgeon.

Healing is a normal biological process that goes on all the time in relation to the amount of energy available for it.

"9. The body has only so much energy available to do all the things it has to do. There is a significant amount of energy consumed in physical movement each day, including working, exercise, eating, digesting, absorbing and assimilating food. Bed rest and fasting allow the body to conserve this energy and use it to repair tissues, restore functions, and 'clean house' in general."

This marked the end of the letter. However, in a burst of missionary zeal, "R. J." concluded: "We would like to extend an invitation to you or any member of your Department to come to the Shangri-La, and spend a few weeks or a month as our personal guest, without charge . . . the idea being that if you could stay here for a while and have the opportunity to live the hygienic way, you would not only be able to observe the remarkable improvement in the health of others, but, more important, you would be able to see the improvement in your own mental and physical well-being. Obviously, this would enable you to make a much wiser decision as to the relative merit of the Natural Hygiene program."

There was no response to Mr. Cheatham's generous invitation.

OPERATION "CO-OP"

Despite his normally soft-spoken, low-key approach, Mr. R. J. Cheatham was a man of action. This was evident in how he organized himself, how he applied himself to his duties and responsibilities, and how he established his order of priorities. And it was this sense of priority that brought him early to the birth of a striking idea that was to influence the lives of thousands.

As one of the most faithful devotees of Dr. Herbert M. Shelton, the founder of the Hygienic movement, Mr. Cheatham was passionately committed to the system of health that had given him back his life. More than anything else, he wanted to see the organization grow. Observing that lack of funds prevented concrete action by the Society on the national level to solve the compelling problem of founding a bona fide Natural Hygiene educational institution, "R. J." decided on a course of his own that was at least a step forward: in a burst of inspiration, he gave birth to his "co-op" plan. It was hardly a total solution to the vexing problem, but at least it meant that hundreds of interested, searching young men and women would have an opportunity, firsthand, to learn about the natural way of life at the grassroots level.

The Shangri-La Natural Hygiene Institute became for them a "Living

Workshop," where, as "co-ops," they learned by doing; where they could study Natural Hygiene by participating in the full range of activities of the program. As their contribution to the arrangement, they were assigned Hygiene-related work on the Institute grounds, such as gardening, landscape maintenance, food preparation, and other similar activities. They were also provided with room and board free of charge. The Workshop was for a period of four months, and, when this stint was over, they were free to move along, spreading the good word wherever their paths would lead—and/or continue their education in parallel fields, which indeed many did to their lasting benefit.

Altogether, the Shangri-La "trip" proved a most rewarding educational experience. For many who might otherwise have been unable to afford any comparable learning program at similar institutions, it was a fortunate opportunity. At the same time, some student-guests were able during this "apprentice" period to surmount a host of problems that many had brought with them; to purify and build health physically and mentally, using the breathing space provided at the "Shang"—as many called the Institute—for a new look at life, at themselves, and at their futures.

The co-ops were given the run of the grounds and provided with all the privileges and facilities accorded regular paying guests, intermingling with them as one large, harmonious group. The curriculum also included special classes and training sessions, which, over the four-month period, would thoroughly indoctrinate them in every component of the holistic Hygiene modality. A key library of must reading material and books was also provided, consonant with this course, and dealt with such adjunctive health areas as sprouting, organic gardening, the preparation of hygienic meals, and exercise programs. These young people also received an opportunity to smooth out the rough edges of their natural shyness, improving their communication and public speaking, not only through the daily association with the regular guests, but also by participating in a regularly scheduled lecture program that reinforced learning and retention.

Thus, over the years, hundreds of co-ops and literally thousands of guests from all over the world were involved in a cooperative health-giving experiment where there was a rich culturing and mutual sharing of common experiences. Collaborating in this dynamic ferment, all could observe, firsthand: (1) the health-building results achieved by the application of nature-oriented principles in prevention, and (2) the remarkable recuperative powers of the sick body in action, in a favorable environment.

It was an exciting new-age setting—a dynamic school of education in an exploding field of natural health sciences. Proof that this new lifestyle filled a gap was in the fact that, even to this day, many co-op "alumni" and guests alike make periodic pilgrimages back to the Shang's fount of wisdom to add a few more "goodies" to their expanding storehouse of knowledge of the human organism and its vital self-healing forces.

TIGHT SHIP

With all this seething activity, one's curiosity is piqued to ask: What was Mr. Cheatham's direct involvement in all this? Really—the truth, now—was he one of those high-flying spellbinders, capitalizing on a good thing by exploiting the paid help while he exposed himself to the rigors of the French Riviera? Hardly! Not Mr. Cheatham! As the old cliché goes: like green manure, he was all over—so much so that one was often led to conjecture whether the law of physics—that one body cannot occupy two places at the same time—applied to him.

For one—as Health Director his entire morning was fully occupied with daily consultations. This did not exclude Saturdays, Sundays or holidays, because he was always on call. But even this was not quite enough for some guests who insisted on private meetings with "R. J.," because they derived a special lift from a more intimate discussion of their problems in his well-appointed library. Then there were the perpetual rounds of evening lectures, four or five a week. He personally undertook full responsibility for the conduct of the co-op educational program, which included training seminars and occasional gab and gripe sessions. Also, arduous housekeeping duties for an operation accommodating around a hundred guests at any one time. As for the purchase of supplies and materiel—whether cement, lumber, window sashes, air conditioners, land fill—or nuts, bolts, and screws—Cheatham was your man. Food and kitchen? The gardens and fruit orchard? Right again! Cheatham! Ongoing construction, maintenance and repairs? Cheatham! How about correspondence? Reams and reams ground out every day, and often far into the night, dictating into his pain-wracked recording machine.

By nature, Mr. Cheatham could not or would not delegate authority, except for a few administrative office functions, and so the full burden for planning, management, and supervision fell squarely upon his own shoulders. He tried hard more than once to employ a full-time assistant manager, but finding a qualified candidate—one who was also compatible —proved impossible, and so he remained burdened and oppressed—a lonely pilot at the helm, guiding his craft twenty-four hours round the clock, in fair weather and foul.

Nothing seemed to escape his notice. His successful background in sales management had taught him that one should *keep the pot boiling*, but, at the same time, the instructions also enjoined that one must *watch the pot*! And watch it he did, perhaps not so wisely, but too well, as it turned out. Watching the pot came naturally to a man who had learned in the Navy how to run a "tight ship." And this he indeed did, with remarkable dedication and zeal.

Despite all, had it not been for the invaluable assistance of a few key staff members, it would have been beyond even his capabilities to execute such a rigorous schedule. The loyal "in-group" of supporters included Helen Knigge, his miracle girl Friday, shining star of administration; Jessie Alm, a fireball accountant with a penchant for public relations, who acted as goodwill ambassador, spreading salve and good cheer all around; Marion Losch, a veteran stalwart who covered that rat's nest of turmoil—the steaming-hot front desk; and Bert Henry in maintenance, a genius at repairs, who, with rubber bands, paper clips, and a wad of gum could hold the Leaning Tower of Pisa together with his left hand, while at the same time putting out brush fires with his right.

Behind every successful man there is a devout, loving woman, and so, behind Mr. Cheatham, hovering in the background, but always pitching in when the going was difficult, was Mrs. Frances Cheatham, who not only fulfilled her role as loving wife and devoted mother of nine children infinitely well, but often pitched in as a full-time partner during the rough days.

THE DYNAMICS OF CHANGE

It appears obvious that Mr. Cheatham's taxing regime violated fundamental Natural Hygiene principles. It was the beginning of a process that acted to reverse the some twenty-nine-odd years of strict obedience to its laws. From 1975—two years preceding his death—he began to compromise with, or ignore, the cardinal precepts that he himself had preached and thundered from his Natural Hygiene pulpit. Instead of eight or ten hours of sleep a day, a one-hour nap at midday, and, going to bed with the setting sun, he himself now took perhaps five or six hours of sleep. He did find time for a bit of sun, but only occasionally now, because of the press of affairs in an ever-growing, expanding situation. He became a psychological prisoner of new work habits, which, interlocked with an iron will, became so ingrained as to defy extrication from the dilemma. There was no relief from the strain of a superhuman workload. Mental poise and tranquility went by the boards—transformed from necessities into luxuries. Decisions! Decisions! Decisions! There was no surcease from them, and from their morbid emergent character.

Mrs. Frances Cheatham watched anxiously, as did all of his intimate staff, noticing "R. J.'s" progressive loss of energy and driving power, despite his valiant attempts to conceal these weaknesses. And—to compound the problem—during this most critical period, he insisted on going on several classic Hygienic fasts, i.e., just drinking distilled water! His rationalization was that these fasts were healing measures, and, because he was indeed a stubborn and strong-willed individual, it proved impossible to gainsay him. Even should the fast have had some modicum of justification at this point, it was not carried out according to the rules, which underlined the necessity for maximum rest and relaxation. All day long, the stressful business problems were still being brought to his bedside; he still continued his dictation of correspondence, and attended other chores, so that it all proved self-defeating.

Fasting, today, occupies the number-one slot in the healing regime of Natural Hygiene. It must be stated, however, that this is of new vintage, having no validity among the majority of the early medical pioneers of the movement, certainly not under the stark, straitened conditions of grave physiological disorder and deterioration, when the body must husband every bit of its remaining strength. Needless to say, this type of fasting is completely discredited also by Drs. Gerson, Issels, and Leroi.

It was inevitable that Mr. Cheatham's vital reserves should eventually crumble and fail. On July 14, 1977, he succumbed to malignant melanoma—the condition he had overcome twenty-nine years before. Notwithstanding the manner of his demise, his almost twenty-nine years of robust, radiant health stand unchallenged as a testimony to his faith and practice of Natural Hygiene.

THE WAYFARER

In tribute to this remarkable man, Rafael J. Cheatham, the author was privileged to deliver the Eulogy on the sad occasion of his passing. In closing, it seems appropriate to use some portions from the Eulogy to convey the spirit and soul of this totally dedicated human being:

"As a man of deep compassion, Mr. Cheatham tirelessly sought to bring knowledge to the unenlightened, comfort to those in distress, and hope of renewal to the afflicted, so that they could carry on life's journey with light and love in their hearts. He was a shining example of truth in action.

"Mr. Cheatham created Shangri-La, an oasis in the midst of a desert of harassed and stress-filled lives. It is an island of security where the wayfarer can rest for a while, away from the oppressive fumes of noxious cigarettes, where—to quote Mr. Cheatham—'people are breathing.' It is a wholesome retreat from the loud and raucous noise of traffic snarls, of jangling telephones, and blaring TV commercials. It is a place to take stock of oneself; to examine the bear-traps of our self-indulgences, to calculate the penalties we must pay for further transgressions and abuse of our bodies; or, conversely, the rewards of changing our style of life. Here at Mr. Cheatham's Shangri-La we learn to recapture, if even for a moment, the joy of being alive, of being ourselves—without artificial stimulation.

"Although Mr. Cheatham was not what you would call a strictly devout or formal religious, his true nature realized that the body is the temple of God, and that we must keep it pure—an injunction as imperative as any one of the ten commandments handed down to Moses on Mount Sinai. How else can we explain Mr. Cheatham's total commitment to the system of Natural Hygiene? Of his devoted efforts to purify this Holy Temple, and to make it a fitting home for the Spirit of God, which is within all of us? As a devout natural hygienist, he lighted many candles which brightened up the darkness, bringing health and happiness, physical and spiritual rewards to all those who found their way to Shangri-La.

"During his illness, on one of my visits to the hospital, I tried, as always, to be of good cheer. I remember speaking of the fruitful twenty-nine years of life which he had enjoyed after his first struggle against malignant melanoma—when the doctors had given him—at best—only five years to live. I sought to encourage him by saying that 'lightning can, and does, often strike twice in the same place,' meaning, of course, that he would recover from his present illness. Mr. Cheatham just looked up at me and with a strange foreknowledge said, 'Not this time, Jack.' He seemed so positive and certain that I felt chagrined.

"And yet, one should not draw the conclusion from this comment that he ever gave up hope. Not Mr. Cheatham. He remained that bold warrior to the very end, a real tiger of courage and strength in the face of every adversity, when the worst was staring him in the face. He surely, in those sad days of trial, pain, and travail, set an example of courage which would be difficult to follow, and which would have led other weaker spirits to throw in the sponge. But, withal, perhaps somewhere deep inside, he sensed that his work was done.

"We mourn his loss, but here, too, we would be remiss in our own faith and spiritual attunement to think or believe that the physical transition as the end of everything. In the Grand Plan of the Divine, it is only the beginning. The soul and spirit have their new work to do also, but on another plane. Mr. Cheatham's hopes and dreams will continue to attend us, and to manifest themselves through the hearts and minds of those who in prayer, faith, and memory keep communion with him.

"With this noteworthy heritage written down in the Scroll of Life, surely our Lord will open wide his doors to admit such a noble soul to the generous rewards due this faithful servant, who so dutifully looked after so many of God's children. Amen."

SHANGRI-LA TODAY

There is no other simon-pure Natural Hygiene institution or clinic in the world that carries on and fulfills the underlying hygienic laws and precepts as completely as does the Shangri-La Natural Hygiene Institute, which Mr. Cheatham founded, and which became his whole life—until his death on July 14, 1977. The handful of practitioners in America and other countries who practice Hygiene, have, most of them, austere and limited facilities, unable, regrettably, truly to maintain a total Hygienic program, across the board. Shangri-La is the only full-blown operation that fulfills the holistic precepts of the science.

Perhaps the others most familiar on the American scene today are Virginia Vetrano (working with Dr. Herbert M. Shelton), Dr. David J. Scott, Dr. Christopher Gian-Curcio, and Dr. William L. Esser, all of whom started out as doctors of chiropractic. Except for Dr. Vetrano, however, none of them maintains a year-round, in-patient operation.

One of the more exciting new generation personalities to emerge on the hygienic front today is an outstanding naturopathic doctor and full-time practitioner of the art, Dr. Jeffrey L. Fine. Dr. Fine was health director of the Shangri-La Natural Hygiene Institute for about two years, but he is now affiliated with the Health Education Center in Fort Lauderdale, Florida. He brings a refreshing and charismatic young talent to the modern scene, with a total metabolic approach to the healing arts, reinforcing the learning process through a well-knit educational program—which includes lectures, graphics, and films. He has also added an important spiritual dimension to all of his consultations and lectures, emphasizing the necessity for a changing of attitudes and a raising of the consciousness above and beyond the physical parameters that have dominated this movement heretofore. This fleshing out of the parameters has changed the nature and long-term effect of what has been a predominantly physiologically oriented modality, improving the quality of life—giving it deeper meaning—so that what is learned is also experienced emotionally, and thus has a lasting effect—not just upon the participants but ultimately upon their families, friends, and society as well.

* * * * * * *

Note:
   Dr. Fine is now Director of FineWay House in a self-contained wing of the well-known Colonnades Hotel, which he calls a "Natural Health Learning Center," and which "combines both a complete program of rejuvenation in a close-knit, supportive environment and all the facilities of a high-class beach resort.

   "The program consists of delicious vegetarian meals, fasting -- yoga, relaxation and meditation classes -- our complete health education program plus medical supervision; while, at the same time and at no extra cost to our guests, the resort facilities include 16 acres with 1500 feet of white sandy beaches on Singer Island in Palm Beach Shores; the healing benefits of ocean air and salt water; our own secluded area, nine tennis courts, saunas, shuffleboard and all other amenities of a great, old-world beach hotel."

   Dr. Fine states: "I will be personally supervising both juice and water fasts and giving a full program of lectures on the dynamics of health and consciousness as I have been for the past 8 years. I will also provide private consultations on your health program."

21

The Hygienic Connection

Sir Arthur Conan Doyle, M.D., was a masterful raconteur of detective tales, featuring the immortal Sherlock Holmes, the greatest private eye of all time, complete with deerstalker cap, meerschaum pipe, and magnifying lens. The caliber of Holmes's exploits and his ingenious logic was of such rare vintage as to stir the wits of the most challenging minds—the veteran readers of whodunits. Doyle's special delight was to keep his reader hanging on by his eyelids as he maintained an excruciating suspense until the final denouement, this last being painfully slow in the telling and so adroitly tormenting that Sherlock Holmes, his protagonist, stands easily accused of a special brand of literary sadism. This is starkly obvious when one observes the reader's jaw hanging slack, his breath and pulse quickening, and his forehead dripping perspiration, as Holmes deliberately drags out the painful climax—first, by exasperatingly lighting up his dreadful pipe, drawing heavily on it once or twice—pretending trouble with the flame; then taking a few deep comfortable puffs before—finally—exhaling a fog of vile-smelling tobacco smoke as he settles back deeper into the cushions of the easy chair of his Baker Street apartment in London's West End.

Had Sherlock Holmes ever overplayed this hand beyond endurance (he did come close once or twice), it is entirely conceivable that even the imperturbable Dr. Watson, his closest friend and confidant, would have succumbed to the strain; and Holmes would have been forever lost to posterity—a victim to one or more of those deadly poisons known only to physicians—an exotic potion that would vanish without a trace, leaving the greatest unsolved mystery of all since, (1) the most formidable crime-solver of them all—Holmes—would be dead, and (2) the last person the police would ever suspect in such a nefarious plot would be Holmes's most intimate friend!

Well, this has really taken us the long way around to make a point—although a most important one in the Natural Hygiene story—for it is here that the denouement takes place that completes the intricate mosaic, without which a subtle cloud of puzzlement may still tend to wrinkle the brow—as with the sometimes fuzzy ending of a mystery story. We would now like to illuminate the underlying message that lends coherence and strength to all the premises, and justifies the efforts and the sacrifices of those whose selflessness in thought, word, and action nobly set the edifice in place.

Gerson, the superb master of the art of healing, provided the golden key to health—nutrition. If we set aside those medicaments (medical therapeutics) and methods that he employed only to bring his patients through the crisis period, we are left holding in our hands the ultimate key in the ensuing convalescence and cure period. As we have amply noted, as a preventive regime, a modified Gerson dietary program could be followed such as he used for recovering and recovered patients.

If we understand clearly the weaknesses of the Hygienic system, particularly with respect to its dogmatic position re food selection and food combining, as heretofore discussed, we see that many of its philosophical concepts, as well as its specific program constituents, are in harmony with the underlying tenets of the Gerson modality, and, of course, with the Ganzheitstherapie of Drs. Josef Issels and Rita Leroi. Eliminating such discords as may exist with the Gerson dietary regime, the Hygienic system can play an incisive role throughout the entire spectrum of health, from prevention to cure—within the context of Gerson's or any other therapeutic program of clinical management. It can be of decided value, too, even when traditional methods are being exclusively employed.

Transcending all the doctrine is the beating heart of a revolutionary premise: that Natural Hygiene is not just a bridge to span the yawning chasm of disease, but organic connective tissue—a life-giving substratum that can in fact be potently employed at any point in the continuum from health to disease. The alert and concerned practitioner can introduce its precious components into the spectrum at any point, and favorably influence the health process and/or course of the disease, assuring incisive help and/or more rapid recovery of the patient. This represents an invaluable contribution that should allow Hygiene an honored and respectable place in the ministry of healing.

As we carefully investigate its philosophy and methods, we find ourselves indeed standing on the edge of illuminating truth. Hygienic alchemy has not uncovered any long-sought wonder drug—nor has it ever searched for one. But—it has seemingly stumbled upon a wildly unimagined equivalent: In our minute examination of hypotheses, premises, and practice, we have chanced upon a therapeutic concept, a catalytic module, a process—so to speak—that can be introduced within the configuration of any preventive health or healing modality to lend it strength, sustenance and succor, even in the most urgent crises—when utilized with timeliness and discretion in the pathological condition. It underlines and fleshes out Dr. Max Gerson's life-giving nutritional therapy with its adjunctive therapeutic inputs; Issels's medicative and immunological agents; and Dr. Leroi's Iscador modality, with its giant doses of psycho-spiritual support. Yes, even the hardcore mechanistics of orthodox medicine—surgery, radiation, and chemotherapy—are well advised to include the mores implicit in the hygienic formulary into their medical dialogues with the chronically ill and terminal patient—or, for that matter, with any ailing human being.

This immediately raises the Natural Hygiene profile to a higher dimension—from science to art. It can play its most beneficial role at the lower end of the spectrum—in prevention, employing every module in the course, advancing in the continuum from good health, through the first intimation of illness and then, in progressive stages, through minor affliction to chronic disease pathology. Without exception, in clinical management, some part of the Hygienic program units can be applied with suitable modifications along this entire continuum, even the terminal stage of cancer—depending upon the specific disease state and the condition of the individual patient's physiological and psychological resources.

There is little room for doubt that the giants in medicine, whose paths we have followed—Drs. Josef Issels, Max Gerson, and Rita Leroi—did follow, to the maximum degree possible, the tenets embodied in the Hygienic System, although in each case there were human and logistical factors present that prevented fullest application. In Max Gerson's case, he was simply one man alone, with a superhuman caseload, oppressed by sometimes subtle and tormenting circumstances, and even open harassment by the medical Establishment. He accomplished his daily miracles within physically narrow confines—his Nanuet Clinic being no more than a converted private home. With no staff to speak of, except for an occasional nurse or two, suffering man-made impediments that often prevented his obtaining such simple services as laboratory testing of tissue samples and radiological access, virtually without funds (while still treating indigent patients free of charge), he could do no more than he did within his logistical and human limitations. Under these straitened conditions, spiritual input was his best substitute for any missing ingredients, and became a precious complement, under the circumstances, to his innovative and effective therapeutic regime, founded on the bedrock of nutrition.

Dr. Josef Issels was able to incorporate the Hygienic system to a greater degree, having space and staff, i.e., Alpine-fresh air, pure water, an ample ration of daily sunshine, adequate facilities for rest and relaxation, and indeed more than abundant exercise, as his patients scampered out like squirrels to climb mountains. His nutritional program, too, was good, although not as highly refined as Gerson's, and his hearty, earthy concern for his friends, the patients, shouted his love from every pore.

A sad commentary, reflecting upon their own system of hospital care, was made by the visiting British team that inspected the Ringberg-Klinik, indicating that the "skilful and kindly terminal care" demonstrated at the clinic, coupled with its unheard-of 1:2 staff to patient ratio, was something devoutly to be wished—and which they hoped one day would come to characterize the hospitals and clinics in England. It underlined the full-blown character and effectiveness of Issels's Ganzheitstherapie.

As for Dr. Rita Leroi of the Lukas-Klinik, her bright countenance alone radiated an assurance and comfort that was sublimely healing in itself—enough for even those of little faith to know that, at least for now, the dark door had been closed, and that, from this point on, the hand of the Lord was upon them. The Lukas-Klinik was enveloped by a spiritual aura that radiated healing vibrations, and, there, apart from the medical elements, the full range of activities included most if not all of the Hygienic mores. Clinical management in the Lukas-Klinik mounted a maximum holistic program whose successful results were proof enough of its effectiveness.

All three masters of the healing arts were alert to all that might and could be done under ideal conditions. It was the mark of noble souls always on the eternal quest for truth—that their minds and hearts were open always, and hungry for this inner productive innovation. This inner motivation alone worked its many wonders, because it was the spiritual essence of being, which acted as a potent counterforce to establish providential balance where any error of omission might occur. There can be no better evidence of the fact that their systems worked than in the hardcore survival and recovery rates of those patients whom they treated with such deep concern and a very special brand of courage.

Over and above what was evident to the eye, tangible to the laboratory technicians staring through their lenses at blood and serum samples, and even what was felt vibrating in the air around them, was the fact that these three practitioners of human and humanistic medicine shared the sufferings of each patient they attended—as if the life were their very own. It seemed at times that these wounded physicians were indeed channels for the flow of divine grace, and that its supreme expression— that greater love—was in the simple fact that so often, even in the most desperate cases, the miracle of healing took place.

We can think of no greater contribution that can be made in our times than to impress this holistic concept upon the medical profession. They are—for better or for worse—our front-line contingent in today's battles against disease and death. It is our fervent prayer therefore that they may recall to their hearts the morality and ethic of their own Oath of Hippocrates, and invoke its principles in their daily rounds. Let them forgo for once the blandishments of wealth and power; let them note and dedicate themselves to the examples we have presented of dedicated, fully committed, and successful peers who place the welfare of their patients above their pretty pride and demoralizing self-interest, which is gnawing at the vitals of our nation.

In our much-vaunted technological world, American genius is recognized as second to none. Just to mention an unbelievable first, enough to psych anyone out: Project "Very Large Array" (VLA), a seventy-eight-million-dollar bundle of the National Radio Astronomy Observatory, using ultrasensitive electronics in radio astronomy, has built a "telescope" with "arms" thirteen miles long and "ears" eighty-two feet wide, weighing two hundred and thirteen tons each. Its assignment: to intercept radio waves generated by celestial bodies in remote galaxies—tens of trillions of miles distant. Radio waves diminish with distance, yet this incredible astronomical "eye" can measure these infinitely feeble transmissions from any one of these heavenly bodies, even though "the total energy of all the signals that have struck all the antennas of all the radio astronomers in the world since 1948, when the science really began to take off, is still equal to *no more than the impact of a few snowflakes striking the Earth*"!

Yet, for all this—with more than five billion dollars already invested in cancer research, and additional billions allocated to environmental problem-solving by industry and government—we can't clean up our air space, purify our water, stop the poisoning of our food—or prevent cancer.

22

Conclusion: Rodents and Roaches

Larry Agran, in *The Cancer Connection,* says: "It is not surprising that the common view, now decades old, is that a cure for cancer must certainly be within our grasp. But the grim reality is otherwise. Despite the billions of dollars poured into cancer research in the United States and throughout the world, it is unlikely that there will be any sudden breakthrough in the near future. There will be no universal cure, no single vaccine against cancer. Certainly not in this decade. Probably not in this century. And possibly never."

This view is underlined by Dr. Frank J. Rauscher, Jr., former Director of the National Cancer Institute, who told the Congress of the United States in a 1974 report: "It is important to understand that research is not likely to produce a single dramatic means to prevent or cure all of the hundred or more forms of cancer. Progress in science and medicine is a step-by-step process that takes time—time often measurable in years."

No amount of rhetoric will dispel the grim fact that cancer is on the rise, ranking second only to heart disease as the major cause of death in the United States. "During the last twenty-five years of intensive pursuit of cancer cures," Agran comments, "the survival rates for the most comon types of cancer—lung cancer, breast cancer, and cancer of the colon—have remained almost unchanged. In the period 1950 to 1959, only 8 of every 100 victims of lung cancer survived five years after diagnosis. In 1975, the five-year survival rate was 9 out of 100. For the 89,000 women in 1975 who were told they have breast cancer, the five-year survival rate is expected to be 64 percent, a slight improvement over the 60 percent survival rate that existed two decades ago. With cancer of the colon—the most common of all major cancers, involving 100,000 new cases each year—the five-year survival rate was 44 percent between 1950 and 1959. Today it is still about 44 percent"!

There have been some limited advances made for victims of Hodgkin's disease, leukemia, and a few other rare forms, but these are at the distant edges of the giant struggle against the major killers. For example, Hodgkin's disease accounts for only one percent of all cancer cases, and leukemia for only three percent.

Cancer statistics reflect more than just an increase in the American population or of the greater proportion of older people in our population.

Even after adjusting for these factors, the evidence is clear: the incidence of malignancies is on the rise—across the board—in all age categories, especially among the very young. Cancer is endemic, and, if the ongoing statistical curve continues at its present unabated rate, it will ultimately infect every man, woman and child in America. And, because there is no reliable report of divine amnesty being granted to any select group, medical doctors and their families are not likely to be excluded. Surely, in the light of this depressing prospect, the most serious consideration should be given to the work of the three great pioneers whose methods of treatment have been so effective. Is this not more desirable and less threatening than today's grim game of Russian roulette, where more and more the odds have so skyrocketed that almost every chamber in the gun now carries a deadly bullet?

God is not dead, but it may well be the medical Establishment that stands in dire need of resuscitation. All the disarming rhetoric aside, it does not have a workable plan; it does not even have a process, except for an archaic, moldering one, which—on the record—is a colossal failure.

The facts are crystal-clear: Our three great lamplighters, Gerson, Issels, and Leroi, did treat and cure cancer, proving that nutrition and nature-oriented treatment works, that Ganzheitstherapie is not just a theory but a viable science. And, if Hygienic principles and methods are added as full-time partners, we can begin to cope with and control a plague that is today utterly out of control—although stubborn pride aborts the medical conscience from admitting it.

Let the medical community bend to the evidence, to the proof, to the necessities. It had better abandon its old bones and relics, and join the people. Let there be an end to considering the physician as sacrosanct, infallible, and above reproach—like Caesar's wife. There is, in all this, less claim to plaudits than to censure, when a hierarchy protects its bunglers by a dispensation of privileged immunity behind a medical Chinese Wall, where mistakes are neatly labeled and then buried, a privilege hardly accorded any other profession.

A healthy dose of reproach might very well be in order when we take a look at the number of "impaired physicians" working at their lasts! The American Medical Association states that "suicides are two and one-half times more common in the ranks of physicians than the general population average." As for alcoholism among medical doctors, this is observed twice as frequently as narcotic addiction. According to a survey by the AMA, "One to two percent of the physicians are markedly affected by drug dependence. . . . Seven to eight percent are now, or will become alcoholics. . . . Alcoholism seems to be the most frequently encountered illness, constituting at least half of the sick physician pathology. . . . Some observers would place it as high as two-thirds. If we were to settle on sixty percent, then the aggregate number of doctors disabled by their alcoholism, drug dependence, or mental illness, would approximate seventeen thousand, or from five to six percent of the total physician population." With the percentage of impaired physicians as high as one out of every twenty practicing, the quality of care delivered to the patient—whether in routine illness, or in chronic or advanced disease—is highly suspect.

Is it not time for members of this very private club to join with the common people? To step down from their Olympian heights—to stop treating grown-ups like juveniles and mental paraplegics by that studied pose behind a much-vaunted mystique that repels normal, concerned inquiry and criticism—and generates, instead, fear and dread, far removed from the imperatives in such times of crisis? Can we not have done with that unfeeling professional cool, the regal aloofness, and the maddening autocracy?

Let us dispense with sophistry that masks failure as success; with speciousness, which reveals everything but the truth; and with apologists: among the medical bedfellows—the drug and pharmaceutical industries; among the sycophant media; and along other labyrinthine trails where petty interest and profit lead. Is it not time, too, that the billions of painfully extracted tax dollars that have been pouring down numberless ratholes were rescued from the faceless research laboratories where research scientists pursue endless nit-picking trails "leading nowhere, just for show" —hanging on like grim death to a bankrupt symptomatic theory, the limb of which has already been sawed off? Is it not time for Americans who are aware of the travesty, to echo, with former President Kennedy, in his memorable inaugural address, his dictum to the American people against the common enemies of man—tyranny, poverty, and disease: "Ask not what your country can do for you—ask what you can do for your country"?

There surrounds the entire issue a smell, such as moved Marcellus in Hamlet to lift up his nose and remark that "something is rotten in the state of Denmark." This appears no hapless stumbling and bumbling around the truth, but rather begs the question: Are we contending with blind ignorance? With the closed mind? Or is it tragically true that absolute power has corrupted absolutely?

America, with one voice, pleads for an honest reply. If there is any integrity at all in the corridors of power and influence of the medical hierarchy and of the government, then good conscience, at least, demands an answer, if only in decent respect for the 370,000 Americans who will succumb this year to cancer, many of them in agonizing deaths. In the wrenching human tragedy, tens of thousands of families will be bereaved by the death of a father, mother, sister, brother, son, or daughter. For some, the grief may be so heartrending as to prove beyond human endurance. Many of these same pitiable families will face destruction of their basic economic security through loss of the breadwinner and be thrown upon the public providence—a most dismal prospect. In addition to these 370,000 this year, another 55,000,000 Americans who are alive today (one out of every four) will contract this dread disease during their lifetimes, ultimately suffering the same grisly fate.

If it is ignorance that is responsible for medicine's failure, then, out of sheer humanity alone, it is beyond toleration. If due to a closed mind, it should be opened—by the exercise of the maximum force that public pressure can exert; and if it is corruption of mind and spirit that consigns 370,000 Americans annually to an early grave without a fighting chance, then it is time to ask whether this dereliction of duty is not of such a magnitude as to demand the most vigorous public and government intervention on the highest levels.

According to the *Information Please Almanac* for 1978, the total battlefield losses suffered by the United States in all the wars ever fought—from the Revolutionary War up to and including the Viet Nam conflict—were 574,387 lives. Thus, in any two-year period today, deaths from cancer would amount to 740,000, or one and a quarter times all the battlefield losses in the entire history of the United States! Does not this tragic condition rightly call for the exercise of executive action, equivalent to that invoked in the gravest of national emergencies—war?

The Chinese suggest that the journey of a thousand miles begins with the first step. Somewhere, somehow, in our human microcosm there has to be a beginning to charting a course toward nobler, more viable objectives than those that have been manifest among the medical community in the face of the cancer challenge. Would it not dignify this failing, faltering profession if they could rescue their consciences from an ice age grip, and summon up the intestinal fortitude to take the first important step in such a journey?

Drs. Max Gerson, Josef Issels, and Rita Leroi have shown the way, having successfully treated thousands of hopeless patients with terminal cancer, rescuing them from the very jaws of death. Their methods work. Those of the orthodox medical Establishment do not.

The American Medical Association, representing the medical community, is in the top leadership position in our nation. It is charged with primary responsibility in the area of health and disease. If it will not—or cannot—recant its indefensible position in the treatment of this scourge, on such terms and with such measures as are demanded by what is, beyond doubt, a national emergency, then this government of the people should mount such an effort to solve this problem as will be the "moral equivalent of war."

Many of the world's leading scientists are convinced that the name of the game we are playing today is showdown. We're in it up to here, having wagered every chip we own in the center of the table. We don't have to wait for a surprise atomic attack, or an invasion from Mars. This one, we are doing to ourselves! Since man has only been on this earth perhaps one million years, while some furry and other scurrying creatures have been using its facilities for something over twenty million, give or take a few hundred thousand, the law of probabilities suggests that, given man's propensity for self-destruction, it is indubitably possible that we will lose the game, and that the rat or the roach will inherit the earth.

Epilogue: Paths of Glory

When Max Gerson left Berlin on the last train—on the eve of that fateful April Fool's Day in 1933—it seemed he was destined never to return. He of course missed the Medical Congress in Berlin and, as the honored guest, this would, in those days, certainly have been the crowning achievement of his life, a distinction particularly to be savored in his own country, where the laurels endowed would have been ever so much sweeter. Notwithstanding—the mills of the gods ground sufficiently fine in their own inscrutable way.

In the fall of 1952, he was invited to Germany as guest lecturer before a Medical Totality Congress, a gathering of the world's most eminent physicians, to discuss the therapy of "the whole man." He was scheduled as a speaker just for the afternoon session, but, by unanimous acclamation, continued long into the late hours of the evening.

During the question-and-answer period, Dr. Gerson described his therapeutic regime and its practical management. In a nutshell: raw and slowly cooked fruits and vegetables; certain fruit and vegetable juices in large amounts—freshly pressed several times daily; aggressive measures for the elimination of toxic wastes from the body by frequent coffee and other enemas; liver therapy, including: (1) calf's liver juice extracted in a special way and (2) liver injections for the stimulation of the liver's detoxification capability. There were other indicated medications to be adapted and prescribed by the doctor to fit the individual requirements of the patient. These consisted chiefly, but not exclusively, of a limited few vitamins and minerals with high specificity, aimed at incisive biological support of the body's metabolism and its healing systems. After a few weeks, some light proteins such as yogurt and cottage cheese could be added. This was the encapsulated outline of the regime he presented to the Congress.

For Max Gerson attending the Congress, the pages of history were turned back in his mind to those dark days of World War II when the German Wehrmacht was ravaging Europe, and naked terror marched rampant through the corridors of the shuddering nations. The strident, thundering voice of a megalomaniac chilled the blood of millions, as they were promised guns instead of butter.

281

In startling contrast to those days of a world gone mad was the peaceful setting in a fairyland of natural beauty—a mountain resort, where Adolf Hitler disported in his hideaway, a veritable Garden of Eden. There were gay and fragrant bouquets of woodland flowers for his most-loved companion, Eva Braun; and simple food, sweet wine, and chocolates—on which he doted—for himself. For the Führer, the war, in this "Eagle's Nest," was unreal and far away.

It was in this mountain aerie in the heart of Germany's Bavarian Alps that Hitler spent the happiest days of his life, while the world around him was reduced to a shambles as the armies of the Third Reich, responding to his slightest order or whim, made a bloodbath of Europe.

But his path of glory and infamy led to the grave, because, at the end, Reichsführer Adolf Hitler and his mistress, Eva Braun, took their lives when Germany surrendered, April 30, 1945.

The mills of the gods had ground slowly, but exceedingly fine. In the scales of the universal Karmic laws, justice distilled an exquisite nectar of retribution by decreeing that the auspicious international body that brought Dr. Max Gerson to Germany as their honored guest, should, exactly seventeen years after Hitler declared war against the Jews, be held in Hitler's happy mountain retreat—BERCHTESGADEN!

Appendix

DR. MAX GERSON'S COMBINED DIETARY REGIME

Dr. Max Gerson's "Combined Dietary Regime" includes certain medications and is published in its entirety in *A Cancer Therapy*. He emphasizes that "the treatment requires guidance from a physician as there are often complications of 'flare-ups'; and activation of chronic infections or other bodily weaknesses which need special medical attention." Gerson also reiterates that "the dietary regime is the basis of the treatment. The main task is to detoxify the entire system to restore the functions of the liver and the metabolism, i.e., the digestive changes of food from intake to output. Neither the dietary regime alone nor medication alone is effective. The combination is essential for success." And for this, supervision and monitoring by a physician is mandatory. Further, "it is not advisable to start the treatment at all, if for any reason, strict adherence to it is not possible."

We shall first explain the main constituents of the *nutritional* component of the regime, which can also serve as a helpful guide in any basic plan for healthful eating.

Juices: Fruit and vegetable juices—especially apple, carrot, grape, orange, and grapefruit—are among the most important pillars of the diet because they provide the vital oxidizing enzymes that purify the cellular system and improve digestion. Also important is a prescribed green-leaf juice that includes lettuce, red cabbage leaves, beet tops, Swiss chard, escarole, endives, romaine, green pepper, and watercress.

A separate grinder and press for extracting the juices is recommended to preserve the oxidizing enzymes and other valuable nutrients. Except, of course, in the case of orange and grapefruit peels, the skins of fruits and vegetables are to be kept intact for juicing—after washing and scrubbing. Apple cores, however, should be removed.

Gerson's very special method for obtaining the best results from fresh (unfrozen) calf's liver juice also is described.

Fruits, Raw Salads, and Vegetable Soup: An abundance of fresh fruits is included in the diet, as are raw salads and a specially prescribed vegetable ("Hippocrates") soup, the vegetables being cooked slowly, without water, over a low flame.

283

Freshness is crucial, so the juices and raw vegetable salads are to be consumed immediately after preparation. The vegetable soup may be kept refrigerated, but no longer than two days. Some herbs are permitted in the diet for fiavor, like allspice, anise, bay leaf, dill, and fennel, but Gerson voices a strong caution to use these most sparingly because they may counteract the healing reaction. For sweetener (with oatmeal cereal, for example), honey, brown sugar, or unsulfured molasses is suggested. Dried fruits are allowed, but they must be unsulfured and free of any preservatives.

Sample meals are illustrated in the regime.

Utensils: Aluminum is considered harmful, but stainless steel, glass, enamel, earthenware, cast iron, or tin may be used.

Prohibitions: Salt and all salt substitutes are absolutely forbidden, as are refined, salted, bottled, canned, frozen, preserved, smoked, and sulfured foods.

Among a long list of other foods that are verboten, the following are included: alcohol, tea, coffee, cocoa and commercial beverages, candy, milk and milk products, chocolate, and cake. Soybeans and soybean products are excluded from the diet and cucumbers, too, for they have too much salt in them. All berries and pineapples are not permitted because their aromatic acids cause unfavorable reactions. Fats and oils are out, and nuts and avocados, which contain too much fatty acid. Hair dyeing and permanents are abjured; fluorine in toothpaste and gargles and bicarbonate of soda and epsom salts are also on the list.

On the temporarily forbidden list, Gerson mentions milk, butter, cheese, eggs, fish, and meat. As the patient's condition improves, the physician may slowly introduce one or another of these foods into the diet.

Peppermint tea is recommended by Gerson when food is not well tolerated or in the case of indigestion or during a reaction period of "flare-ups," nausea, or gas.

Simple as the above dietary outline may appear, it will still take a special force of will and habit to apply—even under the most favorable conditions. The implementing details are all-important, and these can be found elaborated upon in *A Cancer Therapy.*

As mentioned, complementing the dietary regime is the medication; and this, too, is presented in *A Cancer Therapy* in the form of a "Daily Medication Chart" intended for the physician. The chart sets out the frequency and portions of juices and foods and also the dosage of medications that include potassium solution, lugol, niacin, thyroid, and liver injections. The procedure for preparing and administering several different kinds of enemas, including coffee enemas, is described.

As Gerson explains, contrary to what one may think, when the total regime is activated the food is easily and quickly digested, the sick body needing larger portions and more frequent servings. He urges, "Eat and drink as much as you can, even during the night when awake. At the beginning, some patients may find it difficult to consume all the pre-scribed food and juices. After good detoxification—in about one to two weeks—the metabolism should improve and the appetite increase."

The dietary regime, as explained, is the basis of the treatment. In principle, it excludes most sodium-containing foods, while it helps to refill the tissues with the important potassium that has been lost.

A final word, restating what Gerson never failed to repeat: The treatment requires careful guidance and supervision from a physician.

Suggested Reading

MEDICAL ETHICS AND CLINICAL GUIDELINES

1. *Principles of Medical Ethics,* The American Medical Association, Chicago, Illinois, 1976.
2. "The Institutional Guide to DHEW Policy on Protection of Human Subjects," U.S. Department of Health, Education, and Welfare, DHEW Publication No. (NIH) 72-102, December 1, 1971.
3. "Declaration of Helsinski" and "AMA Ethical Guidelines for Clinical Investigation," American Medical Association, Chicago, Illinois.

SPIRITUAL HEALING

1. Kathryn Kuhlman, *Nothing Is Impossible with God,* Prentice-Hall, Inc., Englewood Cliffs, New Jersey, 1974.
2. Masaharu Taniguchi, Ph.D., *The Human Mind and Cancer,* Seicho-No-Ie Foundation, Divine Publication Department, Tokyo, Japan, 1972.
3. Rudolf Steiner, Ph.D., and Ita Wegman, M.D., *Fundamentals of Therapy—An Extension of the Art of Healing Through Spiritual Knowledge,* Rudolf Steiner Press, London, 1925.
4. Sally Hammond, *We Are All Healers,* Turnstone Books, London, 1973.
5. Barbara Leahy Shlemon, *Healing Prayer,* Ave Maria Press, Notre Dame, Indiana, 1976.
6. Francis MacNutt, O.P., *Healing,* Ave Maria Press, Notre Dame, Indiana, 1974.
7. Harry Edwards, *A Guide to the Understanding and Practice of Spiritual Healing,* Healer Publishing Company, Ltd., Burrows Lea, England, 1974.
8. William S. Reed, M.D., *A Doctor's Thoughts on Healing,* Macalester Park Publishing Company, St. Paul, Minnesota, 1961.
9. Rudolf Steiner, *Spiritual Science and Medicine,* Rudolf Steiner Publishing Company, London, 1948.

NATURAL HYGIENE

1. *The Greatest Health Discovery,* The Natural Hygiene Press, Inc., Chicago, Illinois, 1972.
2. Herbert M. Shelton, *An Introduction to Natural Hygiene,* Health Research, Mokelumne Hill, California, 1922.

TESTIMONIAL WORKS

1. Eydie Mae Hunsberger, *How I Conquered Cancer Naturally,* Production House, San Diego, California, 1975.

2. Jaquie Davison, *Cancer Winner—How I Purged Myself of Melanoma,* Pacific Press, Pierce City, Missouri, 1977.

GENERAL REFERENCES

1. Felix Marti-Ibañez, M.D. (editor), *The Patient's Progress,* MD Publications, New York, 1962.
2. Broadcast, "The American Way of Cancer," CBS television network, October 15, 1975.
3. Caroline Bedell Thomas, "What Becomes of Medical Students: The Dark Side," study of incipient mental illness and emotional disturbance as it affects medical students, Johns Hopkins School of Medicine, Baltimore, Maryland.
4. Dr. Caroline Bedell Thomas and Richard L. Greenstreet, "Psychobiological Characteristics in Youth as Predictors of Five Disease States: Suicide, Mental Illness, Hypertension, Coronary Heart Disease and Tumor," *Johns Hopkins Medical Journal,* January 1973, Vol. 132, No. 1, pp. 16-43.
5. Dr. Caroline Bedell Thomas and Karen R. Duszynski, "Closeness to Parents and the Family Constellation in a Prospective Study of Five Disease States: Suicide, Mental Illness, Malignant Tumor, Hypertension and Coronary Heart Disease," *John Hopkins Medical Journal,* May 1974, Vol. 134, No. 5, pp. 251-270.
6. Jeanne A. Griffith, M.D., Peter J. Fabri, B.A., Merrill S. Kies, and Mark R. Sinibaldi, B.S., "Three Medical Students Confront Death on a Pediatric Ward," Loyola University, Maywood, Illinois. Discusses approach of physician to family of those patients who are dying.
7. Norman Cousins, "Anatomy of an Illness (as Perceived By the Patient)." Deals with psychological aspects and other factors such as humor and vitamin C, in patient's report of recovery from a terminal condition, *New England Journal of Medicine,* 1977.
8. S. J. Hought, *Has Dr. Max Gerson a True Cancer Cure?,* London Press, North Hollywood, California, 1962.
9. John Gunther, *Death Be Not Proud,* Pyramid Books, New York, 1957.

NEW AND ALTERNATIVE METHODS

1. Gordon Thomas, *Dr. Issels and His Revolutionary Cancer Treatment,* Peter H. Wyden, Inc., New York, 1973.
2. O. Carl Simonton, M.D., Stephanie Matthews-Simonton, James Creighton, *A Step-by-Step, Self-Help Guide to Overcoming Cancer for Patients and Their Families.* Deals with the role of the mind in cancer therapy. J. P. Tarcher, Inc., Los Angeles and New York, 1978.
3. Josef Issels, M.D., *Cancer: A Second Opinion,* Hodder & Stoughton, London, 1975.
4. Max Wolf, M.D., and Karl Ransberger, Ph.D., *Enzyme Therapy,* Vantage Press, New York, 1972.
5. Dr. Alonzo J. Shadman, "Who Is Your Doctor and Why?"—a study of the state of medicine today, and of homeopathic approaches to therapy.
6. Lecture, Dr. Otto Warburg, "The Prime Cause and Prevention of Cancer," meeting of Nobel Laureates June 30, 1966, Lindau, Lake Constance, Germany.

7. Dr. Harold J. Reilly and Ruth Hagy Brod, *The Edgar Cayce Handbook for Health Through Drugless Therapy,* Jove/HBJ, Macmillan Publishing Co., Inc., New York, 1975.

8. Donald Law, Ph.D., *A Guide to Alternative Medicine,* Turnstone Books, London, 1974.

9. E. E. Rogers, M.D., *The Philosophy and Science of Health,* The Lee Foundation for Nutritional Research, Milwaukee, Wisconsin, 1949.

10. Alan H. Nittler, M.D., *A New Breed of Doctor,* Pyramid Books, New York, 1972.

11. Study, Chisato Maruyama, M.D., "On the Treatment of Malignant Tumors With an Extract from Tubercle Bacilli (Tubercle Vaccine) [generally called "Maruyama Vaccine" in Japan], with illustrations of the clinical results in 1965-1971," Research Institute of Vaccine Therapy for Tumors and Infectious Diseases, Nippon Medical School, Tokyo, Japan, 1973.

12. Hans A. Nieper, M.D., "The Nieper Approach ('Nieper Regimen') to Biological Cancer Treatment," Silbersee Hospital, Hannover, West Germany, 1975.

13. Hans A. Nieper, M.D., "The Changes and Prospects in the Medical Treatment of Cancer Disease," Silbersee Hospital, Hannover, West Germany, 1975.

14. Kazuhiko Asai, Ph.D., *Organic Germanium, a Medical Godsend,* Kogakusha Ltd., Publishers, Tokyo, Japan, 1977.

15. William F. Koch, M.D., *The Survival Factor in Neoplastic and Viral Diseases,* a study of the phenomena of the free radical, the double bond, and its alpha placed hydrogen atom in the pathogenesis and correction of neoplastic, viral, and bacterial diseases. William F. Koch, 1926.

16. K. Morishita, M.D., *The Hidden Truth of Cancer.* Some new concepts in the basic problems of cancer, blood physiology, the origin of the cancer cell, and the prevention and cure of cancer via natural means. George Ohsawa Macrobiotic Foundation, Publishers, 1471 10th Avenue, San Francisco, California 94122.

17. O. Carl Simonton, M.D., and Stephanie S. Simonton, "Belief Systems and Management of the Emotional Aspects of Malignancy," *Journal of Transpersonal Psychology,* Vol. VII, No. 1, 1975.

18. O. Carl Simonton, M.D., "The Role of the Mind in Cancer Therapy," paper presented at Dimensions of Healing Symposium at UCLA.

19. Nathan Pritikin, F.A.P.M., John Kern, M.D., Robert Pritikin, B.A., Steven M. Kaye, M.D., paper presented November 19, 1975, at the 52nd Annual Session of the American Congress of Rehabilitation Medicine, Atlanta, Georgia.

MEDICAL TREATISES

1. Albert L. Lehninger, "Energy Transformation in the Cell," *Scientific American,* May 1960, Vol. 202, No. 5, pp. 102-114.

2. Alvan R. Feinstein, M.D., *Clinical Judgment,* Robert E. Krieger Publishing Company, Huntington, New York, 1967.

3. J. U. Schlegel, M.D., Ph.D., G. E. Pipkin, Ph.D., G. N. Shultz, M.D., "The Aetiology of Bladder Tumours"; includes treatment with Vitamin C. *British Journal of Urology,* Vol. XLI, No. 6, December 1969.

4. Dr. A. J. Cullinane, "The Theory of Natural Immunity by Reference to the Saline Oxygen Level of the Blood and Plasma—The Effect of the pH Value," Binnegar, Wareham, Dorset, England, 1967.

5. Sir MacFarlane Burnet, "The Mechanism of Immunity," dealing with mechanism of the production of antibodies, *Scientific American*, January 1961, Vol. 204, No. 1, pp. 58-67.

6. Drs. H. B. Jones and A. Grendon, "Environmental Factors in the Origin of Cancer and Estimation of the Possible Hazard to Man," *Fd. Cosmet. Toxicol.*, Vol. 13, pp. 251-256, Pergamon Press, 1975.

7. Harry H. LeVeen, M.D., Simon Wapnick, M.D., Vincent Piccone, M.D., Gerald Falk, M.S., Natis Ahmed, M.D., "Tumor Eradication by Radio Frequency Therapy—Response in 21 Patients," *Journal of the American Medical Association*, May 17, 1976, Vol. 235, No. 20. Deals with the transfer of radiofrequency energy for heating tissues locally.

8. Gerhard N. Schrauzer, "Cancer Mortality Correlation Studies II. Regional Associations of Mortalities with the Consumptions of Foods and Other Commodities," *Medical Hypotheses*, Vol. 2, No. 2, March-April, 1976.

9. G. N. Schrauzer, "Cancer Mortality Correlation Studies, I. Statistical Associations Between Cancers at Anatomically Unrelated Sites and Some Epidemiological Implications," *Medical Hypotheses*, Vol. 2, No. 2, March-April, 1976, University of California at San Diego, California.

10. *Cancer Facts and Figures*, American Cancer Society, 1975.

11. George Crile, M.D. *What Women Should Know About the Breast Cancer Controversy*, Macmillan Publishing Co., Inc., New York, 1973.

12. Edgar Berman, M.D., *The Solid Gold Stethoscope*, Macmillan Publishing Co., Inc., New York, 1976.

13. Charles Gordon Zubrod, M.D., "Minireview, Present Status of Cancer Chemotherapy," *Life Sciences*, Vol. 14, pp. 809-818, 1974.

14. Several studies among Seventh Day Adventists, indicating that the dietary regimes and abstention from smoking, drugs, and so forth, contribute generally to a lower incidence of health problems than the general population average, including cancer of the lung and mouth, coronary artery disease, mental health, and so forth. Loma Linda University, Loma Linda, California.

15. Otto Warburg, "The Oxygen-Transferring Ferment of Respiration," Nobel Lecture, December 10, 1931, Elsevier Publishing Company, Amsterdam, Holland.

16. Otto Warburg, *The Prime Cause and Prevention of Cancer*, Konrad Triltsch, publisher, Wurzburg, Germany, 1967.

17. "Proteolytic Enzymes in Tumor Therapy—Alternative or Adjuvans in the Campaign Against Cancer," Scientific Department of Messrs. MUCOS Emulsionsgesellschaft mbH, Munich, West Germany.

18. "Drugs vs. Cancer," U.S. Department of Health, Education, and Welfare, Publication No. (NIH) 76-786, revised 1976.

19. Dr. Victor Richards, *The Wayward Cell—Its Origins, Nature and Treatment*, University of California Press, Berkeley, California, 1974.

20. Dr. Michael B. Shimkin, "Science and Cancer," U.S. Department of Health, Education, and Welfare, 1969.

21. Max Wolf, M.D., and Karl Ransberger, Ph.D., *Enzyme-Therapy*, Vantage Press, New York, 1972.

22. Dr. Max Gerson, *A Cancer Therapy—Results of Fifty Cases*, Totality Book Publishers, Del Mar, California, 1975.

NUTRITIONAL APPROACHES

1. Dr. Maud Tresillian Fere, *Does Diet Cure Cancer?*, Thorsons Publishers Ltd., London, 1963.

2. Otto Carque, *The Key to Rational Dietetics*, Los Angeles, California, 1930.

3. C. Moerman, M.D., *A Solution to the Cancer Problem*, Vlaardingen, the Netherlands, 1962.

4. Dr. Kirstine Nolfi, *Raw Food Treatment of Cancer*, The Shangri-La Health Resort, Bonita Springs, Florida, 1969.

5. Eugenia M. Zellan, Ph.D., R.D., "Let's Reforge the Link" (study of hospital malnutrition), *Nutrition Today*, March/April 1975.

6. Charles E. Butterworth, Jr., M.D., "The Skeleton in the Hospital Closet" (discusses Iatrogenic malnutrition), *Nutrition Today,* March/April 1974.

7. Maurice E. Shils, M.D., Sc.D., "Nutritional and Dietary Factors in Neoplastic Development," Memorial Hospital for Cancer and Allied Diseases, New York.

8. D. P. Burkitt, M.D., A. R. P. Walker, D.Sc.; N. S. Painter, M.S., "Dietary Fiber and Disease," *Journal of the American Medical Association,* August 19, 1974, Vol. 229, No. 8.

9. Lauren V. Ackerman, M.D., "Some Thoughts on Food and Cancer," *Nutrition Today,* January/February 1972.

10. Bonnie S. Worthington, Ph.D., "Effect of Nutritional Status on Immune Phenomena," School of Public Health and Community Medicine, University of Washington, Seattle (Vol. 65, August 1974); deals with the adverse effects of nutritional deficiencies on antibody production and cellular immunity.

THE IMPAIRED PHYSICIAN

1. Stanley Gitlow, M.D., *The Disabled Physician*, Mount Sinai School of Medicine, New York.

2. *The Impaired Physician,* The American Medical Association, Chicago, Illinois.

3. Reuben Bar-Levav, M.D., "Treating Emotionally Disturbed Physicians," *Michigan Psychiatric Society Newsletter,* Vol. XVIII, No. 5, March/April 1976.

4. Sr. Mary Madonna Ashton, C.S.J., "Motivating the Disabled Doctor: Informal Steps," St. Mary's Hospital, Minneapolis, Minnesota, April 11, 1975.

5. Robert D. Clinger, M.D., Ohio State Medical Association, Columbus, Ohio, paper presented at 7th Annual Medical-Scientific Session, National Alcoholism Forum, Washington, D.C., May 6, 1976.

6. G. Douglas Talbott, M.D., Hank Holderfield, Kenneth E. Shoemaker, M.D., Earnest C. Atkins, M.D., "The Disabled Doctors Plan for Georgia," Medical Association of Georgia.

7. Joseph I. Berman, M.D., "Legal Mechanisms for Dealing with the Disabled Physician in Maryland: Partnership Between the Medical Society and the State Commission on Medical Discipline," April 11, 1975.

8. Lynn Chaikin Epstein, M.D., Caroline Bedell Thomas, M.D., John W. Shaffer, Ph.D., Seymour Perlin, M.D., "Clinical Prediction of Physician Suicide Based on Medical Student Data," *The Journal of Nervous and Mental Disease* 1973.

PSYCHOLOGICAL AND PHILOSOPHICAL WORKS

1. Edmond Bordeaux Szekely, *The Essene Gospel of Peace,* Academy Book Publishers, San Diego, California, 1975.

2. Arnold A. Hutschnecker, *The Will To Live,* Prentice-Hall, Inc., Englewood Cliffs, New Jersey, 1951.

3. J. I. Rodale, *Happy People Rarely Get Cancer,* Rodale Press, Inc., Emmaus, Pennsylvania, 1970.

4. Ralph Crawshaw, M.D., "Humanism in Medicine—The Rudimentary Process," Oregon Medical Association, September 1975.

5. Carl G. Jung, *Memories, Dreams, Reflections,* Vintage Books, New York, 1961.

Index to Case Histories and Methods of Treatment

*(Numbers set in **bold face** refer to pages in this book.)*

1. The case of Lydia Bacher. Gordon Thomas, *Dr. Issels and Revolutionary Cancer Treatment,* pp. 105-107, Peter H. Wyden, Inc., New York (1973), **xi**.

2. "Only the wounded physician heals." Carl G. Jung, *Memories, Dreams, Reflections,* p. 134, Vintage Books, New York (1961), **xii-xiii**.

3. Dr. Issels treated more cases than any other single doctor in medical history. Report to BBC by Professor John Anderson of King's College Hospital, London. Cited by Gordon Thomas, *Dr. Issels and His Revolutionary Treatment,* p. xx, and p. 258, Peter H. Wyden, Inc., New York (1973), **xiii-xiv**.

4. Study of survival, 252 patients. Dr. Josef Issels (paper), "Immunotherapy in Progressive Metastatic Cancer—A Fifteen-Year Survival Follow-Up, *Clinical Trials Journal* (London) 1970, 7, No. 3, 357-366, **xiii**.

5. Study of survival, 370 patients. Dr. Josef Issels, *Cancer: A Second Opinion,* p. 160, Hodder & Stoughton, London (1975), **xiii**.

6. Dr. Robert J. C. Harris, Imperial Cancer Research Fund. In evaluating Issels's methods. Extract appears on p. 263 of Gordon Thomas's *Dr. Issels and His Revolutionary Cancer Treatment,* Peter H. Wyden, Inc., New York (1973), **xiv**.

7. Gordon Thomas, *Dr. Issels and His Revolutionary Cancer Treatment,* pp. 128-129, Peter H. Wyden, Inc., New York (1973), **xiv**.

8. Dr. Josef Issels, *Cancer: A Second Opinion.* Hodder & Stoughton, London (1975), **3**.

9. Hippocrates' obedience to the natural laws and diet. Dr. Felix-Marti-Ibañez; *The Patient's Progress,* pp. 36-39, MD Publications, New York (1962), **16**.

10. Virchow's theories of cellular pathology. Dr. Alvan R. Feinstein, *Clinical Judgment,* pp. 118-119, Robert E. Krieger Publishing Company, Huntington, New York (1967), **17**.

11. Tenth International Cancer Congress, Houston, Texas, 1970. Cited by Dr. Josef Issels, *Cancer: A Second Opinion,* p. 23, Hodder & Stoughton, London (1975). Also cited by Dr. Rita Leroi (article), "Cancer, the Disease of Our Time," *Journal for Anthroposophy,* p. 15, No. 19, Spring 1974, New York, **18**.

12. Mistletoe in Germanic myth and legend. Dr. Rita Leroi (article), "Mistletoe and Its Use in the Treatment of Cancer," *Journal for Anthroposophy,* No. 20, Autumn 1974, New York, **19**.

13. Rudolf Steiner, first indications for therapeutic use of mistletoe. Dr. Rita Leroi (article), "Cancer, the Disease of Our Time," *Journal for Anthroposophy,* No. 19, Spring 1974, New York, **19-20**.

14. Lecture in Brussels re human factors in evaluation of drugs. Dr. Alvan R. Feinstein, cited in 1972/1973 Annual Report, Lukas-Klinik, Arlesheim, Switzerland, **20-21**.

15. Study of 912 patients using Iscador treatment. Dr. G. Kienle, Society

for Cancer Research, Stuttgart, Germany; Annual Report 1973/1974, Lukas-Klinik, Arlesheim, Switzerland, **21**.

16. Postoperative treatment results, seventy-eight lung cancer patients (paper). Dr. M. Lindenmann, "Baumgartner Höhe, Sanitorium, Vienna, Austria"; Annual Report 1972/1973, Lukas-Klinik, Arlesheim, Switzerland, **21-22**.

17. Study of Professor Bickenback of Munich University Hospital (paper), "A Clinical Trial of Iscador." Reprinted from *British Homeopathetic Journal,* Vol. LVII, No. 1, January 1968, **23**.

18. Study of ten case histories using mistletoe extracts. Dr. Alexandre Leroi and Dr. Bernard Wohrmann (paper), "A Non-Toxic, Medical Treatment for Cancer Using Mistletoe Extracts." Institute Hiscia, Society for Cancer Research, Arlesheim, Switzerland (1965), **26-28**.

19. Vester. Carcinostatic activity of protein fractions from mistletoe extract. Society for Cancer Research, Arlesheim, Switzerland, "Directions for the Use of Iscador" (1971), **28-29**.

20. Healing capabilities of Iscador, Dr. Rita Leroi, Lukas-Klinik, "Iscador Treatment of Carcinoma," *British Homeopathic Journal,* Vol. LXI, No. 3, July 1972, **29-30**.

21. Improvements observed with Iscador treatment. Society for Cancer Research, Arlesheim, Switzerland, "Directions for the Use of Iscador" (1971), **30**.

22. Society for Cancer Research, Arlesheim, Switzerland, "Directions for the Use of Iscador," 1971; Leroi, A. u. Leroi-von May, R: Behandlung maligner Blasentumoren mit Viscum album. *Z. Urol.* 51 (9), 555-561 (1958); Leroi, A. u. Leroi-von May R: Iscador-Behandlung maligner Blasentumoren. *Beitr. Erw. Heilk.* 13 (2), 47-66 (1960), **30-31**.

23. American Cancer Society, *Unproven Methods of Cancer Management* (1961), also *Cancer Facts and Figures,* American Cancer Society (1975), **34**.

24. American Cancer Society, *Cancer Facts and Figures* (1975), **34**.

25. American Cancer Society, *Unproven Methods of Cancer Management* (1961), **35**.

26. 77,200 pages of data to license new drug. Letter dated May 3, 1966, Department of Health, Education, and Welfare, Food and Drug Administration, **37**.

27. Dr. Max Gerson, *A Cancer Therapy—Results of Fifty Cases,* Totality Book Publishers, Del Mar, California (1975), **39**.

28. American Cancer Society, *Unproven Methods of Cancer Management* (1961), **39**.

29. Story of the Manhattan Project, *Encyclopaedia Britannica,* **42-43**.

30. *China in the Sixteenth Century—the Journals of Matthew Ricci: 1583-1610,* Random House, New York (1953), **44**.

31. Examples of cancer research projects. "Summary of Project Areas Proposed for the National Cancer Program," U.S. Department of Health, Education, and Welfare, August 1973, **45-46**.

32. Lack of intellectual approaches in clinical problems. Dr. Alvan R. Feinstein, *Clinical Judgment,* p. 27, Robert E. Krieger Publishing Company, Huntington, New York (1967), **46**.

33. Dr. Ralph Crawshaw, "Humanism in Medicine—the Rudimentary Process," *The New England Journal of Medicine,* December 18, 1975, **47-48**.

34. Suicides among medical doctors. Dr. Stanley Gitlow, (paper), Mount Sinai School of Medicine, "The Disabled Physician—His Care in New York State," **52**.

35. Drug dependence of physicians. "The Impaired Physician," Department of Mental Health, American Medical Association (1975), **52**.

36. Research report, "Drugs vs. Cancer," U.S. Department of Health, Education, and Welfare, Publication No. (NIH) 76-786, revised 1976, **54**.

37. Chemotherapeutic side effects. Dr. Victor Richards, *The Wayward Cell—Its Origins, Nature and Treatment,* pp. 206-222, University of California Press, Berkeley, California (1974), **55**.

38. Chemotherapy damages all normal cells. Dr. Victor Richards, *The Wayward Cell—Its Origins, Nature and Treatment,* p. 206, University of California Press, Berkeley, California (1974), **55-56**.

39. Dr. Hans A. Nieper (paper), "The Changes and Prospects in the Medical Treatment of Cancer Disease," Department of Medicine, Silbersee Hospital, Hannover, Germany (1975), **56**.

40. CBS News documentary, "The American Way of Cancer," CBS television network, October 15, 1975, **57**.

41. Autopsies reveal presence of undiagnosed cancer. Dr. Hans A. Nieper, "Critical Survey of the State of Cancer Research," Part 1, Silbersee Clinic, Hannover, Germany (1972), **63-64**.

42. Jane E. Brody, "The Drug War on Cancer," *New York Times Magazine,* pp. 48-58, **64**.

43. Dr. Michael B. Shimkin, "Science and Cancer," 2, p. 4, U.S. Department of Health, Education, and Welfare (1969), **64**.

44. X-ray film damage. Dr. Victor Richards, *The Wayward Cell—Its Origins, Nature and Treatment,* p. 104, University of California Press, Berkeley, California (1974), **65**.

45. Dr. Michael B. Shimkin, "Science and Cancer," p. 97, U.S. Department of Health, Education, and Welfare (1969), **66**.

46. D. H. Lacy, Jr., *Computers,* **67**.

47. Dr. Virginia Livingston, *Cancer: A New Breakthrough,* Reward Books, New York, **69**.

48. Dr. Max Gerson, *A Cancer Therapy—Results of Fifty Cases,* Totality Book Publishers, Del Mar, California (1975), **74**.

49. The Sauerbruch Story. Dr. Ferdinand Sauerbruch, *Master Surgeon,* pp. 167-171, Thomas Y. Crowell Company, New York (1954), **75-77**.

50. Dr. Max Gerson, *A Cancer Therapy—Results of Fifty Cases,* p. 9, Totality Book Publishers, Del Mar, California (1975), **79**.

51. The patient from Bielefeld. Dr. Max Gerson, lecture, Escondido, California (1956); *A Cancer Therapy—Results of Fifty Cases,* p. 403, Totality Book Publishers, Del Mar, California (1975), **84-87**.

52. Dr. Alvan R. Feinstein, *Clinical Judgment,* 41, Robert E. Krieger Publishing Company, Inc., Huntington, New York (1967), **110**.

53. New York County Medical Society not passing upon adequacy of physician's treatment. S. J. Haught, *Has Dr. Max Gerson a True Cancer Cure?,* p. 17, London Press, North Hollywood, California (1962), **111**.

54. Suspension of Dr. Max Gerson—specific charge. S. J. Haught, *Has Dr. Max Gerson a True Cancer Cure?,* p. 10, London Press, North Hollywood, California (1962), **111**.

55. *Principles of Medical Ethics,* The American Medical Association, Chicago, Illinois (1976), **111**.

56. Raymond Gram Swing, American Broadcasting Company network, S. J. Haught, *Has Dr. Max Gerson a True Cancer Cure?,* p. 104, London Press, North Hollywood, California (1962), **112-114**.

57. Hearings, U.S. Senate subcommittee, Seventy-Ninth Congress, Second Session, on S. 1875 (July 2, 1946), **119**.

58. Paramahansa Yogananda, *Autobiography of a Yogi*, Self-Realization Fellowship, Los Angeles, California (1946), **144**.

59. John Gunther, *Death Be Not Proud*, Pyramid Books, New York (1957), **152-56**.

60. Edmond Bordeaux Szekely, *The Essene Gospel of Peace*, Academy Book Publishers, San Diego, California (1975), **167-68**.

61. S. J. Haught, *Has Dr. Max Gerson a True Cancer Cure?*, p. 134, London Press, North Hollywood, California (1962), **170-71**.

62. Biodynamic agriculture. Herbert H. Koepf, *What is Bio-Dynamic Agriculture?*, Bio-Dynamic Farming and Gardening Association, 308 East Adams Street, Springfield, Illinois 62701, **182**.

63. Dietary regime of Lukas-Klinik, Dr. Rita Leroi, "The Lukas-Klinik and the Research Institute Hiscia," lecture at Spring Valley to Anthroposophical Therapy and Hygiene Association, *Journal for Anthroposophy*, New York (1973), **183**.

64. Dr. Roy W. Menninger on factor of stress, *U.S. News & World Report*, May 1, 1978, **184-85**.

65. Paramahansa Yogananda, *Autobiography of a Yogi*, "The Law of Miracles," p. 284, Self-Realization Fellowship, Los Angeles, California (1946), **186**.

66. The Christian Medical Foundation, International, 4821 Memorial Highway, Tampa, Florida 33614, **189**.

67. The story of Karen Emmott, Dr. William S. Reed, Christian Medical Foundation, Tampa, Florida, from *Guideposts*, May 1962, **189-90**.

68. "Dear Patient" letter. Dr. Josef Issels, letter given to patients upon arrival at the Ringberg-Klinik, Rottach-Egern, West Germany, **198**.

69. Dr. Harris's evaluation to BBC team, of Dr. Issels's methods, cited by Gordon Thomas, *Dr. Issels and His Revolutionary Cancer Treatment*, p. 263, Peter H. Wyden, Inc., New York (1973), **199-200**.

70. Patient abuse reported by British visiting team. "A Report on the Treatment of Cancer at the Ringberg-Klinik, Rottach-Egern, Bavaria," p. 16, by Department of Health and Social Security of Great Britain (1971), **200**.

71. Dr. Ralph Cranshaw, "Humanism in Medicine—the Rudimentary Process," *The New England Journal of Medicine* (1975), **200-201**.

72. Gordon Thomas, *Dr. Issels and His Revolutionary Cancer Treatment*, Peter H. Wyden, Inc., New York (1973), **201**.

73. Painting therapy, Lukas-Klinik, Dr. Rita Leroi, "The Lukas-Klinik and the Research Institute Hiscia," lecture at Spring Valley to Anthroposophical Therapy and Hygiene Association, *Journal for Anthroposophy*, New York (1973), **211**.

74. Dr. Franz Alexander, *Psychosomatic Medicine, Its Principles and Application*, cited by Dr. Arnold A. Hutschnecker, *The Will to Live*, pp. 83-84, Prentice-Hall, Inc., Englewood Cliffs, New Jersey (1958), **212**.

75. Pearl S. Buck, *A Bridge for Passing*, p. 160, The John Day Company, New York (1961), **218-19**.

76. Brother Lawrence, *The Practice of the Presence of God*, Fleming H. Revell Company, Los Angeles, California (1895), **219**.

77. James Henry Leigh Hunt, "Abou Ben Adhem," **221**.

78. *The Greatest Health Discovery*, Natural Hygiene Press, Inc., Chicago, Illinois (1972), **227**.

79. Quotations from Dr. Charles E. Butterworth are reproduced with permission of *Nutrition Today* magazine, 101 Ridgely Avenue, Annapolis, Maryland 21404, © March/April 1974), **232-233**.

Index